PRINCIPLES OF
Dermatology

Joe Evans MD

PRINCIPLES OF
Dermatology

THIRD EDITION

◻

DONALD P. LOOKINGBILL, M.D.

Professor of Dermatology
Mayo Medical School

Chair, Department of Dermatology
Mayo Clinic Jacksonville
Jacksonville, Florida

JAMES G. MARKS, JR., M.D.

Professor of Medicine
Chief, Division of Dermatology
Milton S. Hershey Medical Center
Pennsylvania State University
Hershey, Pennsylvania

W.B. SAUNDERS COMPANY

A Harcourt Health Sciences Company

Philadelphia   London   New York   St. Louis   Sydney   Toronto

W.B. SAUNDERS COMPANY
A Harcourt Health Sciences Company

The Curtis Center
Independence Square West
Philadelphia, Pennsylvania 19106

Library of Congress Cataloging-in-Publication Data

Lookingbill, Donald P.

 Principles of dermatology / Donald P. Lookingbill, James G. Marks, Jr.—3rd ed.

  p. ; cm.

 Includes bibliographical references and index.

 ISBN 0–7216–7971–4

 1. Dermatology. 2. Skin—Diseases. I. Marks, James G. II. Title.

 [DNLM: 1. Skin Diseases. 2. Dermatology—methods. WR 140 L863p 2000]

 RL71. L64 2000

 616.5—dc21   99–057051

Editor-in-Chief: Lisette Bralow
Acquisitions Editor: Judith Fletcher
Project Manager: Mary Anne Folcher
Production Manager: Frank Polizzano
Illustration Specialist: Peg Shaw
Indexer: Dennis Dolan

PRINCIPLES OF DERMATOLOGY   ISBN 0–7216–7971–4

Printed in the United States of America

Last digit is the print number: 9   8   7   6   5   4   3   2   1

■ PREFACE

The primary goal of this third edition has not changed from that of the first edition; it is to facilitate dermatologic diagnosis through a clinicopathologic approach to skin disease. Unlike most other introductory manuals, each chapter in our text is based on the appearance of the primary skin process (e.g., pustules) rather than on the etiology (e.g., infection). This arrangement helps to reflect the way in which most patients present in the clinical setting.

We are extremely grateful to our many students and residents who have used the first two editions and provided us with thoughtful feedback over the years. Their suggestions have been incorporated into this new edition. *Principles of Dermatology*, third edition, includes even more larger color illustrations along with therapy tables that should be of use to the primary care physicians who use this book.

We acknowledge and thank Jay Spiegel for typing the manuscript, Judy Fletcher for her good humor and constructive support as editor, and our families for again giving us the time to produce this book.

■ PREFACE TO THE FIRST EDITION

Skin diseases affect virtually everyone sometime during life. Because changes in the skin are so easily recognized by the patient, medical attention is frequently sought. Skin reacts in a limited number of ways, but the neophyte is often bewildered by the appearance of rashes that superficially look alike. This text is meant to be an introduction to cutaneous disorders. It is aimed toward medical students so that they may develop a logical approach to the diagnosis of common cutaneous diseases with an understanding of the underlying clinicopathologic correlations. It has been a most rewarding experience for us to see students on our clinical service at the M.S. Hershey Medical Center grasp the basic principles of skin disease in the short time they spend with us. Their questions, learning experience, and suggestions have been incorporated into this book.

We have purposely not tried to make this an encyclopedia of skin diseases, but have chosen those diseases that are most commonly seen. Uncommon diseases are discussed only to illustrate dermatologic principles or important diseases that should not be missed. There are several up-to-date large textbooks available for those who want to delve into the field more deeply.

We are grateful for the contribution of artwork and clinical slides from audiovisual programs in the series *A Brief Course in Dermatology,* produced and distributed by the Institute for Dermatologic Communication and Education, San Francisco, California, as follows: From *Skin Lesions Depicted and Defined,* Part One, *Primary Lesions,* and Part Two, *Secondary and Special Lesions,* by Richard M. Caplan, M.D., Alfred W. Kopf, M.D., and Marion B. Sulzberger, M.D., and from *Techniques for Examination of the Skin,* by David L. Cram, M.D., Howard I. Maibach, M.D., and Marion B. Sulzberger, M.D.

We wish to acknowledge those people whose efforts contributed greatly to producing this book. Our secretaries, Dianne Safford, Joyce Zeager, and Sharon Smith, spent many hours typing the drafts and final manuscript. Nancy Egan, M.D., and Ronald Rovner, M.D., proofread much of the book and gave many worthwhile suggestions. Schering Corporation supported the cost of the illustrations which were so handsomely drawn by Debra Moyer and Daniel S. Beisel. Lastly, and most importantly, our families gave us the support and time necessary to write this volume.

■ CONTENTS

SECTION 8

DIAGNOSIS BY REGION AND SYMPTOM 341

1

PRINCIPLES OF

DERMATOLOGY

■

INTRODUCTION

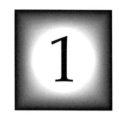

S kin diseases are common. Of the total yearly outpatient visits in the United States, 7% are for dermatologic complaints. Only one third of these patients are seen by dermatologists; most of the remainder are seen by primary care physicians. In a survey of the family practice clinic at the Pennsylvania State University College of Medicine, we found that dermatologic disorders constituted 8.5% of the diagnoses. The incidence is higher in a pediatric practice, in which as many as 30% of the children are seen for skin-related conditions.

Seven percent of all outpatient visits are for dermatologic complaints.

Although thousands of skin disorders have been described, only a small number account for most patient visits. The primary goal of this text is to familiarize the reader with these common diseases. Uncommon and rare skin disorders not covered in this book can be found in one of the comprehensive dermatology texts listed in the references.

Our diagnostic approach divides skin diseases into two large groups: growths and rashes. This grouping is based on both the patient's presenting complaint (often a concern about either a skin growth or a symptom from a rash) and the pathophysiologic process (a growth represents a neoplastic change and a rash is an inflammatory reaction in the skin).

Skin diseases are divided into:
1. Growths
2. Rashes

Growths and rashes are then subdivided according to the component of skin that is affected. Growths are divided into epidermal, pigmented, and dermal proliferative processes. Rashes are divided into those with and those without an epidermal component.

Our approach to skin disease emphasizes the correlations between the clinical appearance of the disorder and the pathophysiologic processes responsible for it. With this clinicopathologic approach, a diagnosis can be reached, and the disease can be better understood and appropriately treated.

REFERENCES

Federman D, Hogan D, Taylor JR, et al.: A comparison of diagnosis, evaluation, and treatment of patients with dermatologic disorders. J Am Acad Dermatol 32:726–729, 1995.

Feldman SR, Fleischer AB, McConnell RC: Most common dermatologic problems identified by internists 1990–1994. Arch Intern Med 158:726–730, 1998.

Johnson ML, Johnson KG, Engel A: Prevalence, morbidity and cost of dermatologic diseases. J Am Acad Dermatol 11:930–936, 1984.

Krowchuk DP, Bradham DD, Fleischer AB: Dermatologic services provided to children and adolescents by primary care and other physicians in the United States. Pediatr Dermatol 1:219–222, 1984.

Pariser RJ, Pariser DM: Primary care physicians' errors in handling cutaneous disorders. J Am Acad Dermatol 17:239–245, 1987.

General Dermatology References

Champion RH, Burton JL, Burns DA, et al.: Rook/Wilkinson/Ebling Textbook of Dermatology. 6th ed. Oxford, Blackwell Scientific Publications, 1998.

Freedberg IM, Eisen AZ, Wolff K, et al.: Fitzpatrick's Dermatology in General Medicine. 5th ed. New York, McGraw-Hill, 1999.

Moschella SL, Hurley HJ: Dermatology. 3rd ed. Philadelphia, WB Saunders, 1992.

Sams WM Jr, Lynch PS: Principles and Practice of Dermatology. New York, Churchill Livingstone, 1990.

Schachner L, Hansen RL: Pediatric Dermatology. 2nd ed. New York, Churchill Livingstone, 1995.

STRUCTURE AND FUNCTION OF SKIN

EPIDERMIS
DERMIS
SKIN APPENDAGES
SUBCUTANEOUS FAT

The skin is a large organ, weighing an average of 4 kg and covering an area of 2 m². Its major function is to act as a barrier against an inhospitable environment—to protect the body from the influences of the outside world. The skin's importance is well illustrated by the high mortality associated with extensive loss of skin from burns.

The major barrier is provided by the epidermis. Underlying it is a vascularized dermis that provides support and nutrition for the dividing cells in the epidermis. The dermis also contains nerves and appendages—sweat glands, hair follicles, and sebaceous glands. Nails are also considered skin appendages. The third and deepest layer of the skin is the subcutaneous fat. The functions of all these components are listed in Table 2–1.

Components of skin:
1. Epidermis
2. Dermis
3. Skin appendages
4. Subcutaneous fat

■ EPIDERMIS

The epidermis is divided into four layers, starting at the dermal junction with the basal cell layer and eventuating, at the outer surface, in the stratum corneum. The dermal side of the epidermis has an irregular contour. The downward projections are called *rete ridges,* which appear three dimensionally as a Swiss cheese–like matrix with the holes filled by dome-shaped dermal papillae. This configuration helps to anchor the epidermis physically to the dermis. The pattern is most pronounced in areas subject to maximum friction, such as the palms and soles.

The cells in the epidermis undergo division and differentiation. Cell division occurs in the basal cell layer, and differentiation occurs in the layers above it.

Cell division occurs in the basal cell layer.

Structure

Basal Cell Layer. The basal cells can be considered the "stem cells" of the epidermis. They are the undifferentiated, proliferating cells. Daughter cells from the basal cell layer migrate upward and begin the process of differentiation. In normal skin, cell division does not take place above the basal cell layer.

TABLE 2–1 ■ SKIN FUNCTIONS

Function	Responsible Structure
Barrier	Epidermis
Physical	Stratum corneum
Light	Melanocytes
Immunologic	Langerhans cells
Tough flexible foundation	Dermis
Temperature regulation	Blood vessels
	Eccrine sweat glands
Sensation	Nerves
Grasp	Nails
Decorative	Hair
Unknown	Sebaceous glands
Insulation from cold and trauma	Subcutaneous fat
Calorie reservoir	Subcutaneous fat

Stratum Spinosum. This layer lies above the basal layer and is composed of *keratinocytes,* which differentiate from the basal cells beneath them. The keratinocytes produce keratin, a fibrous protein that is the major component of the horny stratum corneum. The stratum spinosum derives its name from the "spines," or intercellular bridges, that extend between keratinocytes and are visible with light microscopy. Ultrastructurally, these are composed of desmosomes, which are extensions from keratin within the keratinocyte; functionally they hold the cells together.

> **Keratinization begins in the stratum spinosum.**

Stratum Granulosum. The process of differentiation continues in the stratum granulosum, or granular cell layer, in which the cells acquire additional keratin and become more flattened. In addition, they contain distinctive dark granules, easily seen on light microscopy, that are composed of keratohyalin. Keratohyalin contains two proteins, one of which is called profilaggrin, the precursor to filaggrin. As its name suggests, filaggrin plays an important role in the aggregation of keratin filaments in the stratum corneum. The other protein is called involucrin (from the Latin for "envelope"), and it plays a role in the formation of the cell envelope of the cells in the stratum corneum.

Granular cells also contain lamellar granules, which are visualized with electron microscopy. Lamellar granules contain polysaccharides, glycoproteins, and lipids, which extrude into the intercellular space and ultimately are thought to help form the "cement" that holds together the stratum corneum cells. Degradative enzymes also are found within the granular cells; these are responsible for the eventual destruction of the cells' nuclei and intracytoplasmic organelles.

> **Granular cells contain keratohyalin and lamellar granules.**

Stratum Corneum. A remarkably abrupt transition occurs between the viable, nucleated cells at the top of the granular cell layer and the dead cells of the stratum corneum (Fig. 2–1). The cells in the stratum corneum are large, flat, polyhedral, plate-like envelopes filled with keratin. They are stacked in vertical layers that range in thickness from 15 to 25 layers on most body surfaces to as many as 100 layers on the palms and soles. The cells are held together by a lipid-rich cement in a fashion similar to "bricks and mortar." The tightly packed, keratinized envelopes in the stratum corneum provide a semi-impenetrable layer that constitutes the major physical barrier of the skin.

> **The stratum corneum is the major physical barrier.**

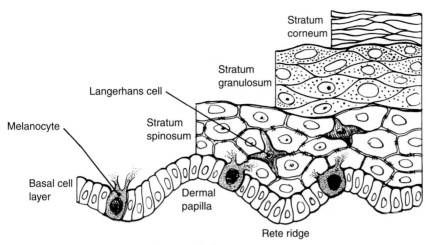

FIGURE 2-1. Epidermis.

The epidermis, then, is composed of cells that divide in the basal cell layer (basal cells), keratinize in the succeeding layers (keratinocytes), and eventuate into the devitalized, keratin-filled cells in the stratum corneum. It takes about 2 weeks for the cells to migrate from the basal cell layer to the top of the granular cell layer and an additional 2 weeks for the cells to cross the stratum corneum to the surface where they finally are shed.

Other Cellular Components

In addition to basal cells and keratinocytes, two other cells are located in the epidermis: melanocytes and Langerhans cells.

Melanocytes. Melanocytes are dendritic, pigment-producing cells located in the basal cell layer. They protect the skin from ultraviolet radiation. Individuals with little or no pigment develop marked sun damage and numerous skin cancers. The dendrites extend into the stratum spinosum and serve as conduits through which pigment granules are transferred to their neighboring keratinocytes. The granules are termed *melanosomes*, and the pigment within is melanin, which is synthesized from tyrosine.

People of all races have a similar number of melanocytes. The difference in skin pigmentation depends on (1) the number and size of the melanosomes and (2) their dispersion in the skin. Sunlight stimulates melanocytes to increase pigment production and more widely disperse their melanosomes.

Langerhans Cells. Langerhans cells are dendritic cells in the epidermis that have an immunologic function. They are derived from the bone marrow and constitute about 5% of the cells within the epidermis. On electron microscopic examination, characteristic "tennis racket"–shaped granules are seen. Langerhans cells are identical to tissue macrophages and present antigens to lymphocytes with which they interact through specific surface receptors. As such, Langerhans cells are important components of the immunologic barrier of the skin.

Langerhans cells are the first line of immunologic defense in the skin.

Dermal-Epidermal Junction

The interface between the epidermis and dermis is called the *basement membrane zone*. With light microscopy, it is visualized only as a fine line. However, electron microscopic examination reveals three layers: (1) the *lamina lucida,* a relatively clear (lucid) zone traversed by delicate anchoring filaments that connect the cell membrane of the basal cells with (2) the *basal lamina;* the basal lamina is an electron-dense zone composed primarily of type IV collagen derived from epidermal cells and (3) *anchoring fibrils,* which are thick fibrous strands, composed of type VII collagen, that complete the connection with the dermis. The basement membrane zone serves as the "glue" between the epidermis and dermis and is the site of blister formation in numerous diseases. Hence, its structure, composition, and immunologic make-up continue to be intensely investigated.

■ DERMIS

The dermis is a tough but elastic support structure that contains blood vessels, nerves, and cutaneous appendages. It ranges in thickness from 1 to 4 mm, making it much thicker than the epidermis, which in most areas is only about as thick as this piece of paper. The dermal matrix is composed of collagen fibers, elastic fibers, and ground substance, which are synthesized by dermal fibroblasts. Collagen and elastic fibers are fibrous proteins that form the strong yet compliant skeletal matrix. In the uppermost part of the dermis (papillary dermis), collagen fibers are fine and loosely arranged. In the remainder of the dermis (reticular dermis), the fibers are thick and densely packed. Elastic fibers are primarily located in the reticular dermis, where they are thinner and more loosely arranged than collagen fibers. The ground substance fills the space between fibers. It is a nonfibrous material made up of several different mucopolysaccharide molecules collectively called proteoglycans or glycosaminoglycans. The ground substance imparts to the dermis a more liquid quality, which facilitates movement of fluids, molecules, and inflammatory cells.

Nerves and blood vessels course through the dermis, and a layer of subcutaneous fat lies below it (Fig. 2–2).

Structural components of the dermis:
1. **Collagen**
2. **Elastic fibers**
3. **Ground substance**

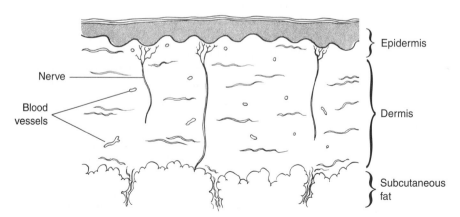

FIGURE 2–2. Dermis and subcutaneous fat.

Nerves. The skin is a major sensory receptor. Without the sensations of touch, temperature, and pain, life would be less interesting and more hazardous. Sensations are detected in the skin by both free nerve endings and more complicated receptors that are corpuscular in structure. The free nerve endings are the more widespread and appear to be more important. The nerve supply of the skin is segmental (dermatomal), with considerable overlap between segments.

Free nerve endings are the most important sensory receptors.

Blood Vessels. The blood vessels in the skin serve two functions: nutrition and temperature regulation. The epidermis has no intrinsic blood supply and therefore depends on diffusion of nutrients and oxygen from the vessels in the papillary dermis. Blood vessels in the dermis also supply the connective tissue and appendageal structures located therein.

The vasculature of the skin is arranged into two horizontal plexuses that are interconnected. The superficial plexus is located at the lower border of the papillary dermis, and the deep plexus is located in the reticular dermis. Temperature regulation is achieved through shunts between the plexuses. Increased blood flow in the superficial plexus permits heat loss, whereas shunting of blood to the deep plexus conserves heat.

Functions of blood vessels:
1. **To supply nutrition**
2. **To regulate temperature**

■ SKIN APPENDAGES

The skin appendages are the eccrine and apocrine sweat glands, hair follicles, sebaceous glands, and nails. Skin appendages are epidermally derived but, except for nails, are located in the dermis.

Eccrine Sweat Glands. For physically active individuals and for people living in hot climates, the eccrine sweat glands are physiologically the most important skin appendage. They help to regulate body temperature by excreting sweat onto the surface of the skin, from which the cooling process of evaporation takes place. Two to 3 million eccrine sweat glands are distributed over the entire body surface, with a total secretory capacity of 10 L of sweat per day. The secretory portion of the sweat apparatus is a coiled tubule located deep in the dermis. The sweat is transported through the dermis through a sweat duct, which ultimately twists a path through the epidermis. Sweat secreted in the glandular portion is isotonic to plasma but becomes hypotonic by the time it exits the skin as a result of ductal reabsorption of electrolytes. Hence, the sweat apparatus is similar to the mechanism in the kidney, that is, glandular (glomerular) excretion is followed by ductal reabsorption.

Eccrine sweat glands help to regulate temperature.

Apocrine Sweat Glands. In humans, apocrine sweat glands serve no known useful function, but they are responsible for body odor. The odor actually results from the action of surface skin bacteria on excreted apocrine sweat, which itself is odorless. Apocrine sweat glands are located mainly in the axillary and anogenital areas. The secretory segment of an apocrine gland is also a coiled tubule located deep in the dermis. However, unlike in eccrine glands, in which the secretory cells remain intact, in apocrine glands the secretory cells "decapitate" their luminal (apical) portions as part of the secretory product. The apocrine duct then drains the secreted sweat into the midportion of a hair follicle, from which it ultimately reaches the skin surface.

Bacterial action on apocrine sweat causes body odor.

Hair Follicle. In most mammals, hair serves a protective function, but in humans it is mainly decorative.

Types of hair:
1. **Vellus (light and fine)**
2. **Terminal (dark and thick)**

Hair follicles are distributed over the entire body surface except the palms and soles. Hair comes in two sizes: (1) vellus hairs, which are short, fine, light colored, and barely noticed; and (2) terminal hairs, which are thicker, longer, and darker than the vellus type. Terminal hairs in some locations are hormonally influenced and do not appear until puberty, for example, beard hair in males and pubic and axillary hair in both sexes.

A hair follicle can be viewed as a specialized invagination of the epidermis (Fig. 2–3) with a population of cells at the bottom (hair bulb) that are even more actively replicating than are normal epidermal basal cells. These cells constitute the hair matrix. As with basal cells in the epidermis, the matrix cells first divide and then differentiate, ultimately forming a keratinous hair shaft. Melanocytes in the matrix contribute pigment, the amount of which determines the color of the hair. As the matrix cells continue to divide, hair is pushed outward and exits through the epidermis at a rate of about 1 cm per month. Hair growth in an individual follicle is cyclical, with a growth (anagen) phase and a resting (telogen) phase. The lengths of the phases vary from one area of the body to another. On the scalp, for example, the anagen phase lasts about 6 years and the telogen phase about 4 months. The maximum length attainable in such a cycle (at 1 cm per month) will be 72 cm. Some individuals can grow hair longer than that, probably because of a prolonged growth phase. However, Rip Van Winkle's beard could not have reached the floor.

Hair growth cycles through growth (anagen) and resting (telogen) phases.

At the end of the anagen phase, growth stops, and the hair follicle enters the telogen phase, during which the matrix portion shrivels and the hair within the follicle is shed. Subsequently, a new matrix is formed at the bottom of the follicle, and the cycle is repeated. At any time, 80% to 90% of scalp hair is in the anagen phase and 10% to 20% is in the telogen phase, thus accounting for a *normal* shedding rate of 50 to 100 hairs per day.

Normally, 50 to 100 hairs are shed from the scalp each day.

As shown in Figure 2–3, the hair follicle is situated in the dermis at an angle. Not shown is an attached arrector pili muscle. When this muscle contracts, the hair is brought into a vertical position, giving a "goose flesh" appearance to the skin.

Sebaceous Glands. Sebaceous glands produce an oily substance termed *sebum*, which may be useful as a skin moisturizer, although this function (or any other)

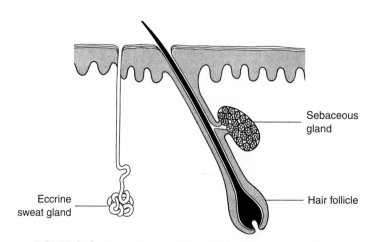

FIGURE 2–3. Sweat gland and hair follicle with sebaceous gland.

has not been proved. In fact, the skin of children and the palmar and plantar skin of adults function well without sebum.

Sebaceous glands are part of the *pilosebaceous unit* and so are found wherever hair follicles are located. In addition, ectopic sebaceous glands are often found on mucous membranes, where they may form small yellow papules called *Fordyce spots*. In the skin, sebaceous glands are most prominent on the scalp and face and are moderately prominent on the upper trunk. The size and secretory activity of these glands are under androgen control. The sebaceous glands in newborns are enlarged owing to maternal hormones, but within months the glands shrink. They enlarge again in preadolescence from stimulation by adrenal androgens and reach full size at puberty, when gonadal androgens are produced.

Sebaceous glands are androgen dependent.

The lipid-laden cells in the sebaceous glands are wholly secreted (holocrine secretion) to form sebum. Triglycerides compose the majority of the lipid found in sebaceous gland cells. From the sebaceous glands, sebum drains into the hair follicle (see Fig. 2–3), from which it exits onto the surface of the skin.

Nails. Nails, like hair, are made of keratin, which is formed from a matrix of dividing epidermal cells (Fig. 2–4). Nails, however, are hard and flat and lie parallel to the skin surface. Located at the ends of fingers and toes, they facilitate fine grasping and pinching maneuvers.

The *nail plate* is a hard, translucent structure composed of keratin. It ranges in thickness from 0.3 to 0.65 mm. Fingernails grow at a continuous rate of about 0.1 mm per day, and toenails grow at a slightly slower rate.

Nail is made of keratin produced in the matrix.

Four epithelial zones are associated with the nail:

1. The *proximal nail fold* helps to protect the matrix. The stratum corneum produced there forms the cuticle.

2. The *matrix* produces the nail plate from its rapidly dividing, keratinizing cells. Most of the matrix underlies the proximal nail fold, but on some digits (especially the thumb) it extends under the nail plate, where it is grossly visible as the white lunula. The most proximal portion of the matrix forms the top of the nail plate; the most distal portion forms the bottom of the nail plate.

3. The epithelium of the *nail bed* produces a minimal amount of keratin, which becomes tightly adherent to the bottom of the nail plate. The pink color of a nail is due to the vascularity in the dermis of the nail bed.

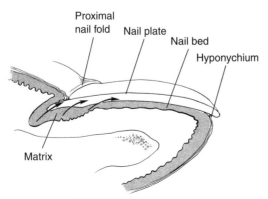

FIGURE 2–4. Normal nail.

4. The epidermis of the *hyponychium* underlies the free distal edge of the nail plate. Stratum corneum produced there forms a cuticle to seal the junction of the distal nail bed and nail plate.

■ SUBCUTANEOUS FAT

Subcutaneous fat:
1. Insulates
2. Absorbs trauma
3. Is a reserve food

A layer of subcutaneous fat lies between the dermis and the underlying fascia. It helps to insulate the body from cold, cushions deep tissues from blunt trauma, and serves as a reserve source of food. Within the subcutaneous fat layer, aggregates of fat cells (lipocytes) are separated by fibrous septa that are traversed by blood vessels and nerves.

R E F E R E N C E S

Dawber R: Diseases of the Hair and Scalp. 3rd ed. Boston, Blackwell Scientific Publications, 1997.

Goldsmith LA: Physiology, Biochemistry and Molecular Biology of the Skin. 2nd ed. New York, Oxford University Press, 1991.

Montagna W, Parakkal P: The Structure and Function of the Skin. 3rd ed. New York, Academic Press, 1974.

Sorer NA, Baden HP: Pathophysiology of Dermatologic Diseases. 2nd ed. New York, McGraw-Hill, 1991.

Zaias N: The Nail in Health and Disease. 2nd ed. Norwalk, CT, Appleton & Lange, 1989.

PATHOGENETIC MECHANISMS OF SKIN DISEASE

IMMUNOLOGIC MECHANISMS
INFECTION
NEOPLASIA
GENODERMATOSES
HORMONAL EFFECTS
NUTRITIONAL DEFICIENCIES
PSYCHODERMATOSES

T he exponential growth of basic scientific medical knowledge in recent decades has dramatically advanced understanding of the pathogenetic mechanisms involved in skin disease. Much of this basic knowledge has been derived directly from skin research, especially in immunology and neoplasia. The visibility and accessibility of skin make it a particularly useful organ to study.

In this chapter, we briefly consider the pathogenetic mechanisms that are most important in skin diseases. These involve immunology, infection, neoplasia, genetics, hormones, nutrition, and psychology. In many skin diseases, a combination of pathogenetic factors is involved. The pathogenesis of specific diseases is discussed in Chapters 6 through 23.

■ IMMUNOLOGIC MECHANISMS

The skin is an end-organ for many immunologically mediated disorders as well as a tool for immunologic research. The skin, however, should *not* be viewed as having only a passive role as an arena where immunologic reactions take place. Rather, the skin should be considered an active player on the "immunologic field of action," which contains immunologic cells (lymphoid and Langerhans cells) and cells (keratinocytes) that produce certain immunity-modulating substances. The interaction among Langerhans cells, keratinocytes, and skin-targeting lymphocytes (Th1 and Th2) has been called the skin-associated lymphoid tissue (SALT). To facilitate immunoregulation and communication among these cells, soluble factors (e.g., cytokines) and cell-surface proteins (e.g., cell adhesion molecules) are produced. The cells within the skin that participate in immunologic reactions and the mediators of inflammation that they produce are listed in Table 3–1. The skin can be viewed as a peripheral arm of the immune system involved in normal homeostasis and host defense.

The skin is an immunologically active organ.

TABLE 3–1 ■ THE SKIN AS AN IMMUNOLOGIC ORGAN

Cells	Inflammatory Mediators Produced
Keratinocytes	With proper stimulation, they synthesize and secrete Interleukins Colony-stimulating factors Transforming growth factors Interferons Eicosanoids Tumor necrosis factor Adhesion molecules
Langerhans cells	They have an antigen-presenting capability, activate T-cells, and secrete Interleukins Tumor necrosis factor Eicosanoids Adhesion molecules
Lymphocytes	A subset of T-cells (Th1 and Th2 CD4+), they have a special affinity for the skin, where they participate in delayed-type immune reactions, e.g., allergic contact dermatitis. They secrete Interleukins Interferons Adhesion molecules Colony-stimulating factors Tumor necrosis factor
Mast cells	They contain vasoactive and chemotactic substances that are particularly important in immediate-type immune reactions. They release Histamine Eicosanoids Enzymes Heparin Cytokines

Immune Reactions

Gell and Coombs divided the immune mechanisms involved in producing tissue damage into four basic types, as outlined in Table 3–2. Many immunologic diseases have skin involvement as well as extracutaneous manifestations. Therefore, the presence of certain skin lesions should serve as a clue to look for systemic problems, for example, purpuric papules in systemic vasculitis.

Type I (immediate) reactions are characterized by the release of vasoactive substances from mast cells or basophils following the reaction of a specific antigen and antibody. The antibody mediating this reaction is usually immunoglobulin (Ig) E but also may be a subset of IgG. The basophil and mast cell possess cell-surface receptors that bind the Fe portion of the IgE molecules. When adjacent membrane-bound IgE molecules are bridged by a specific antigen, vasoactive substances including histamine, serotonin, slow-reacting substance of anaphylaxis (which has been identified as a leukotriene), and prostaglandins are released. Mediator release is manifested cutaneously by hives and systemically by bronchospasm, laryngeal edema, nausea, vomiting, cramping abdominal pain, diarrhea, hypotension, and shock.

Type I (immediate) reactions are immunoglobulin E mediated.

TABLE 3-2 ■ IMMUNE REACTIONS

Type	Name	Mediators	Example
I	Immediate	IgE, histamine	Urticaria, anaphylaxis
II	Cytotoxic	IgG, IgM	Bullous pemphigoid
III	Immune complex	IgG, IgM	Vasculitis
IV	Cell-mediated	T-lymphocytes, lymphokines	Allergic contact dermatitis

Type II (cytotoxic) reactions result in cell damage, lysis, phagocytosis, or stimulation. The antigen is a portion of the plasma membrane or a free antigen or hapten that has been absorbed onto the cell membrane. Circulating IgG or IgM antibodies react with the surface antigen and activate complement, with resultant tissue damage. An example of this type of reaction is bullous pemphigoid. The bullous pemphigoid antigen is part of the basement zone at the dermal-epidermal junction. Circulating autoantibodies affix to the bullous pemphigoid antigen, resulting in activation of complement and in recruitment and degranulation of eosinophils and neutrophils, a process that then produces bullae between the epidermis and the dermis. Direct immunofluorescence of skin in patients with bullous pemphigoid shows deposits of IgG and complement in a linear pattern along the basement membrane zone. Indirect immunofluorescent testing shows circulating IgG bullous pemphigoid antibodies in two thirds of the patients.

> **In type II (cytotoxic) reactions, the antigen is on the cell surface.**

Type III (immune complex) reactions occur when circulating antigen-antibody complexes are deposited in tissue, causing inflammation. The antibody is usually IgG or IgM and combines with an antigen. After tissue deposition, the immune complexes activate complement, resulting in chemotaxis of leukocytes, platelet damage, release of vasoactive substances, and increased vascular permeability. Neutrophils then ingest the immune complexes and release enzymes that cause further tissue damage. For example, in vasculitis, immune complex deposition in postcapillary venules leads to blood vessel damage and clinically results in purpuric papules and nodules. Blood vessels in the bowel, kidneys, lungs, and central nervous system can be affected by the same process.

> **In type III (immune complex) reactions, there are circulating immune complexes.**

Type IV (delayed hypersensitivity) reactions are mediated by sensitized lymphocytes. The interaction between a lymphocyte and a specific antigen results in the release of lymphokines that mediate the reaction. Clinically, allergic contact dermatitis from poison ivy exposure is a common example of cell-mediated immunity. The antigen is contained in poison ivy sap. When the sap comes in contact with the skin, the antigen is absorbed onto the surface of Langerhans cells (skin macrophage) and is presented to sensitized T-lymphocytes (CD4-bearing T-cells). The subsequent release of lymphokines produces papules and vesicles that are typical of allergic contact dermatitis. The reaction is "delayed" in that it usually occurs 24 to 48 hours after exposure to the poison ivy.

> **Type IV (delayed) reactions are T-cell mediated.**

Complement

Complement is a group of normal serum proteins that play an important role in inflammation and host defense. When activated, these proteins augment the immune system, causing cell lysis, alterations in cell membranes, and liberation of mediators of inflammation. Complement is activated by an antibody-antigen reaction (classic pathway) or by contact with a variety of substances such as bacterial

TABLE 3-3 ■ CUTANEOUS MANIFESTATIONS OF COMPLEMENT DEFICIENCIES

Deficient Component	Systemic Disease	Cutaneous Manifestation
Clq, Clr, Cls, C2, C4	Lupus erythematosus–like syndrome	Discoid lupus lesions
C1 inhibitor	Hereditary angioedema	Angioedema
Factor I, C3, factor D	Pyogenic infections	Abscesses
C5, C6, C7, C8	Disseminated gonococcemia	Purpuric pustules

wall lipopolysaccharides (alternative pathway) and is involved in types II and III immunologic reactions.

Patients with complement deficiencies have numerous cutaneous manifestations, as outlined in Table 3–3. Autoimmune syndromes occur in individuals who lack early complement components, and infectious complications develop in people who are deficient in the late components.

Complement deficiencies are rare.

Hereditary angioedema is caused by a deficiency of the C1 inhibitor.

Complement deficiencies are rare but serve to illustrate the importance of complement in immune reactions. An example of an important deficiency is hereditary angioedema, in which patients lack the serum protein C1 esterase inhibitor, which inhibits the activated first complement component. In this dominantly inherited syndrome, failure to downregulate complement activation produces angioedema of the skin, gut, and larynx and may result in death from airway obstruction.

HLA Antigens

The major histocompatibility complex is located on chromosome 6 and is composed of genetic loci—A, B, C, and D, with the D region subdivided into DP, DQ, and DR. These genes code for human leukocyte antigens (HLA), which are glycoproteins and polypeptides present on the cell surface and are responsible for tissue compatibility. HLA antigens are divided into two classes based on structural similarity. Class I comprises HLA-A, HLA-B, and HLA-C antigens, which are present on almost all nucleated cells. Class II comprises HLA-DP, HLA-DQ, and HLA-DR antigens, which are found on B-lymphocytes, activated T-lymphocytes, monocytes, macrophages, and Langerhans cells. The clinical applications of HLA typing are in organ transplantation, paternity testing, and disease associations. Disease association is based on a statistically significant increase or decrease in frequency of HLA antigens in individuals in a defined population who have a given disease compared with controls or unaffected individuals in the same population. Table 3–4 lists the most common skin diseases associated with HLA antigens.

Various theories have been proposed to explain the association between the genes of the HLA complex and disease:

1. A foreign organism has antigenic determinants similar to the HLA antigens, resulting in immunologic cross-reactions with those of the host.
2. The cell-surface antigen controlled by the HLA complex acts as a receptor for an etiologic agent, possibly facilitating disease production.

TABLE 3–4 ■ SKIN DISEASE ASSOCIATED WITH HLA ANTIGENS

Disease	HLA Antigen	% Antigen in Patients	% Antigen in Controls
Dermatitis herpetiformis	B8	77	25
	DR3	95	20
Reiter's syndrome	B27	78	8
Psoriasis	B13	20	5
	B17	26	8
Behçet's disease			
Caucasian	B51	35	11
Japanese	B51	75	31
Pemphigus	A10	61	20

3. A specific immune response in the region of the HLA complex is responsible for the disease process without implying that the HLA gene itself plays a role.

HLA antigens are normal (see Table 3–4); the difference between control subjects and patients is the frequency with which specific antigens are found. In addition, different populations have different frequencies of the same HLA antigens, requiring careful selection of controls. An example is HLA-B5, which normally occurs in 11% of Caucasians and in 31% of Japanese persons.

HLA-associated diseases relate to frequency of antigens in patients versus controls.

Immunodeficiency Disorders

Patients with primary and acquired immunodeficiency diseases frequently present with chronic and recurrent infections, particularly involving unusual opportunistic organisms. Other features that are frequently present in primary immunodeficiency diseases include skin rashes (e.g., eczema), chronic diarrhea, growth failure, and hepatosplenomegaly. AIDS has numerous mucocutaneous manifestations, including oral hairy leukoplakia, Kaposi's sarcoma, severe seborrheic dermatitis and psoriasis, and viral and fungal skin infections (Table 3–5).

■ INFECTION

Pathogenic organisms can reach the skin by either external or internal routes; examples are given in Table 3–6. An external route is more common for cutaneous infections.

Physical, microbial, and immunologic barriers to the invasion of pathogens into the skin are present. The major physical barrier is the stratum corneum, which provides a dry, impermeable surface that is inhospitable to most pathogenic organisms. Increased hydration of the stratum corneum or its traumatic disruption can predispose to microbial invasion.

The skin surface and its appendages also harbor nonpathogenic microorganisms (normal skin flora) that provide ecologic competition for pathogenic microorganisms and produce antibiotics inhibitory to some pathogens. Three classes of resident microbial organisms are recognized:

Cutaneous barriers to infection:
1. **Physical (stratum corneum)**
2. **Microbial (normal skin flora)**
3. **Immunologic (Langerhans cells, lymphocytes)**

TABLE 3-5 ■ IMMUNODEFICIENCY DISORDERS

Disorder	Skin Manifestations
Antibody (B-cell)	
X-linked agammaglobulinemia	Abscesses
	Dermatitis
Cellular (T-cell)	
Congenital thymic hypoplasia	Candidiasis
	Morbilliform rash
AIDS	Kaposi's sarcoma
	Viral and fungal infections
	Seborrheic dermatitis
	Oral hairy leukoplakia
Combined antibody-mediated (B-cell) and cell-mediated (T-cell)	
Severe combined immunodeficiency disease	Candidiasis
Phagocytic dysfunction	
Hyper-IgE syndrome	Abscesses
Chronic granulomatous disease	Dermatitis
Leukocyte adhesion deficiency disease	Cellulitis
	Abscesses

1. Aerobic cocci, of which *Staphylococcus epidermidis* is the most common, thrive best in moist environments such as flexural folds.

2. Anaerobic diphtheroids, of which *Propionibacterium acnes* is the most common, inhabit sebaceous glands and follicles and play a role in the pathogenesis of acne.

3. Yeast organisms of the *Pityrosporum* genus colonize skin that is rich in sebaceous glands. *Pityrosporum orbiculare* is an example. It plays a role in sebor-

Normal skin flora:
Staphylococcus epidermidis
Propionibacterium
Pityrosporum

TABLE 3-6 ■ SOURCE OF SKIN INFECTIONS

Organism	External	Internal
Bacteria	Impetigo	Septic vasculitis
	Folliculitis	Cellulitis
	Abscess and/or furuncle	
	Cellulitis	
Viruses	Wart	Viral exanthem
	Molluscum contagiosum	Herpes varicella-zoster
	Herpes simplex	
Fungi		
Dermatophytes	Tinea	
Candida albicans	Candidiasis	Disseminated candidiasis
Deep fungi	Sporotrichosis	Histoplasmosis
		Coccidioidomycosis
		Blastomycosis
		Cryptococcosis
Spirochetes	Primary syphilis	Secondary syphilis
	Erythema migrans	Tertiary syphilis (gumma)
		Lyme disease
Mycobacteria	"Swimming pool" granuloma (atypical mycobacteria)	Tuberculosis
		Leprosy

rheic dermatitis and is converted to its hyphal form *(Malassezia furfur)* in the disease tinea versicolor.

The immunologic barrier begins in the epidermis with Langerhans cells and lymphocytes, both of which are normally contained in the epidermis. The importance of skin as an immunologic organ has become increasingly apparent in recent years, as is reflected by the acronym SALT (skin-associated lymphoid tissue), which designates the immunologic activity inherent in the skin.

Despite these barriers, some organisms possess special properties that allow them to invade and infect the skin. The skin lesions that result depend on both the nature of these properties and the nature of the host response.

Bacterial Infections

Most bacterial infections of the skin are caused by either *Staphylococcus aureus* or group A β-hemolytic streptococci *(Streptococcus pyogenes).*

Staphylococcus aureus can colonize the skin surface. The organism then gains entry through traumatized stratum corneum or through a hair follicle. The former route causes impetigo; the latter causes folliculitis or a furuncle. The bacteria produce chemotactic factors that attract neutrophils, resulting in pus formation, and enzymes that contribute to the inflammatory response. Certain staphylococcal strains elaborate an epidermolytic toxin that causes intraepidermal separation in bullous impetigo and staphylococcal scalded skin syndrome.

Staphylococcal chemotactic factors produce pus.

Unlike staphylococci, group A streptococci do not colonize skin. The organism is usually inoculated into areas of previously damaged skin (e.g., insect bites and scratches), where infection is established. Streptococcal impetigo (ecthyma) is an example. Streptococci also elaborate various proteolytic enzymes that degrade dermal elements and cause inflammation, as in cellulitis.

Streptococci produce proteolytic enzymes, which cause inflammation.

Viral Infections

Viruses are common causes of skin infection. Three DNA viral families most commonly cause skin disease:

1. Papova, especially human papillomavirus (HPV).
2. Pox, such as molluscum contagiosum virus.
3. Herpes: herpes simplex virus (HSV) and varicella-zoster virus.

With the exception of varicella-zoster virus infection, which is initially acquired by the respiratory route, these "skin" viruses establish infection after direct inoculation into the skin. They then penetrate epidermal cells, where they replicate. Their location in the epidermis and their effect on the host cell vary with the virus. Wart and molluscum contagiosum viruses replicate only in keratinizing cells (i.e., cells in the upper epidermis) and cause *hyperplasia* rather than destruction of the infected cells. Hence, these infections appear as epidermal *growths*. In contrast, HSV has a devastating effect on the host cell. Its replicative cycle occurs over a period of hours and results in lysis and death of the host cell. Clinically, epidermal *vesicles* result.

Papilloma and molluscum contagiosum viruses induce epidermal hyperplasia.

Host immunity is involved in both the acquisition and the involution of these viral diseases. Neutralizing antibodies, lymphocyte-mediated cytotoxicity, and

Herpes simplex virus infection destroys host epidermal cells, causing vesicles.

lymphocyte-produced interferon as well as other lymphokines probably play a role. Immunosuppressed patients are more susceptible to herpes and warts. In immunocompetent hosts infected with herpes, neutralizing antibodies appear to prevent dissemination but not local recurrence. Cell-mediated immunity probably is important in clearing local recurrence of herpes and providing spontaneous regression of warts.

Recurrent HSV infection results from latent virus in sensory or autonomic ganglion cells, where they reside but are not destructive. The intact viral particles are not detectable in these cells, but the viral genome is. During reactivation, the genomes replicate and produce new virus. The viral genomes within ganglion cells are relatively well protected from immunologic influence, and this feature may in part explain their survival.

Fungal Infections

Superficial fungal infections are common.

Superficial fungal infections are common causes of skin disease such as athlete's foot and jock itch. Dermatophytes are the most common cause, followed by infection with *Candida albicans*. Skin involvement also may occur with systemic fungal infection, but these infections are uncommon.

Dermatophytic Infections

Dermatophytes feed on keratin.

Dermatophytes are filamentous fungi that are unique in that they possess enzymes to digest keratin. To these organisms, the stratum corneum does not appear hostile; it appears as food. Infection causes loosening of the stratum corneum, resulting in scale. In addition to stratum corneum, these keratinophilic fungi can infect hair and nails. They grow as hyphae, which are filamentous forms representing cells lying end to end.

The nature of the dermatophyte and the influence of host defense mechanisms help to determine the appearance of the clinical lesion and its clinical course. Slow-growing fungal infections of the uppermost layers of the stratum corneum may not elicit an inflammatory response; for example, chronic tinea pedis results in noninflammatory scaling of the feet. Some dermatophytes are more likely than others to elicit an inflammatory reaction. In general, fungi acquired from animal reservoirs (zoophilic) are more inflammatory than those acquired from human reservoirs (anthropophilic).

The immune response induced by dermatophytes is predominantly cell mediated and can result in spontaneous healing. It may also account for the centrifugal spread frequently seen in dermatophytic infections; that is, the process spreads outward as local immunity develops within the center of the lesion. The finding of negative skin tests within the center of annular dermatophytic lesions has been used to support this hypothesis.

Candidiasis

C. albicans commonly causes external cutaneous infection. *C. albicans* may colonize the mouth, gastrointestinal tract, and vagina. Infection occurs when the yeast forms are transformed into hyphae and pseudohyphae (elongated spores). Conditions and agents favorable to this transition include moisture, steroids, pregnancy, and antibiotics. In the epidermis, the hyphal elements have the ability to activate the alternative complement pathway, resulting in inflammation that is characteristically bright red. Chemotactic factors attract neutrophils, resulting in pustule formation. Cell-mediated immunity is important in the host defense, as is illustrated in chronic mucocutaneous candidiasis. Patients with this disorder are deficient in cell-mediated immunity to *C. albicans,* and this deficiency results in severe and chronic candidal infection of the skin and mucous membranes. Disseminated candidiasis occurs only in severely immunocompromised hosts.

Candida albicans commonly infects skin and mucous membranes.

Candida hyphae activate complement, causing inflammation and pustule formation.

Deep Fungal Infections

Deep fungal infections are much less common than superficial infections. Fungi can infect the skin through direct inoculation, as in sporotrichosis, or by hematogenous spread, as sometimes occurs with cryptococcosis, histoplasmosis, and coccidioidomycosis. The route of entry into the body is determined in part by the physical characteristics of the fungus. *Sporothrix schenckii,* for example, is a soil-living organism that adheres tightly to thorny plants and vegetable matter. It is much less likely to be aerosolized than are the light spores causing histoplasmosis and coccidioidomycosis. Therefore, sporotrichosis is inoculated through skin injury, and histoplasmosis and coccidioidomycosis are acquired by inhalation.

Deep fungal infections of the skin are uncommon.

Clinical presentation depends on the route of inoculation. With direct cutaneous inoculation, ulcerated inflammatory nodules are formed locally and are accompanied by regional lymphadenopathy, the so-called *chancriform complex.* Skin involvement from disseminated disease occurs by hematogenous spread and appears as scattered plaques, nodules, or ulcers, unaccompanied by regional lymphadenopathy. The patient usually is systemically ill.

Spirochetal Infections

Spirochetal diseases characteristically occur in stages, with different clinical manifestations occurring in each stage. In the United States, the two spirochetal diseases affecting the skin are Lyme disease and syphilis. Both begin with skin inoculation of the organism.

In Lyme disease, the spirochete is inoculated from an infected tick, resulting in a skin lesion called *erythema migrans.* In syphilis, the primary lesion is an indurated ulcer, or chancre.

Host immunity against these spirochetes is sufficient to eliminate the local process slowly but is often insufficient to effect a systemic cure. Consequently, after varying periods of latency, secondary and even tertiary systemic stages may occur. Hence, treatment in the primary stage is important.

Spirochetal infections evolve through several clinical stages.

Mycobacterial Infections

Mycobacteria are thick-walled organisms that grow intracellularly and therefore are resistant to antibody destruction. Infection is controlled (often incompletely) by cellular immunity, in which histiocytes play a prominent role. The interplay between the organism and the cellular immune response results in a chronic infection characterized by granuloma formation. Histologically, granulomas are composed of aggregates of epithelioid cells, which are so named because they resemble epithelial cells, but they are in fact altered histiocytes. The skin reaction

Mycobacterial infections are chronic and are characterized by granuloma formation.

in mycobacterial diseases depends on the route of inoculation and the host responsiveness to the organism.

In the United States, cases of mycobacterial skin infection are most often due to atypical mycobacteria, particularly *Mycobacterium marinum*. This is acquired from contact with infected water, hence the term "swimming pool" granuloma. Once inoculated into the skin, the organism elicits a granulomatous response accompanied by reactive epidermal hyperplasia.

Leprosy is a systemic mycobacterial infection that is uncommon in the United States but still present in many parts of the world. The leprosy bacillus has a particular predilection for skin, in which the nature of the lesion depends primarily on the degree of host immunity. Highly reactive hosts produce a vigorous granulomatous response (tuberculoid leprosy) characterized by only a few skin lesions containing rare organisms. Anergic patients develop lepromatous leprosy, in which organisms are abundant and multiple skin lesions result.

■ NEOPLASIA

Etiology of skin cancer:
1. **Ultraviolet radiation**
2. **X-irradiation**
3. **Chemicals**
4. **Viruses**

Skin cancer is the most common human malignancy, with more than 1.2 million new cases occurring in Caucasians in the United States annually. This number equals the combined incidence of all other malignant diseases. Although cancer of the skin usually is easily treated, it causes more than 9,000 deaths per year. Epidemiologically and experimentally, malignant lesions of the skin have played a prominent role in the discovery of the etiology and pathogenesis of cancer. Ultraviolet radiation, x-irradiation, chemicals, and viruses have been implicated, particularly in genetically predisposed individuals.

All these carcinogens appear to act in skin by altering DNA, RNA, and other cellular proteins. Molecular biology has greatly expanded our understanding of carcinogenesis. Normal cellular genes, called *proto-oncogenes* and *tumor suppressor* genes, control cellular growth. The protein products of proto-oncogenes and tumor suppressor genes are growth factors, growth factor receptors, signal transduction components, and regulators of gene transcription. Oncogenes are closely related to normal cellular proto-oncogenes but are altered to cause cancer. Oncogenes have lost their normal constraints, causing uncontrolled cellular growth and, eventually, malignant transformation. These oncogenes are produced by agents that damage DNA. Activation of oncogenes has been implicated in the pathogenesis of skin cancer induced by radiation, chemicals, and viruses. Tumor suppressor genes normally prevent cancers by regulating malignant growth of cells. When inactivated by ultraviolet radiation or HPV, mutations of tumor suppressor genes, PTCH and p53, have been linked to basal cell and squamous cell carcinoma.

Neoplasia genes:
1. **Oncogenes**
2. **Tumor suppressor genes**

The most common cause of skin cancer is *ultraviolet radiation*, which is a complete carcinogen, having both initiating and promoting properties. Experimental, clinical, and epidemiologic data make it one of the most clear-cut causes of human cancer. Sunlight, predominantly in the UVB range of 290 to 320 nm, causes damage to DNA in epidermal cells. This results in mutated oncogenes and tumor suppressor genes causing altered proliferation and replication. Clinically, most skin cancers occur in areas of the body with the most ultraviolet radiation exposure—head, neck, and upper extremities. Patients with the recessively inherited disease *xeroderma pigmentosum* have defective repair processes of ultraviolet-induced

DNA damage and manifest markedly enhanced susceptibility to ultraviolet-induced squamous cell carcinoma, basal cell carcinoma, and melanoma. Epidemiologically, individuals who lack the protection of melanin (albinos or fair-skinned individuals) develop neoplasms of the skin much more frequently than do darkly pigmented individuals. Ultraviolet radiation exposure correlates with increased skin cancer, particularly in farmers, sailors, and populations in latitudes closer to the equator.

In 1924, Block demonstrated that *x-rays* could cause skin cancer in rabbits. This potential was recognized in humans with the development of multiple cutaneous carcinomas in the unshielded hands of dentists and radiologists who then developed chronic radiodermatitis and, later, carcinoma.

Sir Percivall Pott's observation in 1775 that chimney sweeps have a high incidence of scrotal cancer led him to conclude that soot was the cause. Pott's hypothesis of *chemically* induced carcinogenesis was confirmed by Yamagiwa and Ichikawa in 1917. They produced carcinoma on the ears of rabbits after repeated applications of coal tar. The experimental animal models for chemically induced skin cancer have led to some the concepts concerning the basic mechanisms of carcinogenesis. In 1941, Berenblum proposed that carcinogenesis induced by chemicals involves three phases: initiation, promotion, and latency. With benzpyrene (the initiator), he could cause only a few small tumors on the skin of mice. When croton resin (the promoter) was applied along with benzpyrene, the number and size of tumors were markedly increased (progression) after a dormant or latency period. Examples of initiating agents are polycyclic aromatic hydrocarbons, nitrosamines, aromatic amines, and alkylating agents. The initiators are carcinogenic by themselves, and their action is irreversible and mutagenic. Examples of promoting agents are phorbol esters and aromatics. Promoter agents are not carcinogenic alone but must be given after the initiating agent has exerted its effect. Their action is reversible and not cumulative. They do not produce mutagenic effects.

Multiple stages of carcinogenesis:
1. Initiation
2. Promotion
3. Progression

The *viral* etiology of skin cancer, although less well proven in humans, undoubtedly occurs. HPV has been implicated as the cause of cutaneous and cervical carcinoma. Patients with *epidermodysplasia verruciformis*, a rare genetic disorder, develop hundreds of flat warts, and those warts caused by specific types of HPV, particularly HPV-5, are prone to transform into squamous cell carcinoma. The finding of papillomavirus genomes, HPV-16 and HPV-18, in carcinoma of the cervix has provided strong circumstantial evidence for its carcinogenic potential in this setting. The human T-cell leukemia-lymphoma virus (HTLV) is associated with some T-cell cutaneous lymphomas. HTLV was the first human retrovirus to be isolated, and it appears to be related to bovine leukemia virus. Patients with HTLV malignant lymphomas have skin tumors, hypercalcemia, lymphadenopathy, hepatosplenomegaly, and a rapid, fatal course.

Immunologic surveillance of the skin has an important role in allowing the development of carcinoma. Ultraviolet radiation produces selective immune incompetence, which appears to contribute substantially to the development of skin cancers. Short-wavelength ultraviolet light (or UVB) can induce cellular immune defects both at the site of irradiation and systemically. Patients who are immunosuppressed after renal transplantation are at a sevenfold greater risk of developing skin carcinoma than are immunologically normal individuals. Multiple squamous cell carcinomas in the same patient are common. The incidence increases with time from transplantation and in areas of sun exposure.

■ GENODERMATOSES

DNA is the blueprint from which structural and regulatory cell proteins are produced. The unit of DNA coding for a protein—the gene—is composed of exons (transcribed) and introns (spacing) subunits. The information in the DNA is transcribed onto messenger RNA (mRNA). The mRNA leaves the nucleus and attaches to ribosome subunits in the cytoplasm, in which translation of genetic information occurs through transfer RNA (tRNA) with production of polypeptide chains.

Etiology of genodermatoses:
1. **Mutation—enzyme deficiency**
2. **Chromosomal defect**
3. **Unknown**

Genetic disorders are caused by mutations that result in enzyme deficiencies, by chromosomal defects, or by unknown mechanisms. Gene mapping of the human genome has identified the chromosomal loci of many genodermatoses. Mutations usually involve a substitution of one of the DNA bases coding for mRNA. Less often, mutations result from the insertion or deletion of a base or group of bases. Mutations affecting single genes are inherited according to Mendel's law in dominant or recessive and in X-linked or autosomal fashion. *Oculocutaneous albinism*, an autosomal recessive genodermatosis, is caused by a mutation of the gene coding for the pigment-forming enzyme tyrosinase. *Neurofibromatosis type I* is a genodermatosis in which the gene (NF1) resides on the long arm of chromosome 17. The disease is inherited as an autosomal dominant trait, but 50% of index cases are new mutations.

Polygenic or multifactorial disorders are not inherited in a mendelian fashion. Polygenic disorders often impart to an individual a genetic predisposition, but environmental factors also are important in disease expression. Psoriasis is an example of a polygenic genodermatosis in which inheritance cannot be explained on the basis of a single gene locus. In addition to several gene loci, environmental factors such as infection, sunlight, emotion, and physical trauma contribute to the clinical manifestations of psoriasis.

Another group of the genetic disorders involves alterations in chromosomes. These chromosomal disorders result from duplications, deficiency, or translocation of portions of the chromosome. An example is Down's syndrome, in which duplication results in trisomy 21. Recognizing and understanding genodermatoses provide the clinician with information that can be used for better genetic counseling and a rationale for potential methods of treatment and prevention.

■ HORMONAL EFFECTS

Hormones exert regulatory influences on cellular functions, and the skin is not spared (Table 3–7). Most of the pathologic effects on the skin result from increased rather than decreased levels of hormones. The effects of glucocorticoids and androgens are encountered most frequently.

Glucocorticoids

Glucocorticoids cause:
1. **Atrophy and striae**
2. **Purpura**
3. **Steroid acne and hirsutism**
4. **"Moon facies" and a "buffalo hump"**

Increased glucocorticoid secretion from the adrenal glands can be due to a primary process in the adrenal glands or can be secondary to increased adrenocorticotropic hormone (ACTH) secretion by the pituitary glands. Glucocorticoids cause decreased synthesis of collagen and ground substance, resulting in dermal atrophy, striae, and loss of support to the superficial cutaneous blood vessels, a factor that

TABLE 3–7 ■ HORMONES

Disease	Hormone	Cutaneous Manifestations
Cushing's syndrome	Glucocorticoid	Acne Hirsutism Atrophy and striae Purpura Moon facies Central obesity (and "buffalo hump")
Addison's disease	Corticotropin (ACTH)	Hyperpigmentation
Virilizing syndrome	Androgens	Seborrhea Acne Hirsutism Androgenetic alopecia
Acromegaly	Growth hormone	"Dermatomegaly" Acanthosis nigricans
Insulin-resistant diabetes mellitus	Insulin	Acanthosis nigricans
Pheochromocytoma	Norepinephrine	Profuse sweating
Hyperthyroidism	Thyroid hormone (excess)	Warm, moist skin Pretibial myxedema*
Hypothyroidism	Thyroid hormone (deficiency)	Dry, cool skin Myxedema
Renal failure	Parathyroid hormone (excess)	Pruritus

*Often occurs long after the Graves' disease has been treated.

predisposes to purpura. Glucocorticoids augment the effect of androgens in the pilosebaceous unit, with resulting steroid acne and mild hirsutism. The foregoing effects can be caused by topical as well as systemic steroids. Observed but unexplained is the regional variation in subcutaneous fat changes. Patients have increased fat of the face ("moon facies") and the trunk, resulting in central obesity with a "buffalo hump." On the extremities, patients have decreased subcutaneous fat and muscle wasting.

Adrenocorticotropic Hormone—Addison's Disease

Although deficiency in glucocorticoids itself has little effect on the skin, if the deficiency is due to primary adrenal failure, lack of feedback to the pituitary gland results in increased ACTH secretion. This polypeptide is secreted along with melanocyte-stimulating hormone and results in increased pigmentation in the skin and mucous membranes.

Androgens—Virilizing Syndromes

In the skin, androgens exert their major effects on the pilosebaceous unit. These effects include (1) increased sebum production (seborrhea), (2) acne, (3) androgenetic alopecia (male-pattern baldness), and (4) hirsutism. The paradoxic effect of androgens in producing increased hair growth in some areas (e.g., the beard) but decreasing it in others (e.g., the balding scalp) is unexplained.

Androgens cause acne, alopecia, and hirsutism.

The most potent circulating androgen is testosterone, but other secreted androgens of gonadal or adrenal origin can serve as precursors for peripheral testosterone production and so may also be important. In the skin, testosterone is further converted by the enzyme 5-α-reductase to dihydrotestosterone, which is considered to be the most active tissue androgen. Increased 5-α-reductase activity may be important in the pathogenesis of androgenic skin diseases such as acne, androgenic alopecia, and hirsutism.

Growth Hormone—Acromegaly

Excess growth hormone results in "dermatomegaly," in which growth or function of all the skin's components is increased, including the following: (1) epidermal hyperplasia; (2) hyperpigmentation; (3) thickening of the dermis, resulting in induration and furrowing; (4) thickened hair and nails; (5) increased oiliness; (6) increased sweating (hyperhidrosis); and (7) increased growth of hair (hypertrichosis). Acanthosis nigricans, which appears as velvety, hyperpigmented skin in flexural folds, also occurs but is not unique to this disease.

Insulin—Insulin-Resistant Diabetes Mellitus

Patients with diabetes and insulin resistance have high levels of circulating insulin, which frequently binds to insulin-like growth factor receptors in the skin to produce skin thickening and darkening (acanthosis nigricans).

Norepinephrine—Pheochromocytoma

Increased levels of norepinephrine, secreted by a pheochromocytoma, result in paroxysms of hypertension and, often, sweating. The sweating is diffuse, sometimes drenching, and occurs in about two thirds of patients with pheochromocytomas.

Thyroid Hormone Excess—Hyperthyroidism and Graves' Disease

Some of the cutaneous manifestations of excessive thyroid hormone result from the hypermetabolic state, which produces increased heat and results in warm, flushed, moist skin. In Graves' disease, pretibial myxedema also may occur. The cause of the cutaneous mucin deposition in this disease is unknown, although an IgG antibody has been implicated. Pretibial myxedema may not appear until long after Graves' disease has been treated.

Thyroid Hormone Deficiency

The dry, cool skin in hypothyroidism contrasts with that of hyperthyroidism, but the most striking change is the generalized increased thickness of the skin owing to deposition of mucopolysaccharides, which impart to the skin a thickened, "doughy" feel. The cause of cutaneous myxedema is not known, although it is thought to be related in some way to thyroid hormone deficiency.

Parathyroid Hormone

Excessive parathyroid hormone usually is not accompanied by skin manifestations, except for the rare occurrence of metastatic calcification. Secondary hyperparathyroidism, however, occurring in association with renal disease can result in generalized pruritus. The deposition of calcium phosphate salts in the skin is a possible explanation.

■ NUTRITIONAL DEFICIENCIES

The skin, as any other organ, can suffer consequences of nutritional deprivation. As a rapidly dividing tissue, the epidermis has a high nutritional demand, so it is more sensitive to substrate deficiency. Hair is particularly sensitive because the cellular turnover rate in the hair matrix is one of the highest in the body. Accordingly, nutritional deprivation often results in skin desquamation and alopecia. General malnutrition (a prevalent problem in underdeveloped countries) can cause these effects, as can several selective deficiencies (Table 3–8). As noted, three of these disorders have been associated with total parenteral nutrition, in which selective deficiencies have been caused by incomplete formulations of the admin-

**Nutritional deficiencies
often cause:**
1. Skin desquamation
2. Alopecia

TABLE 3-8 ■ NUTRITIONAL DEFICIENCIES

Deficiency	Cutaneous Manifestations
Vitamin A	Dry eyes—corneal scarring Generalized scaling with hyperkeratosis

Vitamin B
  Niacin (pellagra)
  Biotin*
	
	Dermatitis in sun-exposed areas
	Dermatitis with desquamation
	Alopecia

Vitamin C (scurvy)	Imparied wound healing Perifollicular purpura Red, swollen, bleeding gums
Zinc*	Seborrheic dermatitis-like rash Periorificial and acral pustules and bullae Alopecia
Amino acids (glucagonoma)	Glossitis Dermatitis with superficial epidermal necrosis
Essential fatty acids*	Scaling rash starting in flexural folds—generalized Alopecia

*Has been associated with total parenteral nutrition.

istered solutions. With recognition of this problem, it has been generally remedied. Zinc deficiency also occurs in a condition called *acrodermatitis enteropathica*, in which the deficiency results from impaired zinc absorption. Biotin deficiency occurs in two inherited forms in which patients have a deficiency of an enzyme needed to synthesize biotin.

Dermatologic manifestations in these deficiencies also are more prone to occur in areas of skin where increased rates of repair are required. For example, the rash in pellagra occurs in sun-exposed areas, presumably because sufficient vitamin substrate is not available to keep up with the repair of the sun-damaged skin. The glucagonoma syndrome is accompanied by amino acid deficiency, and the skin manifestations occur in areas most prone to trauma, for example, on the tongue, at the angles of the mouth, and in the groin area.

Vitamins A and C have special effects on the skin. Vitamin A regulates keratinization, and its deficiency causes hyperkeratosis and dry, scaling skin. Vitamin C is necessary for normal collagen metabolism. Vitamin C deficiency (scurvy) causes impaired wound healing and perifollicular and gingival bleeding.

■ PSYCHODERMATOSES

In many dermatologic disorders, emotions play an important role as either a cause or a result of the skin disease. Emotions can alter or augment neurally and chemically mediated responses of the skin such as itching, flushing, and sweating. Psychodermatoses can be divided into primary, secondary, or mixed disorders.

Primary psychodermatoses are characterized by emotional disorders that *cause* the changes seen in the skin. Examples are neurotic excoriations, trichotillomania, factitial dermatoses, and delusions of parasitosis. Some of these disorders are discussed in Chapters 9 and 21. Patients characteristically have some of the traits of self-destruction, neurotic behavior, repressed aggression, and obsessive-compulsive personality.

Secondary psychodermatoses are characterized by a skin disease that affects the emotional well-being of the patient. An example is alopecia areata. The hair loss in this disease frequently has a profound effect on the patient's self-image, resulting in depression and anger.

Last, mixed psychodermatoses are characterized by the interplay of emotional and cutaneous diseases. Patients often note disease exacerbation during emotional stress. The disease exacerbation then causes more emotional stress, initiating a vicious cycle. The itch-scratch cycle of atopic dermatitis is made considerably worse during periods of anxiety. Examples of other skin diseases with significant emotional components include acne, psoriasis, and urticaria. Being aware that emotional factors are important in producing and prolonging dermatologic diseases results in a better understanding of the pathogenesis and facilitates the treatment of patients with these disorders.

Psychodermatoses:
1. **Primary—emotions cause skin lesions**
2. **Secondary—skin disease causes emotional changes**
3. **Mixed—vicious cycle of skin and emotional disorder**

R E F E R E N C E S

Immunologic Skin Diseases

Charlesworth EN: Cutaneous Allergy. Cambridge, England, Blackwell Science Publishers, 1996.
Dahl MV: Clinical Immunodermatology. 3rd ed. Chicago, Year Book, 1996.
Jordon RE: Immunologic Diseases of the Skin. Norwalk, CT, Appleton & Lange, 1991.

Katz AM, Rosenthal D, Sauder DN: Cell adhesion molecules: structure, function and implication in a variety of cutaneous and other pathologic conditions. Int J Dermatol 30: 153–160, 1991.
Roitt IM, Brostoff J, Male DK: Immunology. 2nd ed. St. Louis, CV Mosby, 1989.
Soter NA, Baden HP (eds.): Pathophysiology of Dermatologic Diseases. 2nd ed. New York, McGraw-Hill, 1991, pp. 106–108.

Skin Infections

Cobb MW: Human papillomavirus infection. J Am Acad Dermatol 22:547–566, 1990.
Feingold DS, Hirschmann JV, Leyden JJ: Bacterial infections of the skin. J Am Acad Dermatol 20:469–475, 1989.
Hogan PA, Morelli JG, Weston WL: Viral exanthems. Curr Probl Dermatol 2:35–94, 1992.
Roth RR, James WD: Microbiology of the skin: resident flora, ecology, infection. J Am Acad Dermatol 20:367–390, 1989.

Neoplasia

Beattner WA, Takatsuki K, Gallo RC: Human T-cell leukemia-lymphoma virus and adult T-cell leukemia. JAMA 250:1074–1080, 1983.
Bergstresser PR: Ultraviolet radiation produces selective immune incompetence. J Invest Dermatol 81:85–86, 1983.
Buzzell RA: Carcinogenesis of cutaneous malignancies. Dermatol Surg 22:209–215, 1996.
Elder JT: c-Ha-RAS and UV photo carcinogenesis. Arch Dermatol 126:376–382, 1990.
Feldman SR: Oncogenes: the growth control genes. Arch Dermatol 127:707–711, 1991.
Gloster HM, Brodland DG: The epidemiology of skin cancer. Dermatol Surg 22:217–226, 1996.
Hoxtell EO, Mandel JS, Murray SS, et al.: Incidence of skin carcinoma after renal transplantation. Arch Dermatol 113:436–438, 1977.
Quan MB, Moy RL: The role of human papillomavirus in carcinoma. J Am Acad Dermatol 25:698–705, 1991.
Yuspa SH, Dlugosz A: Cutaneous carcinogenesis: natural and experimental. In Goldsmith LA (ed.): Physiology, Biochemistry, and Molecular Biology of the Skin. New York, Oxford University Press, 1991, pp. 1365–1402.

Genodermatoses

Alper JC: Genetic Disorders of the Skin. St. Louis, Mosby–Year Book, 1991.
Harper JI: Genetics and Genodermatoses. In Champion RH, Burton JL, Burns DA, Breathnach SM (eds.): Textbook of Dermatology. 6th ed. Oxford, Blackwell Science, 1998, pp. 357–436.

Hormonal Effects

Braverman IM: Skin Signs of Systemic Disease. 3rd ed. Philadelphia, WB Saunders 1998.
Feingold KR, Elias PM: Endocrine-skin interactions: cutaneous manifestations of adrenal disease, pheochromocytomas, carcinoid syndrome, sex hormone excess and deficiency, polyglandular autoimmune syndromes, multiple endocrine neoplasia syndromes, and other miscellaneous disorders. J Am Acad Dermatol 19:1–20, 1988.
Thiboutot DM: Dermatologic manifestations of endocrine disorders. J Clin Endocrinol Metab 80:3082–3087, 1995.

Nutritional Deficiencies

Barthelmy H, Chouvet B, Cambazard F: Skin and mucosal manifestations in vitamin deficiency. J Am Acad Dermatol 15:1263–1274, 1986.
Hansen RC: Dermatitis and nutritional deficiency. Arch Dermatol 128:1389–1390, 1992.
Miller SJ: Nutritional deficiency and the skin. J Am Acad Dermatol 21:1–30, 1989.

Psychodermatoses

Cotterill JA (ed.): Psychodermatology. Semin Dermatol 2:171–226, 1983.

Gupta MA, Gupta AK: Psychodermatology: an update. J Am Acad Dermatol 34:1030–1046, 1996.

Koblenzer CS: Psychocutaneous Disease. New York, Grune & Stratton, 1987.

Koo JYM, Pharm CT: Psychodermatology: practical guidelines on pharmacotherapy. Arch Dermatol 128:381–388, 1992.

Medansky RS, Handler RM: Dermatopsychosomatics: classification, physiology, and therapeutic approaches. J Am Acad Dermatol 5:125–136, 1981.

PRINCIPLES OF DIAGNOSIS

HISTORY
PHYSICAL EXAMINATION
TERMINOLOGY OF SKIN LESIONS
CLINICOPATHOLOGIC CORRELATIONS
CONFIGURATION OF SKIN LESIONS
DISTRIBUTION OF SKIN LESIONS
LABORATORY TESTS

The approach to a patient with skin disease does not differ markedly from the approach to any other patient. Data are collected from a history and physical examination and sometimes from the laboratory), a differential diagnosis is generated, and the best diagnosis is selected.

In history taking, a modified format is suggested. Instead of beginning with an exhaustive interrogation, it is more efficient to divide the history into a preliminary and a follow-up format.

The most important part of the physical examination is inspection. Dermatology is a visual specialty, and diagnosis rests heavily on skin inspection. Unfortunately, although the skin is the most visible organ of the body, in a routine physical examination it often is the one most overlooked. Skin lesions need to be looked *for*, not *at*. Just as the examiner hears only the subtle heart sounds for which he or she listens, so will a clinician see on the skin only the lesions for which he or she searches. We need to train our eyes to see the skin lesions before us and ultimately be able to recognize them.

We have divided skin disorders into two broad categories: growths and rashes. A *growth* is a discrete lesion resulting from proliferation of one or more of the skin's components. A *rash* is an inflammatory process that usually is more widespread than a growth. For both skin growths and rashes, the most important task is to characterize the clinical appearance of the basic lesion, that is, to identify its morphology. Then the pathophysiologic processes responsible for the clinical lesion must be considered. These clinicopathologic correlations are emphasized in the diagnostic approach presented in this text. For skin rashes, important diagnostic information sometimes can also be obtained by noting the manner in which the lesions are arranged or distributed.

After the history and physical examination have been completed, laboratory tests may be indicated. In dermatology, these are usually simple office procedures that can provide valuable information needed either to confirm or to establish a diagnosis in selected disorders.

Dermatologic diagnosis depends on the examiner's skill in skin inspection.

Steps in dermatologic diagnosis:
1. **History**
2. **Physical—identify the morphology of basic lesion**
3. **Consider clinicopathologic correlations**
4. **Configuration or distribution of lesions (when applicable)**
5. **Laboratory tests**

■ HISTORY

In medicine, the traditional approach is to take the history before doing the physical examination. Some dermatologists prefer to reverse this order. We find it most useful to ask questions both before and after the examination. With this approach, a preliminary history is taken in which several general questions are asked of all patients. Depending on the physical findings, more selective questions may be asked subsequently. For example, a history of sexual contacts would be inappropriate for an 82-year-old invalid complaining of an itching scalp but would be indicated for a patient with an indurated ulcer on the penis.

Preliminary History

In addition to its diagnostic value, a preliminary history also helps to establish rapport with the patient. The short cut of examining the skin without expressing an interest in the person will often be found wanting, especially by the patient. This initial history is composed of two parts that correlate with the chief complaint and the history of the present illness in the standard history format.

Chief Complaint

In eliciting the chief complaint, one can often learn much by asking an open-ended question, such as "What is your skin problem?" This is followed by three general questions regarding the history of the present illness.

History of the Present Illness

The general questions concern onset and evolution of the condition, symptoms, and treatment to date.

The initial history can be abbreviated by asking three general questions:
1. **How long?**
2. **Does it itch?**
3. **How have you treated it?**

1. *Onset and evolution*: "When did it start? Has it gotten better or worse?" Answers to these questions determine the duration of the disorder and how the condition has evolved over time. For most skin conditions, this is important information.

2. *Symptoms*: "Does it bother you?" is an open-ended way of asking about symptoms. For skin disorders, the most common symptom is itching. If the patient does not respond to the general symptom question, you may want to ask specifically, "*Does it itch?*" Questions concerning systemic symptoms (e.g., "How do you feel otherwise?") are not applicable for most skin diseases and so are more appropriately reserved until after the physical examination.

3. *Treatment to date*: The question, "How have you treated it?" results in an incomplete response from almost all patients. For skin disease, one is particularly interested in learning what topical medications have been applied. Many patients do not consider over-the-counter preparations important enough to mention. The same applies for some systemic medications. Providing the patient with specific examples of commonly used topical and systemic medications, such as calamine lotion and aspirin, may jog a patient's memory enough to recall similar products that they may have used. It is important to inquire about medications not only because they cause some conditions, but also because they may aggravate many others. For example, contact dermatitis initially induced by poison ivy may be

perpetuated by contact allergy to an ingredient in one of the preparations used in treatment.

After the skin examination, one may need to return to the treatment question if any suspicion exists that a medication is causing or contributing to the disorder. Interestingly, a patient often recalls using pertinent medication only when he or she is asked the question three or more times.

Finally, at the end of the visit, when one is ready to prescribe medications for the patient, it is helpful to know what medications have already been used. This approach avoids the potentially awkward situation in which a patient replies to your enthusiastic recommendation of your favorite therapy with, "I've already tried that and it didn't work!"

Persistence is often required in eliciting a complete medication history.

Follow-up History

After the initial history and physical examination, it is hoped that one has formulated a diagnosis or at least a differential diagnosis. With a diagnosis in mind, more focused questions may be necessary. This questioning may include obtaining more details about the history of the present illness or may be directed toward eliciting specific information from other categories of the traditional medical history, including past medical history, review of systems, family history, and social history. The following serve only as examples for the use of focused questions.

Past Medical History

After the physical examination, one may want to learn more about the patient's general health. For example, in a patient with suspected herpes zoster, a past history of chickenpox would be of interest. We have discussed how topically applied and systemically administered medications often contribute to skin conditions. Skin findings may encourage further pursuit of these possibilities. For example, in a patient with generalized erythematous rash or hives, systemic drugs should be high on the list of possible causes. Because drugs can cause virtually any type of skin lesion, it is useful to consider drug eruptions in the differential diagnosis of almost any skin disease. It may also be helpful to determine whether the patient has any known allergies, to determine whether any medications are currently being used that could produce a cross-reaction.

Drugs can cause all types of skin rashes.

Review of Systems

In a patient with a malar rash, a diagnosis of systemic lupus erythematosus should be considered, and the examiner will want to question the patient further for symptoms of additional skin or other organ involvement, including Raynaud's phenomenon, photosensitivity, hair loss, mouth ulcers, and arthritis. In a patient with a generalized maculopapular eruption, the two most common causes are drugs and viruses, so the physician will want to inquire about both medication use and viral symptoms such as fever, malaise, and upper respiratory or gastrointestinal symptoms.

Family History

In certain cutaneous conditions, some knowledge of the family history may help in diagnosis. Innumerable inherited disorders have dermatologic expression. The following serve only as examples:

1. In a child with a chronic itching eruption in the antecubital and popliteal fossae, atopic dermatitis is suspected. A positive family history for atopic diseases (atopic dermatitis, asthma, hay fever) supports the diagnosis.

2. In a youngster with multiple café-au-lait spots, a diagnosis of neurofibromatosis is considered. A positive family history for this disorder, substantiated by examination of family members, helps to support the diagnosis of this dominantly inherited disease.

Knowledge of the family's present health also is important when considering infectious diseases. For example, impetigo can occur in several family members, and this knowledge may help in considering the diagnosis; it would certainly be important for treatment. Likewise, in a patient with suspected scabies, it is important to know for both diagnostic and therapeutic purposes whether other family members are itching.

Social History

For persistent skin infections, consider the possibility of AIDS.

In some disorders, knowledge of the patient's social history may be important. For example, a chronic skin ulcer from persistent herpes simplex infection is a sign of immunosuppression, particularly AIDS. Therefore, a patient with such an ulceration should be asked about high-risk factors for acquiring AIDS, including sexual behavior, intravenous drug abuse, and exposure to blood products.

A complete "skin exposure history" is required whenever contact dermatitis is suspected.

Another common occasion for probing into a patient's social history is when the patient is suspected of having contact dermatitis; this aspect of the social history could be subtitled the *skin exposure history*. Patients encounter potentially sensitizing materials both at work and at play. Industrial dermatitis is a leading cause of workers' disability. For chronic hand dermatitis, questions about occupational exposure are important and should be directed particularly to materials and substances the patient contacts either by handling or by immersion. Similarly, a patient presenting with an acute eruption characterized by streaks of vesicles should be queried regarding recent outdoor activities resulting in exposure to poison ivy or poison oak. Contact dermatitis is a common and challenging problem. On the part of the physician, it often requires painstaking efforts in a detective-type search to elicit from the patient an exposure history that fits the dermatitis.

Some harbor the misconception that in dermatology one needs only to glance at the skin to arrive at a diagnosis and that talking with the patient is superfluous. Although this is occasionally true, we hope that the previous examples serve to illustrate that this frequently is not the case. In fact, in some instances (and contact dermatitis is a good example), detailed historical information is essential to establish a diagnosis.

■ PHYSICAL EXAMINATION

The physical examination follows the preliminary history. For the skin to be inspected adequately, three essential requirements must be met: (1) a completely undressed patient, clothed only in an examining gown; (2) adequate illumination, preferably natural light or bright overhead fluorescent lighting; and (3) an examining physician prepared to see what is there.

You should examine the entire mucocutaneous surface, but patients will be more firmly convinced of your sincere interest in their particular problems if you start by examining the affected areas before proceeding with the more complete examination.

At least for the initial examination, the patient needs to be totally disrobed so the entire skin surface can be examined. Busy physicians who tend to overlook this rule will miss much. An occasional patient may be reluctant to comply, saying, "My skin problem is only on my hands; why do you need to look at the rest of my skin?" We tell such patients that we have at least two reasons:

1. Other lesions may be found that "go along with" the lesions on the hands and help confirm the diagnosis. For example, in a patient with sharply demarcated plaques on the palms, the finding of a few scaling plaques on the knees or a sharply marginated intergluteal plaque will help to substantiate a suspicion of psoriasis.

2. An important incidental skin lesion may be found. The finding of a previously undetected malignant melanoma on a patient's back is an example. We studied the yield from a complete skin examination in 1,157 consecutive new dermatology patients and found an incidental skin malignancy in 22 (Lookingbill, 1988). Twenty of these patients had basal cell carcinoma, one had melanoma, and one had Kaposi's sarcoma that served as the presenting manifestation of his AIDS. A subsequent study of 874 patients (Lee et al., 1991) reported an incidental skin cancer detection rate of 3.4%.

The entire skin surface is examined for:
1. **Lesions that may accompany the presenting complaint**
2. **Unrelated but important incidental findings**

For the skin to be examined adequately, it must be properly illuminated. Natural lighting is excellent for this purpose but is difficult to achieve in most offices and hospital rooms. The alternative is bright overhead fluorescent lighting, supplemented with a movable incandescent lamp that is usually wall mounted. One additional illuminator that is often useful is a simple penlight. Either this or the movable incandescent lamp can be used as side lighting to detect whether a lesion is subtly elevated. For this technique, the light is directed onto the lesion from an angle that is roughly parallel to the skin. If the lesion is elevated, a small shadow will be thrown, and the relief of the skin will be appreciated. The penlight also is useful for examining the mouth, an area that is sometimes overlooked but in which one may detect lesions that are helpful in diagnosing a cutaneous disorder.

"Side lighting" helps to detect subtle elevations.

Another piece of examination equipment that is occasionally useful is the Wood's light, a long-wavelength ultraviolet "black" light. Contrary to some popular misconceptions, this light does not enable one to diagnose most skin fungal infections; it only detects fluorescence of affected hairs in some, now uncommon, types of tinea capitis. The Wood's light is, however, still used to accentuate pigmentary alterations in the skin.

Except for provision of adequate illumination, minimal equipment is needed for examining the skin. A simple hand-held lens is not usually necessary. If the diagnosis cannot be made at a 1:1 magnification, enlarging the image is unlikely to improve diagnostic accuracy. However, on some occasions, such as clarifying a burrow in scabies or detecting the Wickham's striae in a lesion of lichen planus, a hand-held lens can be useful. For diagnosing pigmented growths, some dermatologists employ a dermatoscope. This is an illuminated hand-held magnifying device intended to help the clinician to diagnose melanoma clinically.

An adequate examination of the skin should actually be called a mucocutaneous examination so that one is reminded to include an examination of the mouth. Similarly, the scalp and nails should not be overlooked. Because both cutaneous and systemic diseases may be expressed in the nails and nail beds as well as in the mouth, inspection of these areas should be included in every cutaneous examination.

The scalp, mouth, and nails should not be overlooked.

Physical examination depends largely on inspection, but one should not neglect the opportunity to palpate the skin as well. The two major purposes for this are (1) to assess the texture consistency and tenderness of the skin lesions and (2) to reassure patients that we are not afraid to touch their skin lesions—that they do not have some dreadful contagious disease. Nothing is more disquieting to a patient than to be cautiously approached with a gloved hand. For anogenital, mucosal, and all weeping lesions, gloving is necessary and expected, but for most other lesions, the physician learns more and the patient is less frightened if the touching is done without gloves. Palpation is the major method by which we evaluate not only the consistency (e.g., softness, firmness, fluctuance) but also the depth of a lesion. In addition, with palpation, we can determine whether a lesion is tender.

Palpation helps to:
1. Assess texture and consistency
2. Evaluate tenderness
3. Reassure patients that they are not contagious

After the patient is properly gowned and perfectly illuminated, for what do we inspect and palpate? The first and most important step is to characterize the appearance (i.e., identify the morphology) of each skin lesion. After the morphology of a lesion is identified, its clinicopathologic correlation can be considered.

The most important task in the physical examination is to characterize the morphology of the basic lesion.

■ TERMINOLOGY OF SKIN LESIONS

A special vocabulary is used in describing the morphologic appearances of skin lesions. These terms are illustrated and defined in Figure 4–1.

■ CLINICOPATHOLOGIC CORRELATIONS

Determine which of the skin components are involved in the clinical lesion.

The lesions defined in Figure 4–1 result from alterations in one or more of the skin's structural components. For clinical diagnostic purposes, we try to envision what pathologic changes are associated with each clinical lesion (Table 4–1). Scale, lichenification, vesicles, bullae, pustules, and crusts represent epidermal alterations, whereas erythema, purpura, and induration reflect changes in the dermis. Such clinicopathologic correlations form the basis of the diagnostic approach. For example, scaling of a nodule suggests hyperkeratosis of the stratum corneum and, thus, an epidermal growth.

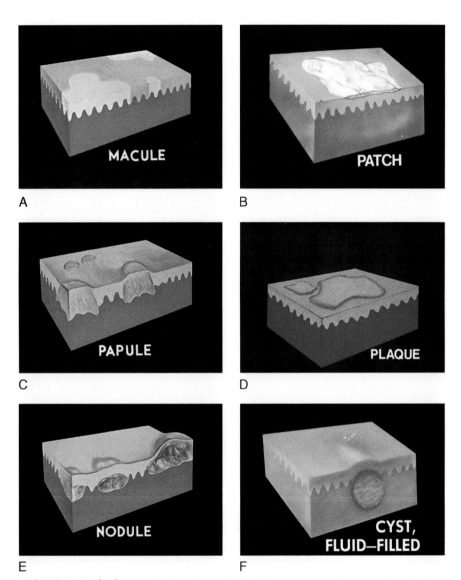

FIGURE 4–1. Skin lesions. **A,** Macule. A flat skin lesion recognizable because its color is different from that of the surrounding normal skin. The most common color changes are white (hypopigmented), brown (hyperpigmented), and red (erythematous and purpuric). **B,** Patch. A macule with some surface change, either slight scale or fine wrinkling. **C,** Papule. A small elevated skin lesion less than 0.5 cm in diameter. **D,** Plaque. An elevated, "plateau-like" lesion greater than 0.5 cm in diameter but without substantial depth. **E,** Nodule. An elevated, "marble-like" lesion greater than 0.5 cm in both diameter and depth. **F,** Cyst. A nodule filled with expressible material that is either liquid or semisolid.

Illustration continued on following page

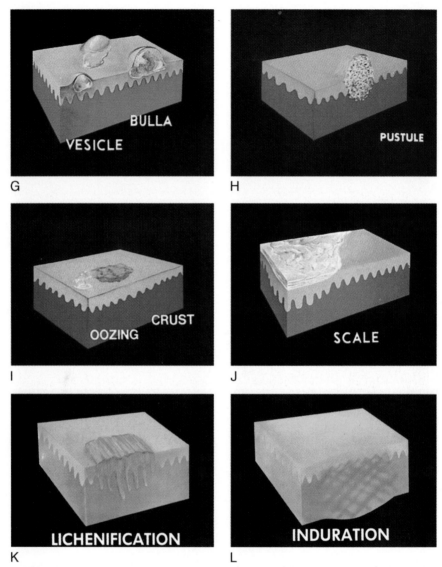

FIGURE 4–1 *Continued.* **G,** Vesicles and bullae. Blisters are filled with clear fluid. Vesicles are less than and bullae are greater than 0.5 cm in diameter. **H,** Pustule. A vesicle filled with cloudy or purulent fluid. **I,** Crust. Liquid debris (e.g., serum or pus) that has dried on the surface of the skin. Crust most often results from breakage of vesicles, pustules, or bullae. **J,** Scale. Visibly thickened stratum corneum. Scales are dry and usually whitish. These features help to distinguish scales from crusts, which are often moist and usually yellowish or brown. **K,** Lichenification. *Epidermal thickening* characterized by (1) visible and palpable thickening of the skin with (2) accentuated skin markings. **L,** Induration. *Dermal thickening* resulting in the skin that *feels* thicker and firmer than normal.

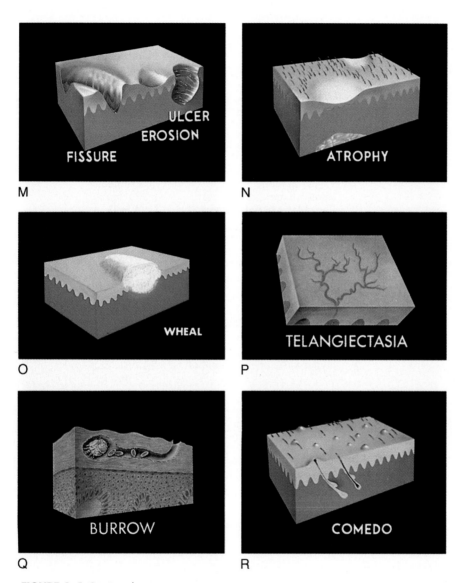

FIGURE 4–1 *Continued.* **M,** Fissure, erosion, and ulcer. A fissure is a thin, linear tear in the epidermis. An erosion is wider but is limited in depth, confined to the epidermis. An ulcer is a defect devoid of epidermis as well as part or all of the dermis. **N,** Atrophy. Loss of skin tissue. With epidermal atrophy, the surface appears thin and wrinkled. Atrophy of the much thicker dermal layer results in a clinically detectable depression in the skin. **O,** Wheal. A papule or plaque of dermal edema. Wheals (or *hives*) often have central pallor and irregular borders. **P,** Telangiectasia. Superficial blood vessels enlarged enough to be clinically visible. **Q,** Burrow. Serpiginous tunnel or streak caused by a burrowing organism. **R,** Comedo (plural, *comedones*). The noninflammatory lesions of acne that result from keratin impaction in the outlet of the pilosebaceous canal.

TABLE 4–1 ■ CLINICOPATHOLOGIC CORRELATIONS

Skin Component	Pathologic Alteration	Clinical Manifestation
Epidermis		
Stratum corneum	Hyperkeratosis	Scale
Subcorneal epidermis	Hyperplasia	Lichenification
	Hyperplasia	Papules, plaques, and nodules
	Disruptive inflammatory changes	Vesicles, bullae, and pustules
	Dried serum	Crusts
Melanocytes	Increased number or function	Pigmented macules, papules, and nodules
	Decreased number or function	White spots
Dermis		
Blood vessels	Hyperplasia or inflammation	Macules, papules, and nodules
	Vasodilatation	Erythema
	Hemorrhage	Purpura
	Vasodilataton with edema	Wheals
Nerves	Hyperplasia	Papules, nodules
Connective tissue	Hyperplasia	Induration, papules, nodules, and plaques
	Loss of epidermis and dermis	Ulceration
Dermal Appendages		
Pilosebaceous units	Hyperplasia	Hirsutism
	Atrophy	Alopecia
	Hyperplasia or inflammation	Comedones, papules; nodules, and cysts
Sweat glands	Hypersecretion	Hyperhidrosis
	Hyperplasia or inflammation	Vesicles, papules, pustules, and cysts
Subcutaneous Fat	Hyperplasia or inflammation	Induration and nodules

Growths are hyperplastic lesions; rashes are inflammatory.

Table 4–2 presents an algorithm for this approach and outlines the organization of the remainder of this book. Most skin disorders can be categorized first as proliferative "growths" (neoplasms) or inflammatory "rashes" (eruptions). The growths and rashes are then subdivided, depending on how they appear clinically and which structural component is involved pathologically.

Growths are subdivided into one of three categories:
1. **Epidermal**
2. **Pigmented**
3. **Dermal or subcutaneous**

Scale and hyperkeratosis are both terms for excess stratum corneum.

Growths

Growths are subdivided into epidermal, pigmented, and dermal or subcutaneous proliferative processes.

Epidermal growths result from hyperplasia of keratinocytes; many of these neoplasms have scaling surfaces. *Scale* accumulates when the rate of stratum corneum production exceeds the rate of shedding. *Hyperkeratosis* is another term used to describe excessive accumulation of keratin, the fibrous protein that makes up the stratum corneum. The term "hyperkeratosis" is most often used with skin growths (e.g., seborrheic keratoses); "scaling" is used to describe both growths and rashes.

Because the normal function of the epidermis is to produce the keratotic stratum corneum, hyperkeratosis may be expected in epidermal neoplasms. These

TABLE 4–2 ■ SCHEMATIC FOR DIAGNOSTICS OF SKIN DISEASES

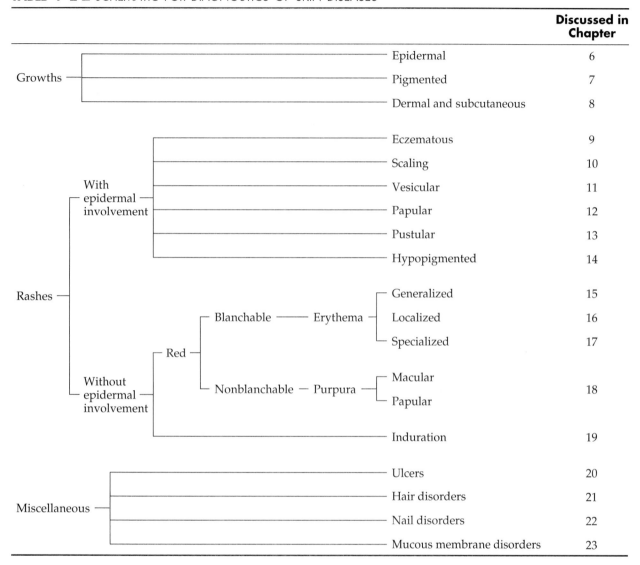

	Discussed in Chapter
Growths → Epidermal	6
Growths → Pigmented	7
Growths → Dermal and subcutaneous	8
Rashes → With epidermal involvement → Eczematous	9
Rashes → With epidermal involvement → Scaling	10
Rashes → With epidermal involvement → Vesicular	11
Rashes → With epidermal involvement → Papular	12
Rashes → With epidermal involvement → Pustular	13
Rashes → With epidermal involvement → Hypopigmented	14
Rashes → Without epidermal involvement → Red → Blanchable → Erythema → Generalized	15
Rashes → Without epidermal involvement → Red → Blanchable → Erythema → Localized	16
Rashes → Without epidermal involvement → Red → Blanchable → Erythema → Specialized	17
Rashes → Without epidermal involvement → Red → Nonblanchable → Purpura → Macular	18
Rashes → Without epidermal involvement → Red → Nonblanchable → Purpura → Papular	18
Rashes → Without epidermal involvement → Induration	19
Miscellaneous → Ulcers	20
Miscellaneous → Hair disorders	21
Miscellaneous → Nail disorders	22
Miscellaneous → Mucous membrane disorders	23

proliferative processes may be benign (e.g., seborrheic keratoses), premalignant (e.g., actinic keratoses), or malignant (e.g., squamous cell carcinoma).

Hyperplasia of the subcorneal epidermis results in elevated lesions of the skin papules, plaques, and nodules. Benign growths originating in the epidermis often appear superficial. Malignant epidermal growths, by definition, have invaded the dermis, and they therefore feel *indurated*, a term used to designate thickening of the dermis.

Malignant epidermal growths usually feel indurated.

Pigmented lesions result from increased melanin production or increased numbers of melanin-producing cells and so may be either macular or papular. Freckles are common examples of hyperpigmented macules that result from increased melanin production. Nevi and melanomas are examples of growths characterized by increased numbers of melanin-producing cells. Nevi that are sufficiently cellular to impart a mass effect are elevated and so clinically appear as hyperpigmented papules, plaques, or even nodules.

Dermal and subcutaneous growths result from *focal* proliferative processes in the dermis or subcutaneous fat. They most often appear as nodules, which are most fully appreciated by palpation. The proliferative elements that form nodules may be either endogenous (e.g., a dermatofibroma that results from the proliferation of dermal fibroblasts) or exogenous to the skin (e.g., a metastasis from an internal malignant disease). Because often no surface markers exist to differentiate one dermal nodule from another, the definitive diagnostic test frequently must be a biopsy. This clinical point deserves emphasis: for undiagnosed skin nodules, particularly firm lesions, malignancy must be suspected, and a biopsy must be performed.

A skin biopsy is often required for the diagnosis of a dermal nodule.

Rashes

For rashes, the first diagnostic step is to determine whether the epidermis is involved. Types of epidermal involvement are listed in Table 4–2. Although some rashes produce several epidermal changes, usually one change is distinctive or predominant.

Eczematous dermatitis is histologically characterized by epidermal intercellular edema (spongiosis), which is manifested clinically by vesicles, "juicy" papules, or lichenification. *Lichenification* represents epidermal hyperplasia clinically expressed as thickened skin with accentuated skin markings. Lichenification is the hallmark of chronic eczematous dermatitis.

Lichenification is the hallmark of chronic eczematous dermatitis.

Epidermal rashes:
1. **Eczematous**
2. **Scaling**
3. **Vesicular**
4. **Papular**
5. **Pustular**
6. **Hypopigmented**

Scaling eruptions are the result of thickened stratum corneum. Scaling rashes can involve either focal areas or the entire cutaneous surface. Examples of the former are more common and are represented by the so-called papulosquamous diseases. These disorders are characterized by scaling (squamous) papules and plaques and patches. Psoriasis and fungal infections serve as examples. Ichthyosis ("fish skin") is an example of generalized scaling.

Scale is usually white or light tan and flakes off rather easily. These features help to distinguish scale from crust. *Crust* is dried serum and debris on the skin surface and usually is darker, most often yellow or brown; it is adherent; and when removed, it reveals a weeping base. The distinction between scale and crust is important because the differential diagnoses are entirely different. Crusts are associated with vesicles, bullae, or pustules.

Scale must be distinguished from crust.

Vesicles and bullae occur when fluid accumulates within or beneath the epidermis. They characterize a relatively small number of important dermatologic disorders, so they are extremely helpful diagnostic findings. Vesicles and bullae occur either intraepidermally or subepidermally. The differential diagnoses are different for intraepidermal and subepidermal blisters, so it is important to try to distinguish them. Clinically, one clue is the fragility of the blister. Because of their more substantial roof, fresh subepidermal blisters are tense and less easily broken, whereas intraepidermal bullae are flaccid and easily ruptured. A biopsy of the *edge* of an early lesion confirms the clinical impression.

Vesicles and bullae are important diagnostic findings.

Pruritic papules are produced by inflammation, predominantly in the dermis. Pustules occur when inflammatory cells aggregate within the epidermis. Pustules may be located superficially in the epidermis, or they may arise from superficial locations in appendageal structures. With purulence, one usually thinks of bac-

Pustules often (but not always) indicate infection.

terial infection. This is an appropriate reflex, and a Gram stain or culture of the contents of a pustule is indicated if a bacterial infection is suspected. However, not all pustular processes are bacterial in origin; viral and fungal infections can also result in pustules, and acne is a common example of a noninfectious cause.

When melanin pigment is lost from the epidermis, white spots result. Because no associated increase in cellular mass occurs, hypopigmented lesions can be expected to be macular (not papular) white spots. Hypopigmentary changes are accentuated under Wood's light examination, whereby previously unnoticed lesions may become apparent and the degree of pigment loss can be roughly assessed. The more pronounced the pigment loss, the whiter the lesion appears under the scrutiny of the Wood's light.

Hypopigmentary changes are accentuated with Wood's light examination.

Dermal rashes without epidermal involvement are either inflammatory or infiltrative; most are inflammatory. Inflammatory eruptions appear red because of vasodilatation of *dermal* blood vessels (the epidermis is devoid of vasculature). Redness in skin lesions can be due to either *erythema or purpura*. It is extremely important to differentiate between the two. With erythema, the increased blood in the skin is contained within dilated blood vessels. Therefore, erythema is *blanchable* (Fig. 4–2). With purpura, blood has extravasated from disrupted blood vessels into the dermis, and the lesion is nonblanchable (Fig. 4–3). The test for blanchability is called *diascopy*. It is performed by simply applying pressure with a finger or glass slide and observing color changes.

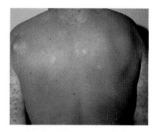

FIGURE 4–2. Erythema is blanchable, as demonstrated with fingertip pressure on the midback.

Erythematous rashes are subdivided into generalized, localized, and specialized (e.g., hives) types. A *wheal*, or hive, is a special type of blanchable, transient, erythematous lesion of the skin. Blood vessels in a wheal are dilated, and fluid leaks from them, causing edema in the surrounding dermis. This fluid is not compartmentalized as in vesicles or bullae but rather is dispersed evenly throughout the dermal tissue. The result is an elevated erythematous lesion, often with central pallor that is due to the intense edema.

Purpuric rashes are subdivided into macular and papular categories. *Macular purpura* is flat and nonpalpable, whereas *papular purpura* is elevated (sometimes subtly) and palpable. This clinical distinction is important because the differential diagnoses and clinical implications are different for the two types. Macular purpura occurs in two settings: (1) conditions associated with increased capillary fragility and (2) bleeding disorders. Macular hemorrhage is not accompanied by inflammation. In papular or palpable purpura, inflammatory changes are present in the vessel walls and are responsible for the elevation of the lesions. Disruption and necrosis of the blood vessels caused by an inflammatory reaction are called *necrotizing vasculitis*. This condition is usually immunologically mediated and can occur in numerous settings, such as sepsis, collagen vascular diseases, and, occasionally, drug reactions. In diagnosis of a patient with palpable purpura, such systemic processes must be excluded.

Macular purpura is usually a sign of a bleeding disorder; papular purpura indicates a necrotizing vasculitis, often systemic.

Rashes resulting from *infiltrative processes* in the dermis are much less common than inflammatory disorders. Clinically, they feel indurated. Induration resulting from increased amounts of collagen is also called *sclerosis*. Scleroderma, an idiopathic disorder of increased collagen deposition, is an example.

Miscellaneous Conditions

Skin ulcers and disorders of hair, nails, and mucous membranes are easily recognizable and grouped as miscellaneous.

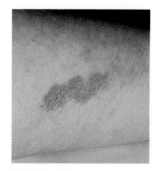

FIGURE 4–3. Purpura is purple and is not blanchable.

Chronic skin ulcers should undergo biopsy to rule out malignancy.

An *ulcer* is totally devoid of epidermis, and some or all of the dermal tissue is missing. Ulcers may extend down to underlying bone, as, for example, in advanced decubitus ulcers. Malignant processes can result in ulcerations that do not heal. For this reason, all chronic ulcers should undergo biopsy.

Too little hair is a much more common dermatologic complaint than too much hair (see Chapter 21). *Alopecia* means hair loss. For diagnostic purposes, it is helpful to classify alopecia as either *nonscarring* or *scarring*. Clinically, the distinction depends on whether follicular openings are visible. The differential diagnoses are different for each of these two categories.

For alopecia, first determine if it is scarring or nonscarring.

Most nail disorders are inflammatory and can affect the nail matrix, nail bed, or periungual skin (paronychia). Inflammation and scaling in the nail bed result in separation of the nail plate from the bed (onycholysis). Fungal infection and psoriasis are the most common causes and are discussed in Chapter 22.

Mucous membrane disorders:
1. **Erosions and ulcerations**
2. **White lesions**

As discussed in Chapter 23, the two most common manifestations of mucous membranes disorders are (1) erosions and ulcerations and (2) white lesions. On mucous membranes, whiteness represents hyperkeratosis, which is white because of maceration from continuous wetness.

■ CONFIGURATION OF SKIN LESIONS

The diagnosis of rash is often aided by considering the configuration of the lesions or their distribution on the body surface. *Configuration* refers to the pattern in which skin lesions are arranged. The four most common patterns are listed in Table 4–3, along with examples of diseases that most often present in these configurations. Occasionally, a configuration is specific for a disease. For example, streaks of vesicles are characteristic of contact dermatitis from poison ivy or poison oak. More often, a configuration is not completely specific for a given disease but may still be helpful in the diagnosis. For example, in psoriasis, scaling papules sometimes develop in streaks as a result of the Koebner reaction, in which lesions of a disorder develop after trauma, such as scratching.

As can be seen from Table 4–3 (Figs. 4–4 through 4–7), configuration considerations are sometimes diagnostically helpful, but morphology takes precedence. The annular impetigo shown in Figure 4–8 illustrates this point. If the crust had been interpreted as scale, the annular lesions would almost certainly have been misdiagnosed as tinea corporis (ringworm). The honey-colored crust, however, should focus attention on the pustular nature of the primary process and should raise the question of bacterial infection. So, for dermatologic diagnosis, the morphology of the primary lesion must be correctly identified before consideration is given to a specific configuration, if one is present. If a conflict appears to exist between the morphology and the configuration, more diagnostic weight should be given to the morphology.

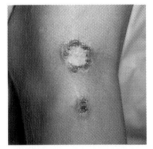

FIGURE 4–8. Annular impetigo. When morphology and configuration (or distribution) appear to conflict, the morphology takes precedence.

■ DISTRIBUTION OF SKIN LESIONS

Many skin diseases have preferential areas of involvement, so the location of the eruption may help in diagnosis. A good example of this is herpes zoster, in which consideration of all three diagnostic criteria (morphology, configuration, and distribution) secures the diagnosis: vesicles in grouped configuration and dermatomal distribution are diagnostic for herpes zoster.

TABLE 4-3 ■ SOME EXAMPLES OF CONFIGURATION

Configuration	Morphology	Disease	Illustration
Linear	Vesicles Papules	Contact dermatitis* Psoriasis† Lichen planus†	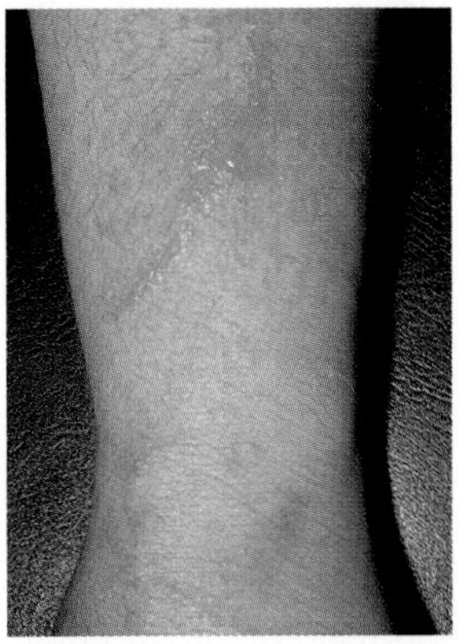 **Figure 4–4.** Contact dermatitis from poison ivy
Grouped	Vesicles Papules	Herpes (simplex and zoster) Insect bites	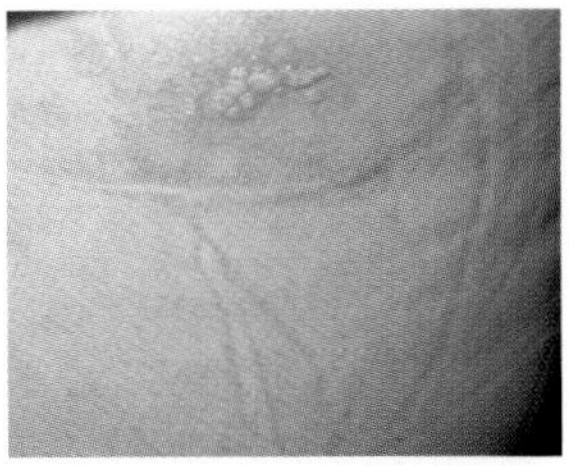 **Figure 4–5.** Herpes simplex
Annular	Scaling	Tinea corporis Secondary syphilis	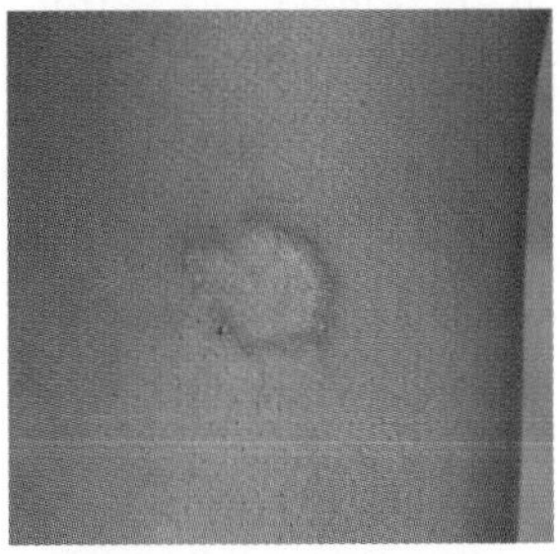 **Figure 4–6.** Tinea corporis
Geographic	Wheals Plaques	Urticaria Mycosis fungoides	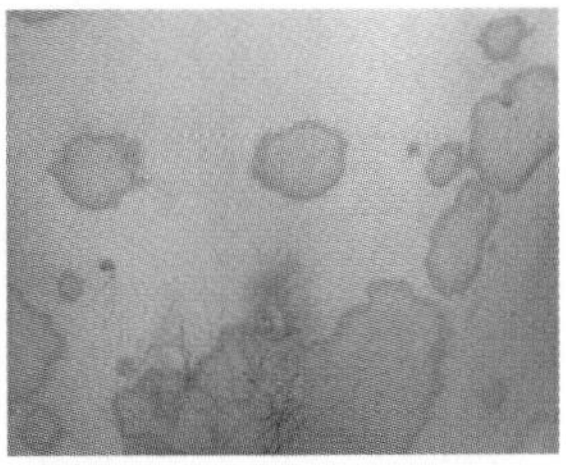 **Figure 4–7.** Urticaria

* Typical for contact dermatitis from a plant resin (e.g., poison ivy).
† The Koebner reaction.

Many skin disorders have favored regional distributions (i.e., a propensity for a particular area of the body) such as on the scalp, face, hands, groin, or feet. Sometimes this propensity can be used as a starting point for developing a differential diagnosis. These "regional" diagnoses are outlined in Chapter 24. For rashes that affect widespread areas, the distribution *pattern* may also aid in the diagnosis. This is particularly true in contact dermatitis, in which the location of the rash on the skin not only may be helpful in leading one to suspect a contact origin but also may provide a clue about the nature of the contactant. For example, a rash on the earlobes and around the neck should lead one to suspect allergic contact dermatitis caused by the nickel present in jewelry.

■ LABORATORY TESTS

In general, laboratory tests serve as important tools that are relied on, sometimes too heavily, as diagnostic aids. Radiographs and blood and urine tests are occasionally helpful for patients suspected of having a systemic disease. For example, an antinuclear antibody test should be ordered in a patient with skin lesions of lupus erythematosus. A serologic test for syphilis is appropriate in a patient with a skin rash in which syphilis is considered to be a possible cause. However, because most dermatologic diseases are limited to the skin, tests for systemic disease are less frequently indicated than are microscopic examinations, cultures, biopsies, and patch tests, which more specifically involve the skin.

As a highly accessible organ, the skin lends itself to direct laboratory examination. Specimen gathering is easy, minimally traumatic, and often highly rewarding diagnostically. Numerous tests can be performed in the office with results immediately available. For other tests, specimens must be sent to the microbiology or pathology laboratory for further evaluation.

Office Microscopic Examinations

Table 4–4 lists some clinical lesions for which microscopic examination of superficial skin specimens is applicable. In most instances, the specimen is obtained

Laboratory tests include:
1. **Microscopic examination**
2. **Cultures**
3. **Biopsy**
4. **Patch tests**

TABLE 4–4 ■ MICROSCOPIC EXAMINATIONS

Clinical Lesion	Test	Finding	Diagnosis
Scale	Potassium hydroxide preparation	Hyphae	Dermatophytic infection Candidal infection
Pustule	Potassium hydroxide preparation	Hyphae and pseudohyphae	Candidal infection
Pustule	Gram stain	Bacteria (usually gram-positive)	Pyoderma (e.g., impetigo)
Vesicle	Tzanck preparation	Multinucleated giant cells	Herpes infections
Pruritic papules ± burrows	Oil mount of skin scraping	Mites and/or eggs	Scabies
Indurated ulcer	Darkfield examination	Motile spirochetes	Syphilis

with a No. 15 scalpel blade and is transferred to a glass slide to be further processed and examined.

Potassium Hydroxide Mount for Dermatophytic Infections

If it scales, scrape it! For undiagnosed scaling lesions of the skin, a fungal origin must be excluded. The best way to do this is with a potassium hydroxide (KOH) preparation of the scale scraping. In experienced hands, this simple test is more sensitive than fungal culture. For those just learning to perform KOH examinations, hyphae are more easily said than seen. The following steps should be followed in performing this examination:

1. *Vigorously* scrape the scale from the edge of the scaling lesion onto a microscopic slide. Use a No. 15 scalpel blade for scraping. Avoid extremely thick pieces of scale, because they are difficult to examine.

2. Place no more than one or two drops of 10% to 20% KOH on the scale before covering with the cover slip.

3. If immediate examination is desired, *gently heat* the slide over an alcohol lamp until the bottom of the slide feels warm. It is preferable to avoid boiling.

4. *Blot* out the excess KOH by firmly pressing a paper towel on top of the cover slip and slide. This important step achieves two purposes. First, it spreads the cells into a thin layer on the slide. A monolayer of cells is desired for the microscopic examination; grossly, this looks like a cloudy film under the cover slip. If chunks are still visible, further heating and pressing are indicated. Second, the blotting removes excess KOH on and around the cover slip; the microscope objective can be permanently etched by contact with KOH.

5. When examining the preparation under the microscope, use *low illumination*. This is most easily achieved by racking the light condenser down all the way. Bright illumination "washes out" the preparation so that hyphae "disappear."

6. Scan the *entire* cover slip under low power (× 10). In the cellular areas, look for the hyphae, which often appear as slightly refractile branching tubes. When suspicious elements are seen, use the high dry objective (× 45) for confirmation (Fig. 4–9).

7. Unlike mucous membrane preparations for candidiasis, in skin scrapings, hyphae are often sparse. *Careful search*, sometimes with multiple preparations, is indicated when one has a high index of suspicion that a lesion may be fungal.

Potassium Hydroxide Preparation for Candidal Infection

In addition to causing scale, candidal infections may cause pustules. Sometimes, the pustules predominate and are a good source of material for KOH examination. The specimen is prepared and examined exactly as outlined earlier. KOH preparations are particularly useful for diagnosing candidal infections because the finding of hyphae or pseudohyphae is diagnostic of *infection* with this organism. Spores are inadequate for diagnosis of infection; yeast organisms, including *Candida albicans*, can colonize skin without infecting it. For this reason, a culture growing *C. albicans* does not necessarily implicate infection, whereas finding hyphal forms on KOH examination does.

Gram Stain

In dermatologic practice, the two most common indications for a Gram stain are (1) to diagnose suspected bullous impetigo by examining the fluid contents of a

If it scales, scrape it!

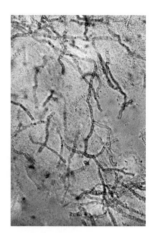

FIGURE 4–9. Unstained potassium hydroxide preparation obtained from a skin scraping. Numerous hyphae are present, many of which are branched.

Hyphae, not spores, are the diagnostic findings in candidal infections.

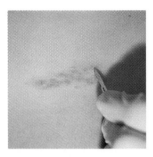

FIGURE 4–10. Scraping the base of a vesicle for a Tzanck preparation.

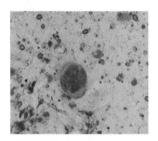

FIGURE 4–11. Multinucleate giant cell.

Specimens for darkfield examinations must be examined immediately.

suspected *intact* bulla and, (2) for a pustular disorder, to establish the cause as bacterial rather than fungal, viral, or sterile. Again, because ruptured pustules can be contaminated with surface bacteria, the contents of an intact pustule should be examined.

Tzanck Preparation

The Tzanck preparation provides an opportunity to make an immediate diagnosis of a herpes simplex or varicella-zoster infection. The preferred specimen is the scraping of the contents and base of a freshly opened vesicle (Fig. 4–10). This material is placed on a glass slide, air dried, methanol fixed, and then stained, usually with either Giemsa or Wright's stain. Toluidine blue stain can also be used. Inclusion bodies are not well seen with these stains, but the finding of multinucleate giant cells is diagnostic for infections with either herpes simplex or varicella-zoster virus (Fig. 4–11).

Scabies Scraping

Finding a scabies mite under the microscope confirms the diagnosis as well as ensures treatment compliance should the patient be skeptical. Burrows produce the highest yield, but because their presence alone is diagnostic, scraping a burrow serves only to dramatize the diagnosis. On close inspection of the burrow, the adult scabies mite sometimes is barely visible as a tiny black speck; under the microscope, it appears more impressive. A scraping may be more helpful when definite burrows are not found, in which case small papules or questionable burrows are scraped. The scraping is done with a No. 15 scalpel blade moistened with oil (any oil) so the skin that is scraped adheres to the blade, from which it can be easily transferred to a drop of oil on a glass slide, covered with a cover slip, and examined microscopically. In scraping, the scalpel blade is held perpendicular to the skin surface. The key to a successful test is to scrape *vigorously*.

Darkfield Examination

Most physicians are not equipped to perform darkfield microscope examinations in their offices; unless the equipment is properly set up and the operator is experienced, the procedure should not be attempted. This examination is most frequently performed in venereal disease clinics, where it can provide immediate diagnosis of syphilis infection. The key to a successful darkfield examination (in addition to having the proper equipment and a trained operator) is in the collection of the specimen. A copious amount of serous fluid must be obtained from the lesion, and this often requires first excoriating a suspected chancre or secondary syphilis lesion with a curette. The serous fluid then is added to a drop of saline, covered with a cover slip, and examined *immediately*. If the specimen is allowed to dry, it will be uninterpretable.

Cultures

The microbiology laboratory can confirm and further characterize pathogens, some of which may be initially identified in an office microscopic examination. Fungi and bacteria are the organisms most frequently sought; viral cultures are becoming more widely obtainable.

Organisms for both superficial and deep fungal infections can be isolated from an appropriate skin specimen. For a superficial fungal (dermatophyte) infection, this specimen is simply a collection of scales scraped from the surface of the lesion. Some physicians prefer to maintain their own fungal cultures in their offices. Small containers with fungal culture media are commercially available, so this can be done conveniently. For deep fungal infections, skin tissue is needed and is most easily obtained with a deep punch biopsy from the active border of the lesion. Tissue should simultaneously be sent to the pathology laboratory for histologic examination to include special fungal stains. If the specimen is sufficiently large, it may be bisected; otherwise, two biopsy specimens should be collected.

Material for bacterial culture should be obtained from intact pustules, bullae, or abscesses. If only crusts are present, they first should be removed so the underlying exudate can be swabbed and cultured. More invasive procedures are required for deeper bacterial infections. For bacterial cellulitis, the responsible organisms can sometimes be retrieved from the involved site by injecting and aspirating 0.5 to 1 mL of nonbacteriostatic saline. Cultures of skin biopsies may also be rewarding, especially for mycobacterial infections of the skin. Some atypical mycobacteria grow only at room temperature, so to handle the skin tissue properly, the laboratory needs not only the specimen but also the clinician's diagnostic considerations.

Material for bacterial culture should be collected from intact pustules, bullae, or abscesses.

Viral cultures must be transported in a viral transport medium, which can be obtained from the viral culture laboratory. For herpes cultures, a vesicle is opened or a crust is unroofed, and the underlying serum is swabbed. The tip of the swab is broken off in the transport medium, and the container is returned to the laboratory for processing. Herpes simplex cultures have a high yield, but herpes varicella-zoster grows either slowly (7 to 10 days) or not at all. An immunofluorescent staining technique for herpes varicella-zoster produces a much higher yield in a much faster time (same day). The test is performed on a vesicle fluid smeared on a special slide, which is returned to the virology laboratory for testing.

Skin Biopsy

In no other organ-based specialty is tissue so easily available for histologic examination as in dermatology. Although a biopsy is not necessary to diagnose the majority of skin disorders, in certain circumstances its value cannot be overemphasized. The following serve only as examples. Already mentioned is the mandate that skin nodules of uncertain origin must undergo biopsy to rule out malignancy. For plaques with unusual shapes and colors, a diagnosis of mycosis fungoides, a cutaneous T-cell lymphoma, may be confirmed with a skin biopsy but sometimes only after multiple biopsies have been taken serially over time. A skin biopsy is usually necessary to secure the exact diagnosis of a primary blistering disorder. In lupus erythematosus, the information obtained from a skin specimen may help to establish the diagnosis.

Occasionally, excisional biopsies are preferred (e.g., for melanomas), but for most skin lesions a punch or shave biopsy is more convenient to perform. For a punch biopsy, a 4-mm instrument is standard, but punches are available in sizes ranging from 2 to 8 mm (Fig. 4–12). The procedure is simple. After the skin is infiltrated with a local anesthetic (Fig. 4–13), the punch is drilled into, and preferably through, the skin (Fig. 4–14). The specimen then is *gently* lifted and is

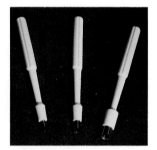

FIGURE 4–12. Disposable punch biopsy instruments. The more commonly used 3-, 4-, and 6-mm sizes are shown.

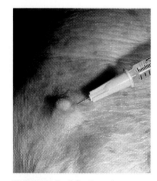

FIGURE 4–13. Local anesthesia is achieved by infiltration with 1% lidocaine.

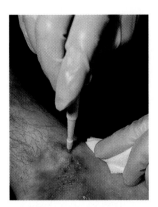

FIGURE 4–14. Punch biopsy. The procedure is performed with a pressing, back-and-forth twisting motion.

snipped off at the subcutaneous fat level (Fig. 4–15). Then, either the skin defect can be closed with a suture or hemostasis can be achieved simply with pressure or absorbable gelatin (Gelfoam) packing.

Note that in the foregoing, gentleness is emphasized. A biopsy specimen will be artifactually damaged, sometimes to the point of being histologically uninterpretable, if it is squeezed too firmly with the tissue forceps. To avoid this problem, one should either lift the specimen gently from below or grasp it by the very edge. With nodules and other dermal processes, it is particularly important that the specimen be of full thickness. For processes involving the subcutaneous fat, even deeper and larger specimens may need to be obtained.

Extremely superficial lesions can undergo biopsy or be removed with a shave technique. A wheal is raised with the anesthetic injection, after which the area is shaved with a scalpel blade maneuvered either parallel to the surface or in a slight "scooping" fashion.

For most skin lesions, adjacent normal skin is not needed, so the biopsy should be obtained from the center of the lesion. The exception is with blistering disorders, in which case the biopsy should be taken from the edge of an early lesion to include a portion of the adjacent, nonblistered skin. This is needed to identify the exact histologic origin of the blister.

For routine histologic processing and for most special stains, the specimen is placed in formalin. For electron microscopy, buffered glutaraldehyde is used. With immunofluorescence testing, the specimen must be either immediately snap frozen or placed in a special buffered transport solution.

Immunofluorescence Tests

For the diagnosis of blistering disorders such as pemphigus, bullous pemphigoid, and dermatitis herpetiformis, immunofluorescence tests on skin (direct) and, sometimes, serum (indirect) are invaluable and are widely used. These techniques detect autoantibodies directed against portions of skin. For example, immunoglobulin (Ig) G antibodies deposited at the basement membrane in pemphigoid are detected by direct immunofluorescence testing using the patient's skin and fluorochrome-labeled anti-IgG antibodies. The same test is also useful in helping to diagnose lupus erythematosus, in which it is called the *lupus band test*. The presence of IgM, IgA, complement, and fibrin can also be detected with appropriate reagents.

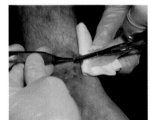

FIGURE 4–15. When removing the specimen, one must take care to avoid damaging the tissue with the forceps.

Electron Microscopy

An electron microscopic examination of skin tissue is less often indicated but is helpful in diagnosing several uncommon disorders, including histiocytosis X and subtypes of the inherited mechanical bullous disease, epidermolysis bullosa.

Patch Tests

Patch tests are used to detect contact allergens.

Patch testing is a valuable tool for identifying responsible allergens in patients with allergic contact dermatitis. These tests detect delayed (type IV) hypersensitivity to contact allergens. Patch tests take several days to develop and hence differ from scratch tests, which evoke immediate (type I) hypersensitivity responses (within minutes) and are much less helpful in dermatology. Either specifically suspected substances may be tested, or an entire battery of allergens may be screened. For either purpose, standardized trays of common sensitizing chemicals are available, each appropriately diluted in solution or petrolatum. These test materials are applied to the skin under occlusive patches that are left in place for 48 hours. The patches then are removed, the sites are inspected, and positive reactions are noted (Fig. 4–16). Because these delayed hypersensitivity responses sometimes take more than 48 hours, a final reading at 96 hours is recommended. If positive tests are found, the last and most important step is to determine their clinical relevance. In itself, a positive patch test does not prove that agent to be the cause of dermatitis. Clinical correlation with an appropriate exposure history also is required. Patch testing should not be done with unknown chemicals because severe irritant contact dermatitis with residual scars can result. Contact dermatitis and patch testing are discussed further in Chapter 9.

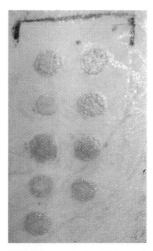

FIGURE 4–16. Multiple positive patch tests at day 2.

R E F E R E N C E S

Barr RJ: Cutaneous cytology. J Am Acad Dermatol *10*:163–180, 1984.

Caplan RM: Medical uses of the Wood's lamp. JAMA *202*:1035–1038, 1967.

Harrist TJ, Mihm MC Jr: Cutaneous immunopathology: the diagnostic use of direct and indirect immunofluorescence techniques in dermatologic disease. Hum Pathol *10*:625–653, 1979.

Helm KF, Marks JG: Atlas of Differential Diagnosis in Dermatology. New York, Churchill Livingstone, 1998.

Lee G, Massa MC, Welykyj S, Choo J, Greaney V: Yield from total skin examination and effectiveness of skin cancer awareness program: findings in 874 new dermatology patients. Cancer *67*:202–205, 1991.

Lookingbill DP: Yield from a complete skin examination: findings in 1157 new dermatology patients. J Am Acad Dermatol *18*:31–37, 1988.

Marks JG, DeLeo VA: Contact and Occupational Dermatology. 2nd ed. St. Louis, Mosby–Year Book, 1997.

McBurney EL: Diagnostic dermatologic methods. Pediatr Clin North Am *30*:419–434, 1983.

Muller G, Jacobs PH, Moore NE: Scraping for human scabies. Arch Dermatol *107*:70, 1973.

Schwarzenberger K: The essentials of the complete skin examination. Med Clin N. Am. *85*:981–999, 1998.

Solomon AB, Rasmussen SE, Varani J, et al.: The Tzanck smear in the diagnosis of cutaneous herpes simplex. JAMA *251*:633–635, 1984.

U.S. Public Health Service: Darkfield Microscopy for the Detection and Identification of *Treponema pallidum*. Washington, DC, U.S. Government Printing Office, publication No. 990, 1962.

Wallace ML, Smoller BR: Immunohistochemistry in diagnostic dermatopathology. J Am Acad Dermatol *34*:163–183, 1996.

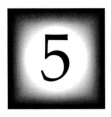

C H A P T E R

5 DERMATOLOGIC THERAPY

■

PRINCIPLES OF TOPICAL THERAPY
DRESSINGS AND BATHS
TOPICAL STEROIDS (GLUCOCORTICOSTEROIDS)
PHOTOTHERAPY
DERMATOLOGIC SURGERY
PATIENT EDUCATION

Because the skin is so accessible, it can be treated with a variety of therapeutic options not available for use in diseases of internal organs. Drugs for dermatologic therapy can be administered topically, intralesionally, and systemically. In addition, physical modalities such as ultraviolet (UV) and ionizing radiation, surgery, laser, and cryotherapy can be easily administered.

At one time, dermatologic therapy was largely based on empiric approaches. However, during the past four decades, much progress has been made in defining the scientific bases for numerous dermatologic treatments, resulting in a well-rounded rationale for choosing specific modalities.

The discussions in this chapter are limited to principles of external therapies unique to the skin. Other, more specific topical therapies (e.g., those used for acne and for fungal diseases), as well as all systemic therapies, are discussed in chapters concerning the diseases in which they are used.

■ PRINCIPLES OF TOPICAL THERAPY

Advantages of topical medication:
1. **Direct delivery to target tissue**
2. **Reduced systemic side effects**

A diverse group of medications is available in topical preparations, including antibiotics, antifungals, corticosteroids, acne preparations, sunscreens, cytotoxic agents, antipruritics, antiseptics, and pesticides. Topical therapy has the distinct advantage of delivering medications directly to the target organ. This route reduces the potential of systemic side effects and toxicity seen with systemic therapy. The disadvantages of topical therapy are that it is time consuming, it can require large volumes of medication, it requires patient education in the technique of using topicals, and, at times, it is not aesthetically pleasing because of staining or greasy preparations.

For a medication to be effective topically, it must be absorbed into the skin. The main diffusion barrier of the skin is the stratum corneum. It is responsible for most of the protection offered by the skin against toxic agents, microorganisms, physical forces, and loss of body fluids.

Percutaneous absorption is influenced by (1) physical and chemical properties of the active ingredient, (2) concentration, (3) vehicle, and (4) variations in type of skin. Cutaneous penetration of an active ingredient is enhanced when it has a low molecular weight, is lipid soluble, and is nonpolar.

Substances move across the stratum corneum by passive diffusion and follow a dose-response curve. The higher the *concentration* applied, the greater is the quantity of medication absorbed.

The *vehicle* is nearly as important as the active agent in the formulation of topical medications. This was realized when investigators found that the release of drugs varied greatly with different vehicles. The more occlusive the vehicle, the greater is the hydration of the stratum corneum and penetration of the medication. In addition, occlusive vehicles increase local skin temperature and prevent mechanical removal and evaporation of the active agent. An ointment is the most occlusive vehicle.

Percutaneous absorption also is influenced by the *location of the skin* to which it is applied. Passive diffusion is slow through the stratum corneum but rapid through the viable epidermis and papillary dermis. Therefore, absorption is generally low on the palm and sole, in which the stratum corneum is thick, and high on the scrotum, face, and ear, in which the stratum corneum is thin. Breakdown of the barrier function of the stratum corneum by diseases, chemicals (soaps or detergents), and physical injury results in increased permeability.

The *selection of a topical preparation* must involve not only the active agent but also its other ingredients. The formulation of many topical medications is complex. A water-based preparation (cream), for example, is composed of numerous ingredients, including the active agent, vehicle, and preservative as well as an emulsifier to bring together the oil and water components of the preparation. As a general rule, it is better to select a commercially formulated preparation that is scientifically compounded than an extemporaneous preparation. The most frequently used vehicles are creams, ointments, lotions, and gels.

Creams are semisolid emulsions of oil in water that vanish when rubbed into the skin. They are white and nongreasy and contain multiple ingredients. Preservatives are added to prevent the growth of bacteria and fungi. *Ointments* (oil-based) are emulsions of water droplets suspended in oil that do not rub in when applied to the skin. They are greasy and clear and do not require preservatives. Ointments are selected when increased hydration, occlusion, and maximal penetration of the active ingredient are desired. *Lotions* are suspensions of powder in water that may require shaking before application. Calamine lotion is the classic example. Itching is relieved by the cooling effect of water evaporation, and a protective layer of powder is left on the skin. Other liquids such as solutions, sprays, aerosols, and tinctures are characterized by ingredients dissolved in alcoholic vehicles, which evaporate to leave the active agent on the skin. These agents are particularly useful for hairy areas. *Gels* are transparent and colorless semisolid emulsions that liquefy when applied to the skin.

Writing a Dermatologic Prescription

Writing a prescription for a topical medication involves more than simply requesting the active ingredient. In addition to the medication, the vehicle, concentration, and amount must be indicated, as well as the instructions for use. Numerous concentrations and usually various vehicles often are available for a given

Percutaneous absorption depends on:
1. Active ingredient
2. Concentration
3. Vehicle
4. Skin type

Elements of a topical prescription:
1. Medication
2. Vehicle
3. Concentration
4. Amount
5. How to apply

topical drug. The physician should indicate which vehicle the pharmacist is to dispense. Patients' compliance often is directly related to their preference of vehicle. Greasy ointments on the face and hands can be unacceptable to the patient and on the trunk or extremities may soak through clothing.

Probably the type of error most frequently made in prescribing a topical drug involves the volume of medication to be dispensed. The size of the area being treated, the frequency of application, and the time between appointments or before predicted clearing of the eruption all must be taken into consideration when writing the prescription. An adequate quantity of medication is necessary to ensure the patient's compliance, successful therapy, and cost savings. Smaller volumes of medication are comparatively more expensive than larger volumes. One gram covers an area approximately 10×10 cm. A single application of a cream or ointment to the face or hands requires 2 g; for one arm or the anterior or posterior trunk, 3 g; for one leg, 4 g; and for the entire body, 30 g. Prescribing 15 g to be applied twice a day to an eruption that involves large portions of the trunk and extremities would be unreasonable; the patient would be required to return for refills twice daily.

The physician needs to know the principles involved in writing a dermatologic prescription. For example, the patient's eruption is moderately severe and requires an intermediate-strength topical steroid such as triamcinolone acetonide. Triamcinolone acetonide is available in three concentrations—0.025%, 0.1%, and 0.5%. A 0.1% concentration is effective for moderately severe eruptions and generally can be used without concern for local or systemic side effects. In this example, it is dispensed in a cream vehicle because the patient prefers a nongreasy preparation that rubs into the skin. The patient is going to use the medication on extensive areas of skin, requiring approximately 10 g per application twice a day. A prescription for 454 g (1 lb) of cream will last almost 2 weeks, and two refills will allow more than enough medication until the next appointment in 4 weeks.

■ DRESSINGS AND BATHS

Dressings are useful as protective coverings over wounds. They prevent contamination from the environment, and many absorb serum and blood.

Dry dressings are used to protect wounds and to absorb drainage. They usually consist of absorbent gauze secured with adhesive tape. Adhesive tape can cause allergic contact dermatitis, in which case hypoallergenic tapes may be used. These are made of an acrylic plastic adhesive mass with a plastic or cloth backing. After surgery, the skin often is painted with an adhesive that contains benzoin, which also may be responsible for allergic contact dermatitis. Dry dressings may be nonadherent or adherent. *Nonadherent dressings* are used for clean wounds. When changed, they should not pull off newly formed epithelium. An example of a nonadherent dressing is petrolatum-impregnated gauze. *Adherent dressings* are used for debridement of moist wounds. The dressings may be dry or wet at first. For dry dressings, gauze is applied and changed regularly. For wet-to-dry dressings, water, saline, or an antiseptic solution is added to the dressing and is allowed to dry. Accumulated debris is removed, although removal may be painful. Discomfort can be reduced if adherent dressings are first moistened (i.e., remoistened) before removal.

Wet dressings are used to treat acute inflammation. They consist of gauze, pads, or towels soaked continuously with water, an *astringent* (drying agent), or

For one application—amount needed:
Face: 2 g
Arm: 3 g
Leg: 4 g
Whole body: 30 g

Types of dressings:
1. **Dry**
2. **Wet**
3. **Occlusive**

an antimicrobial solution. They soothe, cool, and dry through evaporation. In addition, when changed, they remove crusts and exudate. Water is the most important ingredient of wet dressings, but astringents such as aluminum acetate (Domeboro) and antiseptics such as povidone-iodine (Betadine) frequently are added. Impermeable covers such as plastic should *not* be placed over wet dressings because of the maceration that would ensue.

Occlusive dressings made of semipermeable plastic membranes (e.g., Opsite, Vigilon, Duoderm) promote wound healing by maintaining a moist environment. They are frequently used on chronic ulcers, for example, stasis ulcers. The moist environment allows migration of keratinocytes over the ulcer base to proceed more rapidly. In addition, occlusive dressings allow autodigestion of necrotic tissue by accumulation of inflammatory cells. For some wounds, for example, donor graft sites, these dressings also significantly reduce pain.

Baths may be thought of as a form of wet dressing. They are effective in soothing, in decreasing itching, and in cleansing, and they are relaxing. They are used for acute eruptions that are crusting and weeping. They hydrate dry skin, but only if a moisturizer is applied immediately after the bath. Routinely used baths include tar emulsions (Cutar), colloidal oatmeal (Aveeno), and bath oils (Alpha Keri). Baths are limited to 30 minutes to prevent maceration and are repeated once or twice daily.

■ TOPICAL STEROIDS (GLUCOCORTICOSTEROIDS)

Topical steroids have been used for more than 40 years. Perhaps no topical therapeutic modality is used more frequently than these agents. The use of glucocorticosteroids applied directly on diseased skin has resulted in a high therapeutic benefit with relatively little local and systemic toxicity. The mechanism of action of topical glucocorticosteroids is complex and is not thoroughly understood. These drugs usually are used for their antiproliferative and anti-inflammatory effects.

Potency depends on:
1. Steroid structure
2. Vehicle

Potency

The potency of a topical glucocorticosteroid depends on its molecular structure. For example, triamcinolone acetonide is 100 times more potent than hydrocortisone. In addition, the vehicle carrying the steroid is important. For a steroid to be effective, it must be absorbed. Penetration of glucocorticosteroids through the stratum corneum (and, hence, increased activity) is optimized by using nonpolar, lipophilic glucocorticosteroid molecules compounded in vehicles that readily release the steroid.

Vasoconstrictive assay is the most common method to measure potency.

Dozens of different topical glucocorticosteroids have been formulated for use in skin disease, with many of these developed on the basis of potency assays. Measurement of the ability of glucocorticosteroids to induce vasoconstriction or blanching of the skin *vasoconstrictive assay* is the most frequently used method of estimating relative potency. The results of the vasoconstrictor assay parallel those found in clinical studies. Because the vasoconstrictive assay is much simpler to do than complicated clinical studies, it is widely used to screen specific formulations before they are used in clinical trials.

Table 5–1 lists some topical glucocorticosteroids with different potencies. The percentage of the steroid present is relevant only when comparing percentages of

TABLE 5–1 ■ TOPICAL STEROIDS

Potency	Brand Name	Generic Name	Percentage (%)
Lowest	Hytone	Hydrocortisone	1.0
			2.5
Low	Tridesilon	Desonide	0.05
	Aclovate	Alclometasone dipropionate	0.05
	DesOwen	Desonide	0.05
Medium	Valisone	Betamethasone valerate	0.1
	Synalar	Fluocinolone acetonide	0.025
	Westcort	Hydrocortisone valerate	0.2
	Aristocort, Kenalog	Triamcinolone acetonide	0.1
	Cutivate	Fluticasone propionate	0.005
	Elocon	Mometasone furoate	0.1
	Locoid	Hydrocortisone butyrate	0.1
High	Cyclocort	Amcinonide	0.1
	Diprosone	Betamethasone dipropionate	0.05
	Topicort	Desoximetasone	0.25
	Lidex	Fluocinonide	0.05
	Halog	Halcinonide	0.1
Super-high	Diprolene	Betamethasone dipropionate	0.05
	Psorcon	Diflorasone diacetate	0.05
	Temovate	Clobetasol propionate	0.05
	Ultravate	Halobetasol propionate	0.05

the same compound. Thus, triamcinolone acetonide 0.5% is stronger than its 0.1% formulation, but hydrocortisone 1% is much weaker than triamcinolone acetonide 0.1%. In addition, potency depends on the vehicle. The same preparation tends to be more potent in an ointment base than in a cream base because of enhanced percutaneous penetration.

Side Effects

Topical side effects:
1. **Atrophy**
2. **Acne**
3. **Enhanced fungal infection**
4. **Retarded wound healing**
5. **Contact dermatitis**
6. **Glaucoma, cataracts**

Numerous hazards are involved with the use of topical glucocorticosteroids. In general, the more potent the glucocorticosteroid, the greater the likelihood of an adverse reaction.

Local reactions include skin atrophy manifested by telangiectasia and thinned, shiny skin. The intertriginous areas (axilla, submammary, and groin) and face are particularly prone to stria formation and atrophy. Fluorinated steroids (most steroids other than hydrocortisone are fluorinated) are prone to cause acne eruptions of the face called *perioral dermatitis*. Topical steroids promote dermatophytic fungal infections; their effect on cutaneous viral and bacterial infections is less clear. They retard wound and ulcer healing and should not be used on these lesions. Less often, allergic contact dermatitis occurs as a reaction to the vehicle or to the steroid itself. Contact dermatitis should be suspected when the patient's skin condition is made worse by a topical steroid. Although uncommon, ocular side effects, including glaucoma, cataracts, and retarded healing of corneal ulcers, have been reported in association with the application of topical steroids to the eyelids.

Systemic side effects are worrisome but rarely occur. These include adrenal suppression, iatrogenic Cushing's syndrome, and growth retardation in children. These complications have been reported with long-term, extensive use of potent topical steroids, particularly when these agents are used under occlusion. The recent introduction of super–high-potency topical steroids has increased the possibility of hypothalamic-pituitary-axis suppression. These steroids should not be used for longer than 2 consecutive weeks, and the total dosage should not exceed 50 g per week.

Systemic side effects:
1. Adrenal suppression
2. Cushing's syndrome
3. Growth retardation

Guidelines for Topical Steroid Usage

A bewildering array of topical steroids is available in numerous different vehicles. In prescribing a steroid preparation, one should consider several factors before making the selection of potency, vehicle, amount to be dispensed, and frequency of use. It is best to become familiar with one steroid in each class—lowest, medium, and high potency. By using only a few preparations, you will gain an enhanced appreciation of clinical efficacy, frequency of side effects, available vehicles and volumes, and costs. Lowest-potency topical steroids are recommended for dermatoses that are mild and chronic and involve the face and intertriginous regions. More potent steroids—medium and high—are used for dermatoses that are more severe and are recalcitrant to treatment.

Become familiar with one steroid in each potency class—lowest, medium, and high.

After the appropriate potency has been selected, the vehicle should be chosen. Acute and subacute inflammations characterized by vesiculation and oozing are best treated with nonocclusive vehicles in a gel, lotion, or cream. Ointments, because of their occlusive properties, are better for treating chronic inflammation characterized by dryness, scaling, and lichenification. Because of their greasy nature, ointments are less acceptable aesthetically. However, they have less potential for irritation and allergic reaction. Lotions and gels are best used on hairy areas such as the scalp.

Use creams on weeping eruptions, ointments on dry lichenified skin, and gels or lotions on hairy areas.

Another consideration in topical steroid therapy is the frequency of application. The stratum corneum acts as a reservoir and continues to release topical steroid into the skin after the initial application. Applications once or twice a day are usually sufficient. Investigators have observed that chronic dermatoses, especially psoriasis, become less responsive after prolonged use of topical steroids. This phenomenon is called *tachyphylaxis*. This diminished responsiveness after repeated applications has also been observed in vasoconstrictor assays.

Dermatoses may become unresponsive to long-term steroid use.

Finally, the physician should instruct the patient in proper application and to dispense sufficient medication to ensure adequate treatment. A good rule is to use the smallest quantity and the weakest preparation that are effective for a particular eruption. The need for continued treatment should be reviewed periodically.

■ PHOTOTHERAPY

Photobiology and Therapy

The sun emits a broad spectrum of electromagnetic radiation that is both ionizing (cosmic, gamma, and x-rays) and nonionizing (UV, visible, infrared, and radio) (Fig. 5–1). The earth's atmosphere absorbs one third of the solar radiation. Of the

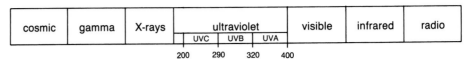

FIGURE 5–1. Electromagnetic spectrum.

radiation that reaches the earth's surface, 60% is infrared, 37% is visible, and 3% is in the UV range. The UV spectrum is between x-ray and visible light and composes the 200- to 400-nm wavelength band. It is subdivided into three groups based on physical and biologic properties: UVC (200 to 290 nm, germicidal spectrum), UVB (290 to 320 nm, sunburn spectrum), and UVA (320 to 400 nm). All the UVC radiation is filtered by the ozone layer, so only UVB and UVA rays reach the earth's surface.

Because light has properties of waves and particles, two theories are used to describe its physics. The wave theory relates the speed of light to its wavelength and frequency; the light spectrum is divided according to its wavelength (nanometers). The quantum theory is based on the existence of a particle of energy (photon) and relates light energy (joules) directly to frequency and inversely to wavelength.

The positive effects of UV radiation include vitamin D metabolism and phototherapy of cutaneous diseases. Numerous diseases are responsive to UV radiation alone or in combination with a photosensitizing drug (photochemotherapy). These diseases include psoriasis, pityriasis rosea, pruritus of uremia, vitiligo, and mycosis fungoides. However, these beneficial effects must be weighed against the potential adverse effects, which include sunburn, aging, and skin cancer.

For therapeutic purposes, sunlight is the least expensive source of UV radiation. However, because of its varying intensity and availability, it often is not the optimal source. To overcome these disadvantages, artificial light sources were developed. Fluorescent bulbs are placed in a light box for office use or are combined in groups of two or four for self-treatment at home. Hot quartz lamps are used less often and only under direct medical supervision in the hospital or office. The enhancement of phototherapy using tar (Goeckerman treatment) is sometimes used to treat psoriasis. More recently, high-intensity UVA fluorescent bulbs were developed and combined with psoralens in the photochemotherapy of psoriasis (PUVA, or psoralens plus UVA). PUVA also is used for selected patients with vitiligo, mycosis fungoides, and alopecia areata. However, close supervision, experience in use, and awareness of adverse effects are necessary for proper administration of UV radiation.

Ultraviolet radiation:
1. **Positive effects—vitamin D, therapeutic**
2. **Negative effects—sunburn, aging, cancer**

Photoprotection

Excessive exposure to solar irradiation results acutely in sunburn and chronically in premature aging and carcinogenesis. These adverse effects may be prevented with the use of topical sunscreens. In addition, sunscreens are beneficial in ameliorating diseases exacerbated by UV radiation, such as lupus erythematosus.

The amount of protection afforded by a sunscreen is measured by its sun protective factor (SPF). The choice of a sunscreen is based on an individual's skin type correlated with the SPF (Table 5–2). The SPF is calculated by comparing the amount of time required to produce erythema (minimal erythema dose [MED])

Sun protective factor = MED with sunscreen/MED without sunscreen

We recommend a sunscreen with an SPF between 15 and 30.

TABLE 5–2 ■ SKIN TYPE AND SUNSCREEN SPF

Skin Type	History and Physical Examination	Sunscreen
1	Always burn—never tan	SPF 30
2	Always burn—then slight tan	SPF 30
3	Sometimes burn—always tan	SPF 15
4	Never burn–always tan	SPF 15

SPF, sun protective factor.

in skin covered with a sunscreen divided by the time required to produce erythema in an unscreened control site. Thus, a sunscreen with an SPF of 10 would allow a person who normally burns in 20 minutes to be exposed as long as 200 minutes before burning occurs.

The two broad categories of sunscreens are chemical and physical. The most widely used chemical sunscreens contain para-aminobenzoic acid (PABA) esters, benzophenones, salicylates, anthranilates, and cinnamates and are available in cream, lotion, or gel vehicles. Physical sunscreens contain titanium dioxide, zinc oxide, or talc in creams or pastes. Sunscreens with benzophenone combined with PABA esters are those most often used to protect against sunburn, which is primarily due to UVB radiation, and, to a lesser degree, to protect against UVA. Many moisturizers that are advertised as having "antiaging" properties contain sunscreens. Investigators have estimated that the lifetime incidence of basal and squamous cell carcinoma would decrease by 78% if an SPF-15 sunscreen were used regularly for the first 18 years of life. Newer sunscreens containing methyoxydibenzoylmethane or avobenzone (Shade UVA GUARD with Parsol) are particularly helpful for patients who have photosensitivities provoked by UVA and for patients who are receiving PUVA therapy.

An additional measure of a sunscreen is its ability to remain effective when the person using it is sweating or swimming. This property is called *substantivity* and has been found to be a function of both the active sunscreen and its vehicle. At present, no universally accepted means of expressing substantivity exists, as there is with SPF. In choosing a sunscreen, phrases such as *water resistant* or *waterproof* indicate a preparation's substantivity.

Sunscreens should be applied 30 minutes to 1 hour before sun exposure and reapplied after swimming and sweating.

Topical sunscreens are not without adverse reactions. PABA may stain clothing yellow and, if in a gel preparation, can sting and cause drying. Less often, allergic contact dermatitis or allergic photocontact dermatitis occurs with use of PABA, PABA esters, benzophenenones, avobenzone, and cinnamates.

■ DERMATOLOGIC SURGERY

Numerous techniques are available for surgery of the skin. The three most common and simplest procedures are elliptical excision, curettage and electrodesiccation, and cryosurgery. For defects that cannot be closed primarily, skin flaps or grafts may be used. A specialized form of cancer surgery, *Mohs' technique,* involves serial excisions of tissue, which are systematically mapped and microscopically examined to define the extent of cancerous invasion and to ensure surgical margins free of tumor. This technique is the most successful means of treating recurrent basal cell and squamous cell carcinomas.

Surgery explanations:
1. Procedure
2. Potential complications
3. What to do after the surgery

Before surgery, the patient should be informed of the procedure chosen, why it is necessary, and what to expect and do after surgery. The potential complications of the procedure including excessive scar formation, infection, bleeding, and nerve injury should also be explained. When properly selected and technically well performed, simple excision, curettage and electrodesiccation, and cryosurgery usually have no significant complications.

Excision

The simple elliptical excision is used for obtaining tissue for biopsy and for the removal of benign and cancerous lesions. The axis of the lesion, cosmetic boundaries (e.g., the vermilion border of the lip), and skin lines should be taken into consideration when planning the excision. Most procedures require a minimal number of instruments, including a needle holder, small forceps, skin hook, small clamp, small pointed scissors, syringe and needle (30 gauge), and No. 15 scalpel blade plus handle. Disposable sterile gloves, eye sheet, and gauze are also necessary.

Lidocaine does not cross-react with procaine hydrochloride.

Numerous antiseptics are available for preoperative preparation of the skin, including 70% isopropyl alcohol, povidone-iodine (Betadine), and chlorhexidine gluconate (Hibiclens). The boundaries of the excision are marked. This is done before injection of local anesthesia because the volume of anesthetic distorts the normal skin contours. The preferred local anesthetic is 1% lidocaine because of the rarity of allergic reactions. In addition, lidocaine, an amide, does not cross-react with procaine hydrochloride (Novocain), an ester. Transdermal anesthesia with a topical anesthetic such as Emla cream can be applied under an occlusive dressing 1 to 2 hours before the procedure to reduce the pain associated with injection.

Normal saline or diphenhydramine hydrochloride (Benadryl) may be used for local anesthesia if lidocaine cannot be used. The addition of epinephrine to lidocaine prolongs its anesthetic effect and reduces operative bleeding. Care should be taken when using epinephrine in the earlobe and digits to avoid ischemic changes secondary to vasoconstriction.

The length of elliptical excision is three times its width.
Suture removal:
1. Face: 5 days
2. Trunk and extremities: 1 to 2 weeks

The length of the ellipse should be three times the width to ensure easy closure. The cut should be made perpendicular to the surface and through the dermis into the subcutaneous tissue. Hemostasis is achieved with pressure, electrodesiccation, or suture ligation. Repair of the wound is easy if an adequate ellipse has been formed, the edges are perpendicular, and skin lines are followed. If the defect is large, the edges may be undermined to reduce closure tension. Buried absorbable suture such as Vicryl is used to close deeper layers. Numerous methods are used for skin closure; use of interrupted sutures with monofilament nylon (Ethicon) is the simplest method. In most cases, 5-0 or 4-0 sutures are adequate for both subcuticular and skin closure. The removal of skin sutures depends on the site, wound tension, and whether buried sutures have been used. In general, facial sutures are removed in 5 days, and trunk and extremity sutures are removed in 1 to 2 weeks. Most wounds are dressed with either sterile adherent bandages or gauze secured with tape. Paper tape with an acrylic adhesive mass should be used in patients with a history of tape sensitivity. Topical antibiotics are not necessary after surgery. The patient is instructed to keep the wound dry for 24 hours, to change the dressings daily, and to return to the clinic if bleeding, purulent drainage, or excessive pain or swelling occurs. Postoperative pain is usually negligible, requiring only acetaminophen.

Curettage and Electrodesiccation

The procedure of curettage and electrodesiccation is most often used for the treatment of selected small basal cell and squamous cell carcinomas. It is a deceptively simple procedure that requires proper selection of tumor and a skilled practitioner. Otherwise, the recurrence rate is unacceptably high. The tumor is prepared and anesthetized with a local anesthetic. The *curette,* an oval instrument with a cutting edge, is used to remove the soft cancerous skin. The tumor margins are determined by "feel," with normal skin having a firm and gritty consistency. After curettage, the base and borders of the wound are electrodesiccated to destroy residual tumor and to provide hemostasis. The wound heals by secondary intention in 2 to 3 weeks.

Curettage and electrodesiccation require experience to avoid high recurrence rate of basal cell or squamous cell carcinoma.

Cryosurgery

Keratoses and warts are frequently treated with cryosurgery. Liquid nitrogen ($-195.6°C$) is the standard agent because it is inexpensive, rapid, and noncombustible. Tissue destruction is caused by intercellular and extracellular ice formation, by denaturing lipid-protein complexes, and by cell dehydration. This treatment requires no skin preparation or anesthesia. Liquid nitrogen application is accomplished with a cotton-tipped stick or a direct spray and usually requires less than 30 seconds. A repeat freeze-thaw cycle results in more cellular damage than a single cycle.

Keratoses and warts are easily treated with liquid nitrogen.

During the procedure, the patient feels a stinging or burning sensation. Subsequently, burning occurs along with tissue swelling. Within 24 hours, a blister often forms in the treated area. If the blister is excessively large or painful, the fluid should be removed in a sterile manner. Otherwise, it is allowed to heal spontaneously.

Treatment of skin cancers with cryotherapy requires an operator experienced with thermocouple devices to ensure adequate freezing for tissue destruction. Postoperative morbidity includes significant tissue edema and necrosis.

■ PATIENT EDUCATION

A dialogue must be established between the physician and the patient. This is begun during the history and physical examination. Once a diagnosis is established, the patient should be told what the disease is, what its cause is, and what to expect from treatment. Patients are frequently hesitant to ask certain questions because they are either afraid or embarrassed. It is important that these unasked questions be answered: Is my disease contagious? Is it cancer? Do I have something wrong internally that is causing my skin problems?

Answer the unasked questions:
1. Contagious?
2. Cancer?
3. Internal?

For therapy to be successful, patient cooperation and compliance are necessary. To ensure this goal, therapeutic options, expected outcome, and potential side effects should be explained. Instructions on how to use topical medications must be demonstrated. All too frequently, too much medication is applied, and it is not rubbed in sufficiently. For example, when applying a white cream, patients should be instructed to apply sparingly and rub it in until it "disappears." If white cream remains on the surface, either too much has been applied or it has not been rubbed in sufficiently. Dressings may be either too wet or too dry or left on too long, resulting in maceration. These pitfalls are avoided when the medication or dressing is applied to the area of dermatitis as a demonstration while the patient is in the office.

Patient instruction sheets augment the spoken word. They inform and instruct patients. Frequently, medical problems and therapies are complex, and the patient fails to understand them. Instruction sheets save time, reinforce what has been told to the patient, answer unasked questions, and provide a reference for the patient to read. Instruction sheets are available from the American Medical Association and the American Academy of Dermatology (telephone, 312–869–3954) and in the book by Dr. E. Epstein, *Common Skin Disorders: A Physician's Illustrated Manual with Patient Instruction Sheets*. Other sources of patient education are support groups, which are listed here:

AIDS
Centers for Disease Control
AIDS Information Clearinghouse
(800) 458-5231
National AIDS Hotline
(800) 342-2437

Alopecia Areata
National Alopecia Areata Foundation
PO BOX 150760
San Rafael, CA 94915
(415) 456-4644

Eczema
Eczema Association for Science & Education
1221 SW Yamhill, Suite 303
Portland, OR 97205
(503) 228-4430

Lupus
American Lupus Society
3914 Del Amo Boulevard, Suite 922
Torrance, CA 90503
(800) 331-1802
(310) 542-8891

Neurofibromatosis
National Neurofibromatosis Foundation
141 Fifth Avenue, Suite 7-S
New York, NY 10010
(800) 323-7938
(212) 460-8980

Psoriasis
National Psoriasis Foundation
6443 SW Beaverton Highway, Suite 210
PO BOX 9009
Portland, OR 97221
(503) 297-1545

Skin Cancer
Skin Cancer Foundation
245 Fifth Avenue, Suite 2402
New York, NY 10016
(212) 725-5176

Tuberous Sclerosis
National Tuberous Sclerosis Association
8000 Corporate Drive, Suite 120
Landover, MD 20785
(800) 225-6872
(301) 459-9888

Vitiligo
National Vitiligo Foundation
PO BOX 6337
Tyler, TX 75711
(903) 534-2925

R E F E R E N C E S

General

Arndt KA: Manual of Dermatologic Therapeutics with Essentials of Diagnosis. 5th ed. Boston, Little, Brown, 1995.

Topical Therapy

Scheuplein RJ: Percutaneous absorption after 25 years: or old wine and new wine skins. J Invest Dermatol *67*:31–38, 1976.

Dressings and Baths

Marks JG, Bainey M: Cutaneous reactions to surgical preparations and dressings. Contact Dermatitis *10*:1–5, 1984.

Topical Steroids

Drake LA, Dinehart SM, Farmer ER, et al.: Guidelines of care for the use of topical glucocorticosteroids. J Am Acad Dermatol *35*:615–619, 1996.

Gilbertson EO, Spellman MC, Piacquadio DJ, et al.: Super potent topical corticosteroid use associated with adrenal suppression: clinical considerations. J Am Acad Dermatol *38*: 318–321, 1998.

Olsen EA: A double-blind controlled comparison of generic and trade-name topical steroids using the vasoconstriction assay. Arch Dermatol *127*:197–201, 1991.

Surber C, Itin PH, Bircher AJ, et al.: Topical corticosteroids. J Am Acad Dermatol *32*:1025–1030, 1995.

Topical corticosteroids. Med Lett *33*:108–110, 1991.

Phototherapy

Johnson EY, Lookingbill DP: Sunscreen use and sun exposure: trends in a white population. Arch Dermatol *120*:727–731, 1984.

Kligman LH, Akin FJ, Kligman AM: Sunscreens prevent ultraviolet photocarcinogenesis. J Am Acad Dermatol *3*:30–35, 1980.

Menter JM: Recent developments in UVA photoprotection. Int J Dermatol *29*:389–393, 1990.

Morison WL, Hadley TP, Gilchrest BA, Stern RS: Photobiology. J Am Acad Dermatol *25*: 327–329, 1991.

Naylor MF, Farmer KC: The case for sunscreens: a review of their use in preventing actinic damage and neoplasia. Arch Dermatol *133*:1146–1154, 1997.

Pathak MA: Sunscreens: topical and systemic approaches for protection of human skin against harmful effects of solar radiation. J Am Acad Dermatol *7*:285–312, 1982.

Robinson JK, Amonette R, Wyatt SW, et al.: Executive summary of the national "Sun Safety: Protecting Our Future" conference: American Academy of Dermatology and Centers for Disease Control and Prevention. J Am Acad Dermatol *38*:774–780, 1998.

Stern RS, Weinstein MC, Baker SG: Risk reduction for nonmelanoma skin cancer with childhood sunscreen use. Arch Dermatol *122*:537–545, 1986.

Sunscreens. Med Lett *30*:61–63, 1988.

Dermatologic Surgery

Kuflik EG: Cryosurgery updated. J Am Acad Dermatol *31*:925–944, 1994.

Ratz JL, Geronemus RG, Maloney ME, et al.: Textbook of dermatologic surgery. Philadelphia, Lippincott–Raven, 1998.

Shriner DL, McCoy DK, Goldberg DJ, et al.: Mohs micrographic surgery. J Am Acad Dermatol *39*:79–97, 1998.

Patient Education

Epstein E: Common Skin Disorders: A Physician's Illustrated Manual with Patient Instruction Sheets. 2nd ed. Oradell, NJ, Medical Economics, 1983.

2

GROWTHS

∎

EPIDERMAL GROWTHS

■

WART
CORN
SEBORRHEIC KERATOSIS
SKIN TAG
MOLLUSCUM CONTAGIOSUM
ACTINIC KERATOSIS
SQUAMOUS CELL CARCINOMA
BASAL CELL CARCINOMA

Neoplasms of the epidermis (Table 6–1) are derived from a proliferation of either basal cells or keratinocytes. Epidermal growths are recognized clinically by a localized thickening of the epidermis that often is accompanied by thickening of the stratum corneum, which is called *hyperkeratosis* or *scale*. Large, indurated, rapidly growing, crusted, or ulcerated tumors suggest a malignant process and should undergo biopsy. Unless injured or irritated, benign growths do not bleed or become crusted or ulcerated.

■ WART

Definition. Warts are benign neoplasms caused by infection of epidermal cells with papillomaviruses. The thickening of the epidermis with scaling and an upward extension of the dermal papillae containing prominent capillaries give them their "warty" or verrucous appearance (Fig. 6–1).

Warts are caused by papillomaviruses.

Incidence. Warts generally occur in healthy children and young adults. Genital human papillomavirus (HPV) infection may be the most common sexually transmitted disease. One percent of sexually active adults are estimated to have genital warts, and an additional 10% to 20% have latent infection. For sexually active young college women, the incidence of infection is high—43%. From 5% to 7% of patients seen by dermatologists are seen for warts.

History. Predisposing conditions make the occurrence of multiple warts more likely. Immunosuppressed patients, such as renal transplant recipients, are prone to the development of warts. Inquiry into the patient's occupation is important because butchers and meat cutters have a significantly higher incidence of common warts. Anogenital warts (condylomata acuminata) affect sexually active in-

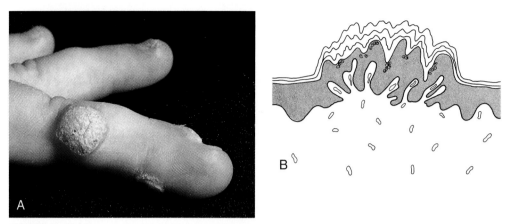

FIGURE 6-1. Wart. **A**, Epidermis—scaling, verrucous papule with interrupted skin lines and black puncta. **B**, Epidermis—thickened, with overlying hyperkeratosis. Vacuolated keratinocytes are present in the granular cell layer.

dividuals, and their occurrence in children should raise suspicions of sexual abuse. However, most patients with warts do not have any of these predisposing conditions.

Common and plantar warts interrupt skin lines and have black puncta.

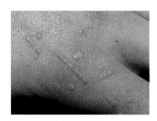

FIGURE 6-2. Flat warts.

Physical Examination. The *common wart* (Fig. 6–1), or verruca vulgaris, is a flesh-colored, firm papule or nodule that has a corrugated or hyperkeratotic surface. It interrupts the normal skin lines and is studded with black puncta. Common warts occur individually, in groups, or in a linear fashion from autoinoculation. The hands and fingers are the usual sites. Involvement around nails frequently results in extension underneath the nail plate. A filiform variant of verruca vulgaris occurs on the head and neck.

A *flat wart* has a subtle appearance (Fig. 6–2). It is a flesh-colored or reddish brown, slightly raised, flat-surfaced, 2- to 5-mm, well marginated papule. On extremely close inspection (a hand magnifying lens may be needed), the surface appears finely verrucous. Multiple lesions commonly affect the hands and face. A linear arrangement of lesions is common.

A *plantar wart* occurs as a single, painful papule on the plantar aspect of the foot. It is covered by a thick callus. When the callus is pared down with a scalpel, the underlying wart is visualized with interruption of skin lines and black puncta. Multiple plantar warts may coalesce in a mosaic configuration or remain discrete in a mother-daughter relationship, with a central large wart surrounded by multiple smaller warts.

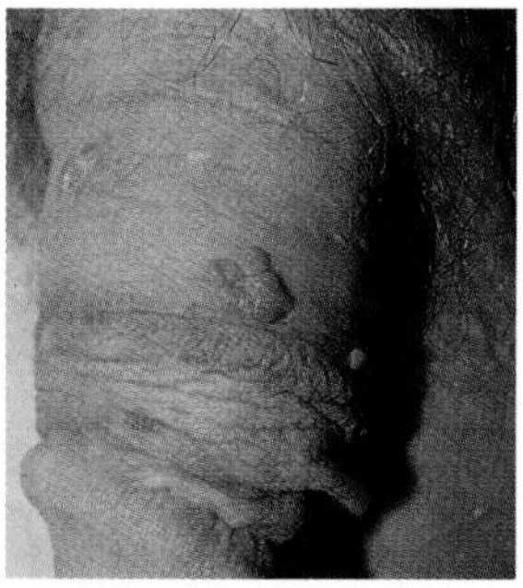

Condyloma acuminatum (venereal wart) (Fig. 6–3) involves the rectum, perineal region, inguinal folds, external genitalia, and, occasionally, urethra and vagina. It is composed of a soft, moist papule and plaque that may be sessile or pedunculated. It has a verrucous surface that often is cauliflower-like. Soaking the genital area for 5 minutes with 3% to 5% acetic acid (white vinegar) causes warts to turn white; then, use of a hand magnifying lens or colposcopy enables better visualization of small genital warts (acetowhitening). Although acetowhitening increases sensitivity of detection, it is not specific for HPV lesions and is not recommended for routine screening because overdiagnosis of external genital warts may occur.

FIGURE 6-3. Condyloma acuminatum.

TABLE 6–1 ■ EPIDERMAL GROWTHS

	Frequency*	Etiology	Physical Examination	Differential Diagnosis	Laboratory Test (Biopsy)
Wart	5.2	Papillomavirus			No
Common			Flesh-colored, scaling, vegetative papule or nodule, skin lines interrupted, studded with black puncta	Corn Squamous cell carcinoma	
Flat			Reddish, smooth, flat, well-demarcated papule	Lichen planus Comedo	
Plantar			Solitary, grouped or mosaic scaling papules, skin lines interrupted, studded with black puncta	Corn Squamous cell carcinoma	
Condyloma acuminatum			Soft, moist, cauliflower-appearing papules or nodule	Squamous cell carcinoma Secondary syphilis	No
Corn	0.4	Friction	Hyperkeratotic papule or nodule with compact clear core	Wart	No
Skin tag	0.5	—	Soft, skin-colored, pedunculated papule	Nevus Neurofibroma	No
Seborrheic keratosis	1.6	—	Tan-brown, greasy, "pasted-on" papule or plaque	Wart Actinic keratosis Nevus Malignant melanoma Pigmented basal cell carcinoma	No
Molluscum contagiosum	0.3	Poxvirus	Translucent papule with umbilicated center	Comedo Nodular basal cell	No
Actinic keratosis	1.7	Sunlight	Ill-marginated, reddish, rough, scaling patch or papule	Squamous cell carcinoma Seborrheic keratosis Superficial basal cell carcinoma	When thick scale or indurated base
Squamous cell carcinoma	0.2	Sunlight Viruses Chemicals	Flesh-colored, hard, crusted or scaling nodule, often ulcerated	Keratoacanthoma Basal cell carcinoma Wart Actinic keratosis	Yes
Basal cell carcinoma	1.7	Sunlight			Yes
Nodular			Pearly nodule with telangiectasia, often has central depression or ulcer	Molluscum contagiosum Squamous cell carcinoma Sebaceous hyperplasia Nevus	
Pigmented			Blue-black plaque or nodule with pearly border	Malignant melanoma Nevus Seborrheic keratosis	
Superficial			Red, scaling, crusted eczematous-appearing patch	Psoriasis Eczema Bowen's disease	
Sclerosing			Whitish, slightly depressed, sometimes crusted plaque	Squamous cell carcinoma Nonhealing scar	

* Percentage of new dermatology patients with this diagnosis seen in the Hershey Medical Center Dermatology Clinic, Hershey, PA.

Differential Diagnosis. A common wart usually is easily recognized. When covered with thick scale, it may be confused with a *callus*, which on paring does not have interrupted skin lines. The diagnosis of *squamous cell carcinoma* should be entertained for a lesion that is resistant to treatment, is enlarging, and is crusted or ulcerated.

A flat wart on the face may be confused with a noninflammatory acne lesion, the "whitehead" or *comedo.* The tops of comedones are smooth and dome-shaped, whereas flat warts have roughened flat tops. When flat warts occur on the hand and forearm, *lichen planus*, an idiopathic inflammatory skin disease, is in the differential diagnosis. Lichen planus papules are red to purple; warts are flesh colored.

Plantar warts and *corns* are often confused because both are painful and have a thick, scaling surface. However, paring down the surface demonstrates the interruption of skin lines and black puncta characteristic of a plantar wart.

Condyloma acuminatum may resemble the verrucous form of squamous cell carcinoma. Lesions that do not respond to treatment must undergo biopsy. *Secondary syphilis* of the anus and genitals (condyloma latum) is ruled out with a darkfield examination and serology. *Seborrheic keratoses* in the genital region also may resemble condyloma acuminatum.

Bowenoid papulosis is an uncommon disorder characterized by erythematous, sometimes pigmented, papules occurring in the genital region of sexually active young adults. Histologically, bowenoid papulosis has the appearance of squamous cell carcinoma in situ. Its relationship with HPV infection has been confirmed by finding HPV DNA in bowenoid papulosis, especially HPV-16. Conservative surgical modalities should be used to treat bowenoid papulosis. Radical, mutilating procedures are unwarranted.

Laboratory and Biopsy. Warts are usually not examined by biopsy unless a suspicion of carcinoma exists. When examined by biopsy, warts demonstrate a thickened epidermis (acanthosis) with overlying hyperkeratosis. Distinctive large keratinocytes (koilocytes) with small pyknotic nuclei surrounded by clear cytoplasm are found in the upper layers of the epidermis. Typing of HPV based on DNA homology is an experimental technique currently available only in research laboratories. HPV has been cultured in human skin transplanted under the renal capsule of nude mice.

Avoid overzealous treatment, which produces scars.

Therapy. Treatment of warts is nonspecific, destructive, and usually painful. A eutectic mixture of local anesthetics (Emla cream) applied topically under occlusion 1 to 2 hours before painful procedures may be beneficial in treating warts in uncooperative children. The goal is destruction of the keratinocytes that are infected with HPV. This may be accomplished with a variety of physical, chemical, or biologic modalities.

The physical modalities include cryotherapy with liquid nitrogen, electrodesiccation and curettage, surgical excision, and laser therapy. Cryotherapy, the most common initial mode of treatment, uses either a cotton-tipped stick or a cryospray unit for application of the liquid nitrogen onto the verruca. A white ice ball develops at the site of freezing and should extend 1 to 2 mm beyond the margins of the wart. After the area has thawed, a second freezing results in greater destruction of the wart. Subsequent blister formation often occurs within 24 hours. After several weeks, the blister dries, and the skin containing the wart peels off. Often, follow-up treatments every 2 to 4 weeks are necessary to eradicate any residual wart. Eradication generally requires two or three office visits. The ad-

---

THERAPY OF WARTS

- Cryotherapy with liquid nitrogen
- Acids:
    Salicyclic
    Trichloroacetic 75%–100% in office
- Cantharidin in office
- Tretinoin 0.1% cream—flat warts
- Podophyllin 25%—genital warts, in office
- Podofilox solution or gel—bid × 3 days/week × 4 weeks—genital warts
- Imiquimod cream—qd × 3 days/week × 16 weeks—genital warts
- Surgical excision, curettage, electrocautery
- Laser
- Interferon
- Bleomycin intralesionally
- 5-Fluorouracil

---

vantages of cryotherapy are that (1) it is quick, (2) it does not require local anesthesia, and (3) the discomfort from the freezing is tolerated well by most patients, except young children. Caution must be used in all the physical modalities, especially surgical excision, because of potential scarring. The scar may be cosmetically unacceptable, or it may be painful if on the plantar surface. Although laser surgery was initially thought to be superior to other surgical procedures in removing warts, this now appears not to be true.

Numerous chemotherapeutic agents are used to treat warts either in the office or at home. The initial treatments include salicylic acid at home or trichloroacetic acid in the office. Common warts may be treated with flexible collodion containing 17% salicylic acid (DuoFilm) or 17% salicylic acid in a polyacrylic vehicle (Occlusal-HP) applied daily. The wart is softened by soaking in water for 5 minutes before application, and any loosened tissue is gently removed. After the acid has been applied, the wart can be covered with adhesive tape. Cantharidin 0.7% (Verr-Canth), a potent blistering agent derived from the blister beetle, is an alternative office treatment that is applied to common warts and covered with tape. After 24 hours, a blister forms beneath the wart. The blister roof dries and peels off, taking with it the wart. Occasionally, cantharidin or cryotherapy may result in formation of a new wart in an annular configuration (ring) at the periphery of the blister.

Tretinoin (Retin-A) is useful in treatment of flat warts; its efficacy probably results from its irritant effect.

Plantar verrucae are treated with daily applications of salicylic acid plaster (Mediplast), 17% salicylic acid in a polyacrylic vehicle (Occlusal-HP), or 17% salicylic acid in flexible collodion (DuoPlant).

Condyloma acuminatum is commonly treated with 25% podophyllin resin (Podocon–25), which can be very toxic and is used only in the clinician's office. Within 4 to 6 hours after application, excess podophyllin should be washed off to prevent excessive local irritation. Caution must be used when applying podophyllin to extensive lesions because severe systemic reactions may result from absorption. The Centers for Disease Control and Prevention prefer cryotherapy

Podophyllin is toxic; do not apply to extensive lesions or use to treat pregnant women.

over podophyllin for treatment of condyloma acuminatum. Podophyllin is a cytotoxic agent and has resulted in renal toxicity, polyneuritis, and shock. Podophyllin must never be used during pregnancy because of potential harmful effects on the fetus. Podofilox, a chemically pure ligand derived from podophyllin, is available as a 0.5% topical solution or gel (Condylox) for patient self-treatment of external genital warts. Application is made twice daily for 3 consecutive days followed by a 4-day rest period. This cycle may be repeated up to four times. The sexual partners of infected individuals should be examined for the presence of genital warts. Female patients with genital warts should have periodic gynecologic exams with Papanicolaou smears. Screening for other sexually transmitted diseases should be considered.

Recalcitrant warts have been treated with 5-fluorouracil topically, bleomycin intralesionally, and interferon topically, intralesionally, and systemically.

Biologic treatments have centered on the induction of immune responses. Imiquimod (Aldara) applied topically induces the cytokines interferon-α, tumor necrosis factor-γ, and interleukins 1, 6, and 8. Squaric acid dibutylester, poison ivy resin, and other allergens have been used to induce allergic contact dermatitis. Presumably, the wart is destroyed by the delayed hypersensitivity reaction that occurs at the site of application of the allergens. Currently, no wart vaccines are available.

Course and Complications. Investigators have estimated that 35% to 65% of warts spontaneously resolve within 2 years. Treatment results in cure rates of as high as 80%.

Papillomavirus is associated with some carcinomas, particularly cervical carcinoma.

Of concern is the relationship between papillomavirus and carcinoma. Papillomavirus-associated cancers occur in humans, cattle, horses, and rabbits and experimentally in rodents. Patients with the rare syndrome *epidermodysplasia verruciformis*, manifested by widespread refractory warts, who are infected with HPV-5 or HPV-8, have progression of their sun-exposed flat warts into squamous cell carcinoma. Furthermore, HPV genomes have been demonstrated within the malignant squamous cells. The epidemiologic evidence for an association between papillomavirus (type 16, 18, or 33) and cervical cancer appears overwhelming. HPV infection of the cervix appears to represent a necessary but not sufficient condition for developing malignancy. Other possible cofactors, such as cigarette smoking, appear to be required for carcinogenesis. HPV typing, however, has not been proven to be beneficial in the diagnosis and management of external genital warts.

Pathogenesis. The contagious nature of warts was observed in ancient times. Jadassohn in the 1800s was the first to prove conclusively the infectious nature of warts. He ground up wart material and inoculated the normal skin of volunteers. After an incubation period of 2 to 3 months, warts developed in the inoculation sites. Ciuffo in 1907 proved the viral nature of warts using ultrafiltration techniques.

The papillomavirus is a double-stranded DNA virus that infects and replicates in keratinizing cells in the epidermis. The HPV virion is an icosahedral particle composed of a viral genome surrounded by a proteinaceous capsid. Progeny HPV virions are assembled and become apparent in the upper layers of the epidermis, especially the stratum corneum and stratum granulosum. Viral genomes are found in lower layers of the epidermis and probably help to explain the chronicity and treatment failure of many warts. The presence of the wart virus stimulates epidermal proliferation, resulting in epidermal thickening and hyperkeratosis. Papillomaviruses have been subdivided into distinct types based on DNA homology. On this basis, more than 80 genotypes have been described. The clinical type of wart had been thought to be determined by local conditions at the site of infection. However, it now appears that different HPV types are responsible for the different clinical lesions—common, flat, plantar, and condyloma acuminatum because good correlation often exists between clinical presentation and HPV type.

The viral and host factors that influence persistence, regression, latency, and reactivation of warts are poorly understood. Serum antibodies to warts have been detected. More important, cell-mediated immunity appears to contribute to the regression of warts; in immunodeficient hosts (e.g., those with organ transplants or epidermodysplasia verruciformis), warts may reactivate or persist.

■ CORN

Definition. A corn is a localized thickening of epidermis secondary to chronic pressure or friction. It most often occurs on the toe (Fig. 6–4). Synonyms are clavus and heloma.

Incidence. Corns are extremely common. Many patients treat themselves or see a podiatrist rather than a physician.

History. The patient seeks medical care because of painful feet when standing or walking. A history of ill-fitting footwear or foot injury may be obtained.

Physical Examination. Corns are white-gray or yellow-brown, well-circumscribed, horny papules or nodules. Paring the surface with a scalpel reveals a translucent core with preservation of skin lines. Hard corns occur on the sole and external surface of the toes, where drying occurs. Soft corns occur between the toes, where sweating results in maceration.

Corns have a clear center and intact skin lines.

Differential Diagnosis. Plantar warts and corns are commonly confused. The simple maneuver of paring the surface and identifying the presence of skin lines with a translucent core confirms that the lesion is a corn.

Laboratory and Biopsy. A biopsy is unnecessary.

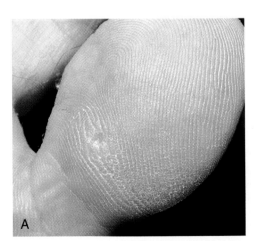

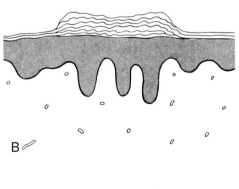

FIGURE 6–4. Corn. **A,** Epidermis—thick, scaling papule or plaque. **B,** Epidermis—thickened, with hyperkeratosis.

THERAPY OF CORN

- Paring down with scalpel
- Softening with salicylic acid plaster
- Reduction of trauma—change of shoes, protective pads, rings, etc.
- Surgery—correction of deformity

Therapy. The goal of treating corns is to provide immediate relief of pain and then to reduce the friction and pressure that have caused the corn. Immediate relief is provided by paring down the hyperkeratotic surface. Softening of hard corns may be accomplished with keratolytic agents such as salicylic acid plasters (Mediplast). Changing ill-fitting footwear and shielding the sites with pads, rings, and orthotic devices reduce mechanical trauma. When these procedures fail, surgical correction of a foot deformity or removal of a bony prominence (exostosis) should be considered.

A corn will persist unless friction and pressure are relieved.

Course and Complications. Persistence of the corn can be expected unless the underlying mechanical problem is reduced or removed. Underlying bursitis from chronic inflammation and sinus formation with infection, osteomyelitis, and gangrene may occur and are particularly worrisome in patients with arteriosclerosis, diabetes mellitus, or peripheral neurologic disorders.

Pathogenesis. Repeated pressure and trauma resulting extrinsically from ill-fitting shoes and intrinsically from an exostosis or other anatomic skeletal defects result in the formation of corns.

■ SEBORRHEIC KERATOSIS

Definition. A seborrheic keratosis is a benign neoplasm of epidermal cells that clinically appears as a scaling, "pasted-on" papule or plaque (Fig. 6–5). It is thought to be an autosomal dominant inherited trait.

Incidence. Seborrheic keratoses usually appear in middle age, with at least a few lesions present in most elderly patients.

History. Many patients remember family members who had seborrheic keratoses. These neoplasms are gradually acquired in middle and later life and grow slowly.

Physical Examination. Seborrheic keratoses vary in size from 2 mm to 2 cm and are slightly to markedly elevated. Color ranges from flesh to tan or brown or, occasionally, black. The keratoses are oval to round, greasy-appearing, "pasted-on," sharply marginated growths. The surface is often verrucous or crumbly in appearance and may be punctuated with keratin-filled pits. The lesions occur on the head, neck, trunk, and extremities, sparing the palms and soles.

Well-marginated, "pasted-on" appearance is distinctive.

Differential Diagnosis. Wart, actinic keratosis, and pigmented growths such as a *nevus, pigmented basal cell carcinoma,* or *malignant melanoma* may be confused with a seborrheic keratosis. The occurrence of multiple similar scaling growths with a

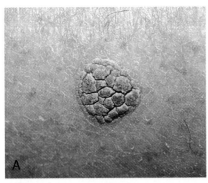
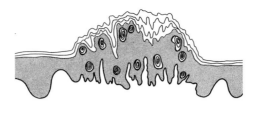

FIGURE 6–5. Seborrheic keratosis. **A,** Epidermis—scaling, well-marginated papule or plaque. **B,** Epidermis—hyperkeratosis with thickened epidermis containing horny pseudocysts.

greasy, well-marginated, "pasted-on" appearance gives the observer the clue that these lesions are seborrheic keratoses. The superficial, exophytic epidermal growth and keratotic surface of a seborrheic keratosis differentiate it from a nevus, a pigmented dermal growth with which it is often confused.

Laboratory and Biopsy. Excisional or shaved biopsy confirms the clinical impression of seborrheic keratosis. This neoplasm is characterized by a uniform, well-demarcated intraepidermal proliferation of small, benign squamous cells. Invaginations of the epidermis form small, keratin-filled pseudocysts.

Therapy. No therapy is necessary for seborrheic keratoses unless they become irritated, are cosmetically unacceptable, or require confirmation that they are benign. Cryotherapy with liquid nitrogen is an efficient and effective means of removal. As an alternative, seborrheic keratoses can be anesthetized and curetted or shaved off. Caution should be used; vigorous treatment may result in scarring. Excisional surgery is seldom needed unless concern about malignancy exists.

Course and Complications. The tendency is to acquire more seborrheic keratoses with age. Sometimes, seborrheic keratoses become irritated from rubbing, clothing, or excoriations. Occasionally, their typical morphologic appearance becomes obscured by inflammation, thus making a biopsy necessary for diagnosis.

The number of seborrheic keratoses increases with age.

Of note is the rare *sign of Leser-Trélat*, the rapid increase in size and number of seborrheic keratoses accompanied by pruritus. This is a cutaneous sign of internal malignancy, usually adenocarcinoma involving the stomach, ovary, uterus, or breast. The extremities and shoulders are the most frequent sites of involvement.

THERAPY OF SEBORRHEIC KERATOSIS

- Cryotherapy with liquid nitrogen
- Curettage
- Shave biopsy/excision

■ SKIN TAG

Definition. A skin tag (acrochordon) is a benign fleshy tumor that is frequently acquired in adult life. It is characterized by a slightly hyperplastic epithelium covering a dermal connective tissue stalk (Fig. 6–6). It appears as a pedunculated, flesh-colored growth.

Incidence. This benign tumor is extremely common in adulthood. The incidence of patients coming into our clinic specifically for skin tags is 0.5%, but as an incidental finding, 50% to 60% of patients older than age 50 have skin tags. A steady increase in frequency occurs from the second decade (11%) to the fifth decade (59%) of life, after which the number of individuals with skin tags remains stable.

History. Most patients ignore skin tags and accept their acquisition as a sign of aging. Some patients request their removal because of irritation or cosmetic appearance.

> **Skin tags appear as fleshy, pedunculated papules.**

Physical Examination. A skin tag is a soft, tan- to flesh-colored, 1- to 10-mm, pedunculated, fleshy papule. It has a smooth or folded surface and frequently appears boggy or filiform. It is found on any skin surface but has a predilection for the axilla, neck, inframammary region, inguinal region, and eyelids. When irritated or injured, it can appear as a necrotic, crusted papule that may not be clinically distinctive and causes concern regarding a malignancy.

Differential Diagnosis. Intradermal nevi may have a boggy, flesh-colored appearance, making them impossible to differentiate from skin tags other than by histologic examination. The acquisition of skin tags in later life would help to differentiate them historically from nevi. *Neurofibromas* can resemble skin tags, but on palpation a neurofibroma can be invaginated into what feels like a "buttonhole" defect in the dermis. Uncommonly, *basal or squamous cell carcinoma* may have the appearance of a skin tag.

> **Large or necrotic skin tags should be sent to pathology.**

Laboratory and Biopsy. Skin tags are covered by a slightly hyperplastic epithelium consisting of hyperkeratosis, papillomatosis, and acanthosis. The underlying dermal connective tissue stalk is composed of loose collagen containing numerous capillaries. Typical multiple, 1- to 5-mm, flesh-colored pedunculated skin tags

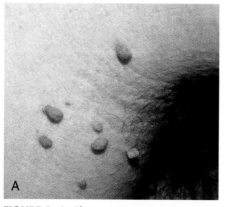
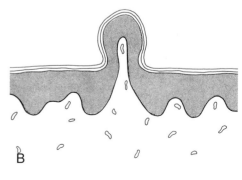

FIGURE 6–6. Skin tag. **A,** Epidermis—mildly thickened. Dermis—soft, pedunculated papule. **B,** Epidermis—mildly thickened. Dermis—loose connective tissue stalk.

THERAPY OF SKIN TAGS

- Snipping off with scissors
- Cryotherapy with liquid nitrogen

need not be submitted for pathologic examination. Larger solitary and necrotic or crusted skin tags should be examined histologically.

Therapy. Skin tags need not be removed unless the patient requests it. The easiest means of removal of skin tags is by quickly snipping them with scissors. This usually requires no local anesthesia, and the crushing action of the scissors results in little bleeding. As an alternative, they may be frozen with liquid nitrogen.

Course and Complications. The number of skin tags increases with age. They normally are of little consequence and require no treatment. Concern has recently been expressed that skin tags may be a marker for the presence of colon polyps in highly selected referral populations presenting for colonoscopy. In the primary care setting, no association exists between skin tags and colon polyps.

■ MOLLUSCUM CONTAGIOSUM

A molluscum contagiosum papule is small, smooth, and characteristically umbilicated.

Definition. Molluscum contagiosum is caused by a DNA poxvirus that infects epidermal cells. Clinically, the lesions appear as smooth, dome-shaped papules that often are umbilicated (Fig. 6–7).

Incidence. Molluscum contagiosum is a common childhood disease. Spread among family members occurs but is uncommon.

History. In adults, venereal transmission is suggested by a history of sexual exposure and the location of lesions in the genital region.

Physical Examination. The papules of molluscum contagiosum are 2 to 5 mm wide, hard, smooth, dome shaped, and flesh colored or translucent. The papules have a central umbilication from which a "cheesy" core can be expressed. They occur singly or in groups, most often on the trunk, face, and extremities of children and on the genitals of sexually active adults. Uncommonly, they become disseminated, resulting in hundreds of lesions. If inflamed, they are difficult to recognize because of secondary erythema and crusting.

Differential Diagnosis. The translucent papule of molluscum contagiosum can resemble *nodular basal cell carcinoma* or a *comedo*. Nodular basal cell carcinomas usually have telangiectasia and occur in sun-exposed skin of older patients. Comedones lack umbilication. An inflamed molluscum contagiosum may appear to be a bacterial infection of the skin.

When in doubt, the diagnosis may be confirmed by expressing the cheesy core and smearing it onto a glass slide for microscopic examination.

Laboratory and Biopsy. The diagnosis usually is clinically obvious. When doubt exists, a simple office procedure is confirmatory. The molluscum papule is removed by curettage and is crushed onto a slide. This unstained material readily reveals numerous oval molluscum bodies when examined with a microscope. A

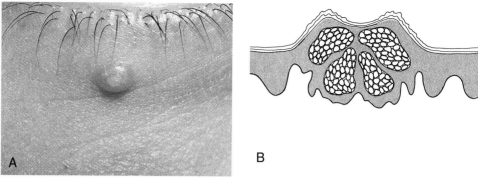

FIGURE 6–7. Molluscum contagiosum. **A,** Epidermis—umbilicated papule. **B,** Epidermis—thickened, contains molluscum.

biopsy usually is not necessary unless the typical features are masked by secondary inflammation.

Therapy. The most reliable means of eradication is by curettage. The molluscum papule composed of many molluscum bodies is scraped off, although with some discomfort and bleeding. The initial treatment is usually cryotherapy with liquid nitrogen. For children who will not tolerate the pain of curettage or cryotherapy, the careful application of the blistering chemical cantharidin (Verr-Canth) can be used in the office or topical salicylic acid preparations (DuoFilm) can be used at home similar to the treatment of warts.

Course and Complications. Spontaneous remission often occurs within 6 to 9 months, although lesions have been known to persist for many years, and more lesions may develop by autoinoculation. Individual lesions can become secondarily inflamed and may resemble furuncles. Involvement of the eyelids is uncommon but may result in chronic conjunctivitis. The development of hundreds of lesions with little tendency for involution should alert the clinician to consider immunocompromise. Molluscum contagiosum is one of the most common cutaneous findings in AIDS and AIDS-related complex, infecting 9% of these individuals. In the AIDS patient, molluscum contagiosum is often recalcitrant to treatment and causes significant morbidity and disfigurement.

Pathogenesis. Although it is difficult to produce lesions after experimental inoculation, molluscum contagiosum is certainly contagious. Intimate physical contact such as occurs in Turkish baths, wrestling, and sexual intercourse has resulted in transmission of the disease.

The molluscum contagiosum virus replicates in the cytoplasm of the keratinocyte, with resulting large intracytoplasmic inclusion bodies (molluscum bodies) and proliferation of the epidermis. The center of the papule ultimately disintegrates, forming a crater and releasing molluscum bodies.

Spontaneous involution results from a host immune response that is presumed to be cell mediated. The stimulus that provokes this response after many months of inactivity is unknown, as with warts.

THERAPY OF MOLLUSCUM CONTAGIOSUM

- Cryotherapy with liquid nitrogen
- Salicylic acid
- Cantharidin
- Curettage

■ ACTINIC KERATOSIS

Definition. Actinic (solar) keratosis is a precancerous neoplasm of the epidermis caused by the ultraviolet portion of sunlight. A nonrecommended synonym is senile keratosis. The abnormal keratinocytes in actinic keratoses are confined to the epidermis and constitute a premalignant change. The proliferation of these abnormal cells is clinically manifest as a rough, scaling patch or papule (Fig. 6–8).

Incidence. The incidence of actinic keratoses varies with (1) skin pigmentation, (2) geographic location, and (3) amount of sun exposure. Thus, the incidence of actinic keratoses is high in Caucasians who have light skin, in the southern United States where there is an abundance of natural sunlight, and in those who engage in frequent outdoor activity. In our clinic, 1.7% of new patients were seen because of actinic keratoses, but the incidence would be higher in the "Sunbelt." Moreover, in many patients, actinic keratoses are an incidental finding.

Light skin and abundant sun exposure may result in actinic keratoses.

History. Risk factors can usually be elicited in the history. The patient may have a genetic predisposition. Fair-skinned Caucasians have the least amount of protective pigment. A family history of skin cancer or an Irish or Anglo-Saxon heritage is frequently obtained. Second, the geographic location where the patient has lived directly influences the amount of ultraviolet light exposure. As one moves

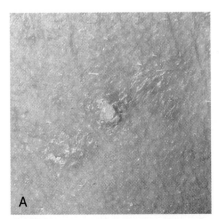
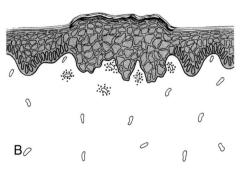

FIGURE 6–8. Actinic keratosis. **A,** Epidermis—scaling, ill-marginated patch or papule. Dermis—erythema. **B,** Epidermis—atypical keratinocytes in lower epidermis. Dermis—chronic inflammation.

toward the equator, the ultraviolet light intensity increases dramatically. Last, the occupational and recreational activities of the patient with reference to sun exposure provide another clue. Farmers, sailors, and others with occupations that require working outdoors have a high amount of ultraviolet light exposure. Similarly, persons who spend many hours at the poolside or on the beach are at higher risk.

An actinic keratosis is rough, scaling, and ill marginated; it is often easier felt than seen.

Physical Examination. Actinic keratoses are 1- to 10-mm, reddish, ill-marginated patches and papules that have a rough, yellowish brown, adherent scale. Their ill-defined margins make them indistinct to the casual observer. Their rough-textured surface is often easier to feel than to see. They occur in sun-exposed areas: the face, dorsum of the hands and forearms, neck, and upper back and chest. They generally are found on ultraviolet-damaged skin that has a yellowish hue, wrinkles, and freckled pigmentation.

Differential Diagnosis. An actinic keratosis must be differentiated from other epidermal tumors. Most often, it is confused with a *seborrheic keratosis*. The well-demarcated, "pasted-on" appearance of a seborrheic keratosis differentiates it from an actinic keratosis. *Bowen's disease* (in situ squamous cell carcinoma) is a larger plaque with margins that are well defined, in contrast to the margins of an actinic keratosis. Hypertrophic or indurated actinic keratosis (Fig. 6–9) cannot be differentiated with certainty from *squamous cell carcinoma* and should undergo biopsy. *Superficial basal cell carcinoma*, which resembles Bowen's disease clinically, is occasionally confused with actinic keratosis.

Indurated actinic keratoses should undergo biopsy to rule out carcinoma.

Laboratory and Biopsy. Actinic keratosis is characterized histologically by a partial-thickness dysplasia of the epidermis. One sees hyperkeratosis with underlying irregular hyperplasia of mildly dysplastic keratinocytes. A chronic inflammatory response is present in the dermis. All thick and indurated actinic keratoses should undergo biopsy to rule out squamous cell carcinoma.

Use sunscreens to prevent more actinic damage.

Therapy. Prevention by reducing sunlight exposure is the most effective form of therapy. Patients who are sensitive to the sun or have developed actinic keratoses should wear protective clothing such as broad-brimmed hats and long-sleeved shirts when outside. Sunscreens with a sun protective factor (SPF) of 15 to 30 should be used on exposed skin. The regular use of sunscreens prevents the development of new actinic keratoses as well as hastens the resolutions of those that already exist. Avoiding sun exposure during midday (10:00 a.m. to 2:00 p.m.), when ultraviolet radiant energy is most intense, is recommended. Patient awareness and education should begin in childhood.

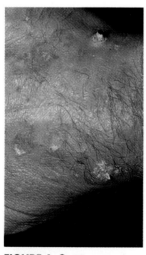

FIGURE 6–9. Hypertrophic actinic keratosis.

THERAPY OF ACTINIC KERATOSIS

- Sun protection
    Sunscreen SPF 15–30
    Hat and long-sleeved shirt
    Avoidance of intense midday sun (10:00 a.m.–2:00 p.m.)
- Cryotherapy with liquid nitrogen
- 5-Fluorouracil 5% cream bid $\times$ 2–3 weeks

Topical chemotherapy with 5-fluorouracil (Efudex cream 5%) is the most common means of treating multiple actinic keratoses. 5-Fluorouracil inhibits DNA synthesis by blocking the enzyme thymidylate synthase. When 5-fluorouracil is applied to normal skin, little reaction occurs, but when it is applied to sun-damaged skin, those areas with actinic keratoses become inflamed. The medication is applied to the involved areas twice daily. Erythema develops within several days. Subsequently, within 2 to 4 weeks, the actinic keratoses become painful, crusted, and eroded, at which time the medication is stopped. Patients need to be warned about the discomfort and cosmetically unsightly effects of 5-fluorouracil, which are temporary and resolve after discontinuing treatment. Because of the marked amount of inflammation that can occur, small regions may be treated at a time in patients with extensive actinic keratoses. A few patients become allergic to 5-fluorouracil. Patients with severe actinic damage can be expected to require treatment every 1 to 2 years.

Cryosurgery with liquid nitrogen is an alternative therapy, most useful when only a few lesions are present. Thick, hypertrophic actinic keratoses are also better treated in this manner. Freezing can be accomplished in a manner similar to that described for warts. Avoid overzealous treatment of thin actinic keratoses because of possible scarring.

Course and Complications. In patients with chronically sun-damaged skin, the acquisition of more actinic keratoses can be expected. Some actinic keratoses spontaneously disappear (up to 26%), although others may develop into squamous cell carcinoma. The number that do develop into squamous cell carcinoma appears to be small, less than 1 in 1,000 within 1 year. Metastases from squamous cell carcinomas arising in actinic keratoses are uncommon.

Pathogenesis. Actinic keratoses are produced by ultraviolet radiation-induced damage to keratinocyte DNA. This results in unrepaired or error-prone repaired DNA. Abnormal replication occurs that causes abnormal epidermal cellular hyperplasia. The cells within an actinic keratosis are arranged in a disorderly way and have increased mitoses and an abnormal chromatin pattern. Other precancerous keratinocytic neoplasms similar to actinic keratoses are caused by artificial ultraviolet light, x-irradiation, or polycyclic aromatic hydrocarbons.

Actinic keratosis has the potential of developing into a squamous cell carcinoma.

■ SQUAMOUS CELL CARCINOMA

Definition. Squamous cell carcinoma is a malignant neoplasm of keratinocytes. It is locally invasive and has the potential to metastasize. It appears clinically as a scaling, indurated plaque or nodule that sometimes bleeds or ulcerates (Fig. 6–10). The etiology of squamous cell carcinoma includes ultraviolet radiation, x-irradiation, and chemical carcinogens such as soot and arsenic.

Incidence. Squamous cell carcinoma is the second most common skin cancer, with nearly 200,000 new cases diagnosed each year in the United States. The incidence of squamous cell carcinoma varies greatly with reference to ethnic group, geographic location, and occupation. It is most common in men more than 60 years old who have light skin and abundant sunlight exposure. Closer to the equator, the incidence increases. The incidence of squamous cell carcinoma is 5 times greater in New Orleans than in Chicago. In Tucson, Arizona, the incidence is 100 per 100,000. The incidence rate of squamous cell carcinoma has risen threefold from the 1960s to the 1980s. In renal transplant patients, squamous cell carcinoma is 3.5 times more frequent than basal cell carcinoma and greater than 250 times

Squamous cell carcinoma is the second most common skin cancer.

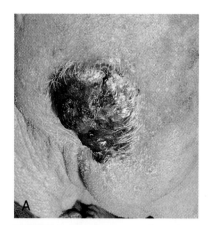 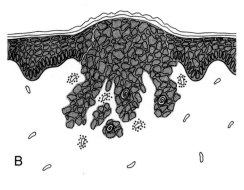

FIGURE 6–10. Squamous cell carcinoma. **A,** Epidermis—scaling, crusted nodule. Dermis—erythema, induration. **B,** Epidermis—hyperkeratosis, atypical keratinocytes. Dermis—invasive tumor, inflammation.

more frequent than in the general population. Nine years after renal transplantation, patients have a more than 40% incidence of squamous cell carcinoma.

History. The patient's history of sunlight exposure in occupational and recreational activities is important in determining the risk of developing squamous cell carcinoma. A family history of skin cancer and a personal history of fair skin and sunburning are additional predisposing factors. The history of a chronic, nonhealing, bleeding growth or ulcer should arouse suspicion of squamous cell carcinoma.

Most squamous cell carcinomas occur on the head, neck, and arms.

Physical Examination. Squamous cell carcinoma occurs most often in sun-exposed skin. It also develops on the mucous membranes and in sites of chronic injury such as burn scars, irradiated sites, erosive discoid lupus erythematosus, and osteomyelitis sinuses. The occurrence of squamous cell carcinoma varies with anatomic location: head and neck, 81%; upper extremities, 16%; trunk, 1.5%; and legs, 1.3%. The tumor nodule is hard, is erythematous to flesh colored, and has a smooth or verrucous surface. The central portion may be hyperkeratotic, ulcerated, or crusted. Deep invasion results in fixation to underlying tissue. Squamous cell carcinoma of the lip involves the lower lip in 90% of cases and usually arises from a chronically damaged epithelium secondary to actinic exposure or smoking.

Chronic ulcers should undergo biopsy to exclude malignancy.

Differential Diagnosis. Squamous cell carcinoma can be differentiated clinically or by biopsy from a *keratoacanthoma, hypertrophic actinic keratosis, wart, basal cell carcinoma,* and *seborrheic keratosis.* All persistent ulcers or crusted lesions must undergo biopsy to rule out squamous cell carcinoma.

Bowen's disease (Fig. 6–11) is squamous cell carcinoma in situ of the skin. It appears as an erythematous, scaling, crusted, well-marginated patch. Squamous cell carcinoma in situ of the glans penis is referred to as erythroplasia of Queyrat and appears as a red, velvety, moist patch.

Keratoacanthoma is a rapidly growing neoplasm of the epithelium that is biologically benign but histologically resembles a squamous cell carcinoma (Fig. 6–12). Keratoacanthoma is a round, flesh-colored nodule that characteristically grows rapidly (within 4 to 6 weeks) and has a central keratin-filled crater. Most keratoacanthomas spontaneously involute within 6 months. However, because some may be difficult to differentiate from squamous cell carcinoma, excision or other destructive treatment is recommended.

Laboratory and Biopsy. Any lesion suspected of being squamous cell carcinoma should undergo biopsy. Squamous cell carcinoma consists of malignant epidermal cells that invade the dermis. It is graded according to the degree of atypicality of the tumor cells, with grade 1 predominantly mature, whereas grades 2, 3, and 4 are less well differentiated. Grade 4 tumors may be difficult to differentiate from malignant melanoma because their spindle-shape cells lack intercellular bridges.

The biopsy of squamous cell carcinoma in situ *(Bowen's disease)* reveals a thickened epidermis consisting of atypical, poorly oriented, dysplastic cells that lie completely within the epidermis. *Keratoacanthoma* has a large, central keratin-filled crater surrounded by well-differentiated epidermal cells that sometimes appear dysplastic, thus making it difficult to distinguish from a squamous cell carcinoma.

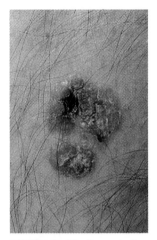

FIGURE 6–11. Bowen's disease (squamous cell carcinoma in situ).

Therapy. Excision is the treatment of choice, although a well-differentiated small squamous cell carcinoma occurring in actinically damaged skin may be effectively treated with curettage and electrodesiccation. These surgical techniques are reviewed in Chapter 5. Large and recurrent poorly differentiated tumors, as well as those occurring on the mucous membrane and in scars, should be treated by scalpel excision with narrow margins (3 to 5 mm) that are checked histologically to be free of tumor or by the Mohs' technique. Nonsurgical therapy such as ionizing radiation is useful in selected patients. Sun protective measures such as the use of sunscreens, protective clothing, and avoiding midday ultraviolet light exposure are important for prevention of future squamous cell carcinomas.

Course and Complications. The course of squamous cell carcinoma is variable. Those carcinomas most likely to metastasize are relatively large and poorly differentiated and invade more deeply and occur in damaged skin or on mucous membranes. Two percent of all squamous cell carcinomas of the skin metastasize. Those that arise in actinic keratoses are less aggressive, with a metastasis rate of 0.5%. Much higher rates of metastasis, up to 9.0%, occur in squamous cell carcinoma arising in chronic leg ulcers, burn scars, radiodermatitis, osteomyelitis sinuses, and the mucous membrane of the lips, glans penis, and vulva. When metastasis occurs, it is usually through the lymphatics to the regional lymph nodes. Prophylactic lymph node dissection is not done unless the patient has lymphadenopathy.

Squamous cell carcinoma arising in actinic keratosis has a low metastatic potential.

Pathogenesis. Sir Percivall Pott in 1775 was the first to describe occupationally induced cancer and to relate cancer to an etiologic agent. He described the occurrence of squamous cell carcinoma of the scrotum in chimney sweeps and suggested that its cause was chronic soot exposure. In 1809, Lambe related squamous cell carcinoma to arsenic in drinking water. The relationship between ultraviolet

---

THERAPY OF SQUAMOUS CELL CARCINOMA

- Excision
- Curettage and electrodesiccation
- Mohs' micrographic surgery
- Radiation

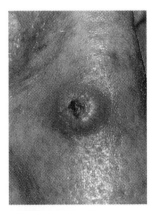

FIGURE 6–12. Keratoacanthoma.

radiation and squamous cell carcinoma was suggested in 1875 by Thiersch. Frieben in 1902 described the occurrence of squamous cell carcinoma after exposure to x-rays.

Experimentally, Yamagiwa and Ichikawa in 1915 were the first to produce squamous cell carcinoma in mice and rabbits after the topical application of coal tar. Several years later, in 1924, Block induced squamous cell carcinoma in rabbits after x-irradiation. Using mice repeatedly exposed to ultraviolet radiation, Findley in 1928 was the first to produce ultraviolet radiation-induced carcinoma.

All these carcinogens—ultraviolet radiation, x-irradiation, coal tar, and arsenic—are active in the skin, initiating malignancy by altering cellular DNA, RNA, and proteins. In addition, ultraviolet radiation also alters the immune system, making the host more susceptible to these tumors. Chronic immunosuppression, as occurs in organ transplant patients, is also associated with increased frequency of squamous cell carcinoma, especially in sun-damaged skin.

■ BASAL CELL CARCINOMA

Definition. Basal cell carcinoma is a malignant neoplasm arising from the basal cells of the epidermis (Fig. 6–13). Although these cancers rarely metastasize, their potential for local destruction attests to their malignant nature. Ultraviolet radiation is the cause of most basal cell carcinomas in humans. Four clinically and histopathologically distinct types of basal cell carcinoma are recognized: nodular, pigmented, superficial, and scarring (sclerotic).

Basal cell carcinoma is the most common skin cancer. These lesions rarely metastasize.

Incidence. Basal cell carcinoma is the most common human malignant disease; it affects more than 800,000 persons annually in the United States. In Queensland, Australia, 4.6% of adults aged 20 to 69 years had skin cancer, mostly basal cell carcinoma. In Tucson, Arizona, the annual incidence is 315 per 100,000 population. Two percent of the new patients in our clinic are seen for basal cell carcinoma. The increased frequency in adult Caucasians is related to sun exposure.

History. The patient with basal cell carcinoma seeks medical attention because of a new growth, especially if it is a nonhealing, easily bleeding lesion. There may be a personal or family history of skin cancer. The risk of basal cell carcinoma is higher in patients with light skin, in those who live in southern latitudes, and in

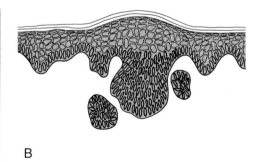

FIGURE 6–13. Nodular basal cell carcinoma. **A,** Epidermis—pearly papule. Dermis—induration. **B,** Epidermis—thickened. Dermis—invasive buds and lobules of basaloid cells.

those who work or play outdoors. Frequently, these patients have a history of sunburning easily and tanning poorly.

Physical Examination. The usual patient with basal cell carcinoma has fair skin, blue eyes, blonde or red hair, and actinic-damaged skin manifested by freckles, yellow wrinkling, and actinic keratoses. Basal cell carcinoma occurs in sun-exposed skin, particularly the head and neck.

The *nodular type* (see Fig. 6–13) of basal cell carcinoma is the most common. It is a "pearly," semitranslucent papule or nodule that often has a central depression or crater, telangiectasia, and a rolled, waxy border. When ulceration and crusting occur, the lesion is referred to as a *rodent ulcer*. Nodular basal cell carcinoma occurs most frequently on the face, especially the nose.

Pigmented basal cell carcinoma (Fig. 6–14) is a shiny, blue-black papule, nodule, or plaque. The pigment is often speckled, and a pearly, rolled margin can be seen if the tumor is viewed from the side.

Superficial basal cell carcinoma (Fig. 6–15) occurs most frequently on the thorax. It is a red, slightly scaling, well-demarcated eczematous appearing patch. Centrally, it may become slightly eroded and crusted, subsequently leaving an atrophic, slightly depressed center. Its shape is oval to round, with a characteristic thread-like, pearly, rolled border. It is often referred to as multicentric superficial basal cell carcinoma because it skips islands of normal skin, similar to the way a forest fire may surround a stand of trees yet leave it unburned.

The *scarring (sclerotic or morpheaform) basal cell carcinoma* is an atrophic, white, slightly eroded or crusted plaque that often looks like a scar. It is frequently depressed and is the least common and most aggressive type of basal cell carcinoma.

Differential Diagnosis. Nodular basal cell carcinoma and *sebaceous hyperplasia* are sometimes difficult to differentiate clinically. Sebaceous hyperplasia is the proliferation of sebaceous glands surrounding a hair follicle that appears as a 1- to 3-mm, yellowish papule with overlying telangiectasia and a central pore. The yellowish coloration and central pore help to differentiate it from a basal cell carcinoma. Other epithelial growths that resemble a nodular basal cell carcinoma include a *nonpigmented nevus, molluscum contagiosum,* and *squamous cell carcinoma.*

Pigmented basal cell carcinoma can be confused with a *seborrheic keratosis, pigmented nevus,* and, most important, *malignant melanoma.* The pearly, rolled border of pigmented basal cell carcinoma helps to differentiate it from a malignant melanoma. If doubt exists, an excisional biopsy should be performed.

Superficial basal cell carcinoma resembles a patch of *dermatitis.* It can be confused with *psoriasis, nummular dermatitis,* and *Bowen's disease.* A persistent solitary lesion and lack of response to topical steroids clinically differentiate superficial basal cell carcinoma from dermatitis or psoriasis. A skin biopsy is the only way to differentiate it from Bowen's disease.

Any *nonhealing scar-like lesions* should undergo biopsy to rule out a scarring basal cell carcinoma or a *squamous cell carcinoma.*

Laboratory and Biopsy. The diagnosis of basal cell carcinoma should be confirmed by either shave biopsy or punch biopsy. The technique of skin biopsy is reviewed in Chapter 4. The tumors are made up of uniform cells that resemble the basal layers of the epidermis. They have a uniform large, oval, blue nucleus with indistinct cytoplasm. The tumor extends from the epidermis into the dermis as nodular or cystic structures, bands, or strands or as buds from the epidermis. The nodular areas have peripheral palisading with retraction from the surrounding stroma.

"Pearly" appearance is the most characteristic feature of a basal cell carcinoma.

Types of basal cell carcinoma:
1. **Nodular**
2. **Pigmented**
3. **Superficial**
4. **Scarring (sclerotic)**

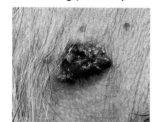

FIGURE 6–14. Pigmented basal cell carcinoma.

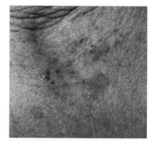

FIGURE 6–15. Superficial basal cell carcinoma.

Nonhealing scars should undergo biopsy to exclude carcinoma.

The cells in some basal cell carcinomas have a "squamoid" appearance, which makes them difficult to differentiate from squamous cell carcinoma. The infiltrative, morpheaform, micronodular, and mixed histologic subtypes of primary basal cell carcinoma are more aggressive and are more difficult to eradicate.

Therapy. Treatment of basal cell carcinoma should be individualized according to the location of the lesion, the histopathologic type, the age of the patient, the general health of the patient, the size of the basal cell carcinoma, and whether it is primary or recurrent. Recurrence of basal cell carcinoma is particularly related to location on the nose or ear, size greater than 2 cm, and histologic pattern of micronodular, infiltrative, and morpheic types. Treatment modalities include scalpel excision, curettage and electrodesiccation, radiotherapy, cryotherapy, and topical 5-fluorouracil. When *properly* selected, each modality has a cure rate of greater than 90%. Surgical modalities are those most frequently used, and their techniques are reviewed in Chapter 5.

Excision with primary suture closure is the most frequently used form of therapy and allows for histologic assessment of surgical margins. When the wound is large, grafts or tissue transposition flaps may be used to achieve closure. Excision is good for most basal cell carcinomas, but it is the treatment of choice for large basal cell carcinomas, recurrent tumors, sclerosing types of basal cell carcinoma, basal cell carcinomas in high-recurrence areas such as the nose or ear, and basal cell carcinoma that extends into the subcutaneous tissue. A specialized form of excision using detailed mapping of the extent of the tumor with histologic orientation is the *Mohs' micrographic surgical technique.* This meticulous procedure is most often used for recurrent basal cell carcinoma and primary tumors with a high risk of recurrence.

Curettage and electrodesiccation is a therapeutic modality frequently used by dermatologists. The clinical margins of the tumor are defined by vigorous curettage until the firm, fibrous consistency of normal dermis is felt. This is followed by electrodesiccation. The entire procedure of curettage and electrodesiccation is repeated twice more. The resultant wound heals by secondary intention over a 2- to 3-week period, with excellent cosmetic results in most cases. Experience is needed to obtain good cure rates. Curettage and electrodesiccation should not be used for basal cell carcinomas greater than 2 cm wide, for tumors with poorly defined clinical borders, for sclerosing basal cell carcinomas, for recurrent basal cell carcinomas, or in certain anatomic locations such as the nasolabial fold, scalp, and eyelids.

Radiation therapy is reserved for elderly patients because the subsequent chronic radiodermatitis that occurs years after the therapy may be cosmetically

---

THERAPY OF BASAL CELL CARCINOMA

- Excision
- Curettage and electrodesiccation
- Mohs' micrographic surgery
- Radiation
- Cryotherapy
- 5-Fluorouracil topically for multiple superficial basal cell carcinomas

unacceptable and because of the potential for developing a new primary cancer in the radiotherapy site. Radiation therapy is used when the patient refuses surgical treatment or has a large tumor that would be difficult to treat surgically.

Cryosurgery with liquid nitrogen is reserved for those clinicians experienced in its use for cancer therapy. The margins and depth of the tumor must be estimated clinically. Cryoprobes are used to monitor the depth of the freeze. After surgery, marked tissue reaction occurs with edema, tissue necrosis, weeping, and crusting.

Topical chemotherapy with *5-fluorouracil* is, in general, inappropriate for treating skin cancer. It should not be used on deep or recurrent tumors. It is occasionally used in patients who have multiple superficial, multicentric basal cell carcinomas that otherwise would require numerous surgical procedures. Treatment is continued for weeks until marked inflammation and erosion occur. Residual areas suspected to have tumor must undergo biopsy, and another therapeutic modality must be used if basal cell carcinoma persists.

Prevention of further sun-induced damage to the skin is mandatory. Sun protection includes the regular use of sunscreens with an SPF of 15 to 30, protective clothing (hat and long-sleeved shirt), and avoidance of midday sun (10 a.m.– 2 p.m.)

Course and Complications. Because its course is frequently indolent, a basal cell carcinoma is often ignored. It may enlarge locally and can invade underlying tissues, resulting in significant morbidity and mutilation. Vital structures such as an eye, a nose, or an ear may be totally lost.

Basal cell cancer rarely metastasizes, presumably because of stromal dependence. The metastatic rate is estimated to be less than 0.003% (1 in 52,000 cases in one series). The excessively large, ulcerated, locally destructive, and recurrent basal cell carcinoma is most likely to metastasize. Regional lymph nodes, lung, and bone are the most likely tissues involved. Routine follow-up every 12 months of patients with basal cell carcinomas is recommended because 35% of these patients will develop another basal cell carcinoma within 5 years.

Pathogenesis. The most common factor related to the development of basal cell carcinoma is ultraviolet radiation. Other factors to be considered are arsenic ingestion, genetic predisposition, x-irradiation, and chronic irritation. The origin of basal cell carcinoma is a pluripotential primordial epithelial cell in the basal layer of the skin or, less often, a cutaneous appendage such as the hair follicle.

■ UNKNOWN (Fig. 6–16)

This 55-year-old Caucasian man was seen in the dermatology clinic because of a nodule on his nose. It had been present for the past year and was growing slowly. His occupation was farming. He had a history of tanning poorly and numerous sunburns. His past medical and dermatologic history was otherwise negative.

What is your differential diagnosis?

This pearly nodule with telangiectasia and a central depression is characteristic of a nodular basal cell carcinoma. The surrounding skin is thickened and furrowed and has a yellowish hue typical of sun damage. Also to be considered in the

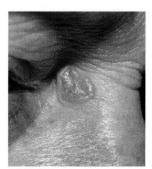

FIGURE 6–16. Unknown.

differential diagnosis is a squamous cell carcinoma. The lesion's relatively recent onset rules out a flesh-colored nevus, and its size makes sebaceous hyperplasia unlikely.

How would you treat it?

Excisional surgery was chosen to remove this tumor, because it was thick and could have invaded the subcutaneous tissue. Histology confirmed the clinical diagnosis of basal cell carcinoma.

What precautions should the patient take in the future?

This patient should prevent further sun damage to the skin. He should wear protective clothing, including a broad-brimmed hat and a long-sleeved shirt, when working outside. In addition, he should use a sunscreen with an SPF of 15 or greater. He should be seen again in the clinic for periodic examinations because his chances of developing skin cancer in the future are high.

Important Points

1. The recent acquisition of a pearly nodule may indicate a skin cancer.
2. Basal cell carcinoma is treatable and rarely metastasizes.
3. Precautions should be taught to prevent excessive ultraviolet radiation exposure, because this is the most common etiologic agent of basal cell carcinoma.

REFERENCES

Wart

Androphy EJ: Human papillomavirus. Arch Dermatol 125:683–685, 1989.
Beutner KB: Human papillomavirus infection. J Am Acad Dermatol 20:114–123, 1989.
Beutner KB, Spruance SL, Hougham AJ, et al.: Treatment of genital warts with an immune-response modifier (imiquimod). J Am Acad Dermatol 38:230–239, 1998.
Chuang TY: Condylomata acuminata (genital warts): an epidemiologic view. J Am Acad Dermatol 16:376–384, 1987.
Cobb MW: Human papillomavirus infection. J Am Acad Dermatol 22:547–566, 1990.
Ho GYF, Bierman R, Beardsley L, et al.: Natural history of cervicovaginal papillomavirus infection in young women. N Engl J Med 338:423–428, 1998.
Lee AN, Mallory SB: Contact immunotherapy with squaric acid dibutylester for the treatment of recalcitrant warts. J Am Acad Dermatol 41:595–599, 1999.
Lowy DR, Ju WD: Pathophysiology of cutaneous viral infections: papillomaviruses. In Soter NA, Baden HP (eds.): Pathophysiology of Dermatologic Diseases. 2nd ed. New York, McGraw-Hill, 1991, pp. 441–452.
Majewski S, Jablonska S: Human papillomavirus-associated tumors of the skin and mucosa. J Am Acad Dermatol 36:659–680, 1997.
Quan MB, Moy BL: The role of human papillomavirus in carcinoma. J Am Acad Dermatol 25:698–705, 1991.

Corn

Yale I: Podiatric Medicine. Baltimore, Williams & Wilkins, 1974, pp. 94–130.

Seborrheic Keratosis

Eads TJ, Hood AF, Chuang TY, et al.: The diagnostic yield of histologic examination of seborrheic keratoses. Arch Dermatol *133*:1417–1420, 1997.

Holdiness MR: On the classification of the sign of Leser-Trélat. J Am Acad Dermatol *19*: 754–757, 1988.

Stern BS, Boudreaux C, Arndt KA: Diagnostic accuracy and appropriateness of care for seborrheic keratoses. JAMA *265*:74–77, 1991.

Skin Tag

Banik R, Lubach D: Skin tags: Localization and frequencies according to sex and age. Dermatologica *174*:180–183, 1987.

Eads TJ, Chuang TY, Fabre VC, et al.: The utility of submitting fibroepithelial polyps for histological examination. Arch Dermatol *132*:1459–1462, 1996.

Gould BE, Ellison C, Greene HL, Bernhard JD: Lack of association between skin tags and colon polyps in a primary care setting. Arch Intern Med *148*:1799–1800, 1988.

Molluscum Contagiosum

Felnan YM: Molluscum contagiosum. Cutis *33*:113–117, 1984.

Goodman DS, Teplitz ED, Wishher A, et al.: Prevalence of cutaneous disease in patients with acquired immunodeficiency syndrome (AIDS) or AIDS-related complex. J Am Acad Dermatol *17*:210–220, 1987.

Lynch PJ, Minkin W: Molluscum contagiosum of the adult. Arch Dermatol *98*:141–143, 1968.

Myskowski PL: Molluscum contagiosum: new insights, new directions. Arch Dermatol *133*: 1039–1041, 1997.

Postlethwaite B: Molluscum contagiosum: a review. Arch Environ Health *21*:432–452, 1970.

Actinic Keratosis

Callen JP, Bickers DR, Moy RL: Actinic keratoses. J Am Acad Dermatol *36*:650–653, 1997.

Drake LA, Ceilley RI, Cornelison RL, et al.: Guidelines of care for actinic keratoses. J Am Acad Dermatol *32*:95–98, 1995.

Marks R: The role of treatment of actinic keratoses in the prevention of morbidity and mortality due to squamous cell carcinoma. Arch Dermatol *127*:1031–1033, 1991.

Naylor MF, Boyd A, Smith DW, et al.: High sun protection factor sunscreens in the suppression of actinic neoplasia. Arch Dermatol *131*:170–175, 1995.

Schwartz RA: Premalignant keratinocytic neoplasms. J Am Acad Dermatol *35*:223–242, 1996.

Thompson SC, Jolley D, Marks R: Reduction of solar keratoses by regular sunscreen use. N Engl J Med *329*:1147–1151, 1993.

Squamous Cell Carcinoma

Bernstein SC, Lim KK, Brodland DG, et al.: The many faces of squamous cell carcinoma. Dermatol Surg *22*:243–254, 1996.

Chaung T-Y, Popesen NA, Su W-PD, Chute CG: Squamous cell carcinoma. Arch Dermatol *126*:185–188, 1990.

Dinehart SM, Pollack SV: Metastases from squamous cell carcinoma of the skin and lip. J Am Acad Dermatol *21*:241–248, 1989.

Dinehart SM, Nelson-Adesokan P, Cockerell C, et al.: Metastatic cutaneous squamous cell carcinoma derived from actinic keratosis. Cancer *79*:920–923, 1997.

Drake LA, Ceilley RI, Cornelison BL, et al.: American Academy of Dermatology guidelines of care for cutaneous squamous cell carcinoma. Am Acad Dermatol Bull *9*:6–9, 1991.

Glass AG, Hoover RN: The emerging epidemic of melanoma and squamous cell skin cancer. JAMA *262*:2097–2100, 1989.

Johnson TM, Rowe DE, Nelson BR, Swanson NA: Squamous cell carcinoma of the skin (excluding lip and oral mucosa). J Am Acad Dermatol *26*:467–484, 1992.

Kwa BE, Campaua K, Moy BL: Biology of cutaneous squamous cell carcinoma. J Am Acad Dermatol *26*:1–26, 1992.

Weinstock MA, Bogaars HA, Ashley M, et al.: Nonmelanoma skin cancer mortality: a population-based study. Arch Dermatol *127*:1194–1197, 1991.

Basal Cell Carcinoma

Drake LA, Ceilley RI, Cornelison RL, et al.: American Academy of Dermatology: guidelines of care for basal cell carcinoma. J Am Acad Dermatol *26:*117–120, 1992.

Federman DG, Concato J, Caralis PV, et al.: Screening for skin cancer in primary care settings. Arch Dermatol *133:*1423–1425, 1997.

Goldsmith LA, Koh HK, Bewerse BA, et al.: Full proceedings from the national conference to develop a national skin cancer agenda. J Am Acad Dermatol *35:*748–756, 1996.

Green A, Beardmore G, Hart V, et al.: Skin cancer in a Queensland population. J Am Acad Dermatol *19:*1045–1052, 1988.

Miller SJ: Biology of basal cell carcinoma. J Am Acad Dermatol (part I) *24:*1–13, 1991; (part II) *24:*161–175, 1991.

Orengo IF, Salasche SJ, Fewkes J, et al.: Correlation of histologic subtypes of primary basal cell carcinoma and number of Mohs stages required to achieve a tumor-free plane. J Am Acad Dermatol *37:*395–397, 1997.

Pollack SV, Goslen JB, Sherertz EF: The biology of basal cell carcinoma: a review. J Am Acad Dermatol *7:*569–577, 1982.

Robinson JK: Risk of developing another basal cell carcinoma: a 5-year prospective study. Cancer *60:*118–120, 1987.

Robinson JK: What are adequate treatment and follow-up for nonmelanoma cutaneous cancer? Arch Dermatol *123:*331–333, 1987.

Sexton M, Jones DB, Maloney ME: Histologic pattern analysis of basal cell carcinoma: study of a series of 1039 consecutive neoplasms. J Am Acad Dermatol *23:*1118–1126, 1990.

Thissen MRTM, Neuman MHA, Schouten LJ: A systemic review of treatment modalities for primary basal cell carcinomas. Arch Dermatol *135:*1177–1183.

Wallberg P, Kaaman T, Lindberg M: Multiple basal cell carcinoma. Acta Derm Venereol *78:*127–129, 1998.

PIGMENTED GROWTHS

FRECKLE
LENTIGO
MELASMA
NEVUS
MALIGNANT MELANOMA

T he skin has one pigment-forming cell—the melanocyte. Melanocytes are dendritic cells found in the basal layer of the epidermis. Nevus cells, a type of melanocyte, are found in the basal layer of the epidermis as well as in the dermis, are arranged in nests, and do not have dendritic processes. Melanocytes contain tyrosinase, the enzyme necessary for pigment (melanin) synthesis, and are thought to be derived from a progenitor cell in the neural crest.

Pigmented growths (Table 7–1) are a result of an increased number of melanocytes, nevus cells, or pigment deposition. Although malignant melanoma is uncommon, diagnosis of this malignant lesion is important because it can be recognized early, when it is curable.

■ FRECKLE

Definition. A freckle (ephelis) is a hyperpigmented macule found in sun-exposed areas of skin (Fig. 7–1). The amount of melanin in the basal area of the epidermis is increased without an increase in the number of melanocytes.

Incidence. Freckles are a common incidental finding during a skin examination and are rarely a reason, in and of themselves, for seeking medical attention.

History. Freckles usually appear before 3 years of age and darken after ultraviolet light exposure. The patient has a history of sunburning easily.

Sunlight darkens freckles.

Physical Examination. The freckled individual typically has a fair complexion and reddish or sandy hair. Hundreds of freckles occur on sun-exposed skin. They are 1- to 6-mm, irregularly shaped, discrete brown macules.

Freckles occur only in sun-exposed areas.

Differential Diagnosis. Lentigo and *junctional nevus* can look like a freckle. *Actinic lentigo* does not darken with sun exposure and is acquired later in life. In contrast, freckles darken after sun exposure and are present from early childhood. *Lentigo simplex* is acquired in childhood, but the lentigines are not confined to sun-exposed

91

TABLE 7-1 ▪ PIGMENTED GROWTHS

	Frequency*	History	Physical Examination	Differential Diagnosis	Laboratory (Biopsy)
Freckle	—	Appear before 3 years	Tan macule, sun-exposed skin	Junctional nevus Lentigo Seborrheic keratosis	No
Lentigo	0.2	Acquired any age	Brown macule	Junctional nevus Freckle Seborrheic keratosis	If uneven color
Melasma	0.2	Adults	Brown macules on face	Postinflammatory hyperpigmentation Freckle	No
Nevus	2.8	Not acquired past third decade	Flesh- or brown-colored macule or papule, smooth or verrucous surface	Melanoma Seborrheic keratosis Skin tag Neurofibroma Dermatofibroma Basal cell carcinoma Lentigo Freckle	If change
Melanoma	0.3	Recent acquisition Itches Bleeds Growing			Excision
Superficial spreading			Irregular surface, border, color	Nevus Seborrheic keratosis Hemangioma Pigmented basal cell carcinoma	
Lentigo maligna			Irregular surface, border, color	Actinic lentigo Seborrheic keratosis	
Acral lentiginous melanoma			Irregular surface, border, color	Nevus Tinea nigra palmaris	
Nodular			Blue-black nodule	Blue nevus Pyogenic granuloma Angioma Dermatofibroma	

* Percentage of new dermatology patients with this diagnosis seen in the Hershey Medical Center Dermatology Clinic, Hershey, PA.

skin. *Junctional nevi* and freckles are acquired in childhood. Darker pigmentation and lack of change after sunlight exposure favor a diagnosis of junctional nevus.

Laboratory and Biopsy. Ordinarily, freckles do not undergo biopsy.

Freckles are better admired than treated.

Therapy. Freckles should be accepted as normal. Prevention by sunlight avoidance is effective but not practical.

Pathogenesis. Ultraviolet radiation induces an increase in melanin pigment in the basal layer of the epidermis without an increase in melanocytes.

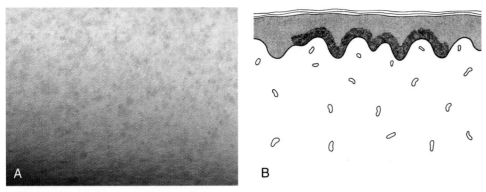

FIGURE 7–1. Freckles. **A,** Epidermis—brown macule. **B,** Epidermis—melanin pigmentation in basal layer.

■ LENTIGO

Definition. A lentigo (plural, lentigines) is a hyperpigmented brown macule caused by an increased number of melanocytes. Two types are recognized: lentigo simplex lesions arise in childhood and are few in number, whereas actinic (solar) lentigines (Fig. 7–2) arise in middle age and are numerous in sun-exposed skin.

Incidence. Lentigo simplex is uncommon. Actinic lentigines are found on more than 90% of Caucasians after the age of 70 years, but they seldom cause a patient to seek medical advice.

History. Lentigo simplex may be congenital or may arise in childhood. It has no relation to sun exposure. Conversely, actinic lentigo is acquired in middle age, does not fade, and occurs in sun-exposed skin. Patients often call actinic lentigo "liver spots."

Physical Examination. Lentigo is a uniform, brown or brown-black macule. Lentigo simplex is sharply marginated and occurs anywhere on the body and mucosae. These lesions are usually few in number.

Actinic or solar lentigo is a tan or brown macule, ranging in size from several millimeters to several centimeters, with distinct borders. The lesion occurs in sun-exposed areas of the body—on the dorsum of the hands, neck, head, and shoulders.

Differential Diagnosis. In childhood, the differential diagnosis of lentigo includes junctional nevus and freckle. In adults, seborrheic keratosis and lentigo maligna are included in the differential diagnosis. The most important of these is lentigo maligna, which appears as an irregularly colored (varying shades of brown and black), irregularly bordered macule on sun-exposed regions of the body. A lentigo maligna is an in situ malignant melanoma.

Types of lentigo:
1. **Simplex—few, congenital or in childhood**
2. **Actinic—many, sun-exposed skin, in middle age**

Lentigo is a brown macule with uniform color.

THERAPY OF FRECKLES

- None

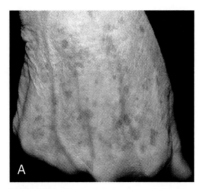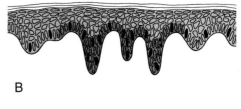

FIGURE 7–2. Actinic lentigo. **A,** Epidermis—brown macule. **B,** Epidermis—increased basal layer pigmentation resulting from increase in melanocytes and melanin; rete ridges are elongated.

Laboratory and Biopsy. Biopsy is seldom indicated. If biopsy is performed, the histologic picture is characterized by an increased number of melanocytes within the epidermis as well as increased pigmentation within the keratinocytes. The rete ridges may be normal or elongated.

Therapy. No therapeutic intervention is required, except for cosmetic purposes. Preparations containing hydroquinone are generally ineffective. Mild freezing with liquid nitrogen is sometimes effective. Laser destruction of these pigmented lesions is also effective. For multiple actinic lentigo, tretinoin cream 0.1% (Retin-A) applied daily is effective in lightening these photoaging spots. Irritation, however, is common, thus requiring less frequent application (every other or every third day) or use of a less concentrated cream (0.025% or 0.05%). Sunscreens with a sun protective factor (SPF) of 15 to 30 should be used to prevent the development of more actinic lentigo.

Course and Complications. Lentigo has no malignant potential. The *multiple lentigines syndrome*, a rare but distinctive syndrome, is characterized by hundreds of lentigines on the trunk, head, and extremities, including the palms and soles. It is dominantly inherited and also called the *LEOPARD* syndrome (*L*, lentigines; *E*, electrocardiographic abnormalities; *O*, ocular hypertelorism; *P*, pulmonary stenosis; *A*, abnormal genitalia; *R*, retarded growth and development; and *D*, deafness).

Peutz-Jeghers syndrome is a dominantly inherited trait that is distinctive because of numerous lentigines occurring around the mouth and eyes as well as on the lips, oral mucosa, hands, and feet in association with gastrointestinal polyps. Intussusception, hemorrhage, and malignancy are complications of these polyps.

Syndromes with numerous lentigines:
1. **LEOPARD**
2. **Peutz-Jeghers**

■ MELASMA

Definition. Melasma (chloasma) is patchy macular hyperpigmentation of the face (Fig. 7–3). It usually affects women. The melanocytes in melasma produce more melanin in response to multiple factors, including ultraviolet radiation, genetic predisposition, and hormonal influences.

THERAPY OF LENTIGO

- Cryotherapy
- Laser
- Tretinoin cream 0.1% daily or less frequently
- Sunscreen SPF 15–30

Incidence. Melasma is more common in women and in darkly pigmented ethnic groups. The frequency of new patients presenting in our clinic with the chief complaint of melasma is 0.2%, but it is a common incidental finding.

History. Displeasure with one's self-image causes a patient to seek medical attention. Adults acquire melasma in association with sunlight exposure, pregnancy (chloasma, the "mask of pregnancy"), and the use of birth control pills.

Sunlight, pregnancy, and birth control pills exacerbate melasma.

Physical Examination. Macular brown patches of melasma occur symmetrically on the face. They are sharply delineated and involve the malar eminences, forehead, upper lip, and mandible. The brown pigmentation is often patchy within the macule, giving it a reticulated appearance.

Differential Diagnosis. Postinflammatory hyperpigmentation and *freckles* are pigmented macules. For the former, patients have a history of prior dermatitis. Freckles are smaller and more numerous and involve the trunk and extremities in addition to the face.

Laboratory and Biopsy. No laboratory tests are necessary.

Therapy. Hydroquinone, a bleaching agent, is most frequently used to treat melasma. A 2% concentration is available over the counter, whereas 4% hydroquinone cream (Eldoquin-Forte) requires a prescription. It is applied twice daily to affected areas. Sunscreens with an SPF of 15 to 30 should be used prophylactically. If after several months no lightening occurs, tretinoin cream 0.1% (Retin-A) may be cautiously applied daily in addition to the use of hydroquinone and a sunscreen. Less commonly used treatments include azelaic acid (Azelex) and chemical peels.

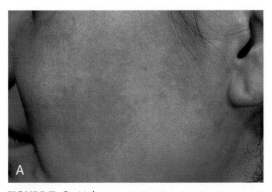 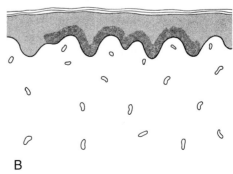

FIGURE 7–3. Melasma. **A,** Epidermis—brown macule. **B,** Epidermis—melanin pigmentation in basal layer.

THERAPY OF MELASMA

- Hydroquinone cream 4% twice daily
- Sunscreen SPF 15–30
- Tretinoin cream 0.1% daily or less frequently
- Azelaic acid cream 20%
- Chemical peels

Course and Complications. Melasma fades post partum, with sunlight protection, and with discontinuation of birth control pills. However, it may take months to years for normal skin color to return.

Pathogenesis. The melanocytes in the areas of involvement are increased in number as well as in activity, producing a greater number of melanosomes. Hormonal factors have been implicated because of the association with pregnancy and birth control pills, but melasma is infrequently found in menopausal women who receive estrogen replacement. Plasma measurements of ß-melanocyte-stimulating hormone are normal.

■ NEVUS

Types of nevi:
1. **Junctional**
2. **Compound**
3. **Intradermal**

Definition. A nevus (mole) is a benign neoplasm of pigment forming cells, the nevus cell. Nevi are congenital or acquired. A junctional nevus is macular, with nevus cells confined to the base of the epidermis. Compound (Fig. 7–4) and intradermal nevi are papular, with nevus cells in the epidermis and dermis and in the dermis only, respectively.

Incidence. Nevi should be considered a normal skin finding. The average number of nevi per person is 15 to 40 for Caucasians and 2 to 11 for blacks. In our clinic, 3% of new patients are seen because of concern about nevi that have become irritated, have changed in color or size, or are cosmetically unattractive.

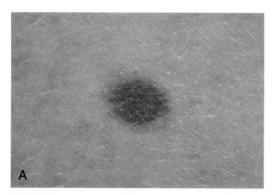
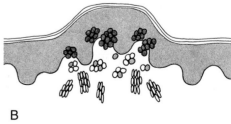

FIGURE 7–4. Compound nevus. **A,** Dermis—brown papule. **B,** Epidermis—pigmented nevus cell nests in lower epidermis. Dermis—pigmented nests of round nevus cells in upper dermis; bundles of spindle-shaped nevus cells in lower dermis.

History. Most nevi are acquired after 6 months of age and before the age of 35 years. Thereafter, one sees progressive decline in number, so that nevi are infrequent by age 80. Moles usually appear singularly, rarely in crops. It is common to have darkening in color, itching, and development of new nevi during pregnancy and adolescence. Otherwise, symptomatic nevi should be regarded suspiciously.

Physical Examination. Nevi vary greatly in appearance and coloration. Individually, they are uniform in color, surface, and border. They are flat or elevated, smooth or verrucoid, polypoid or sessile, and pigmented or flesh colored. Their coloration is orderly, with shades of brown and occasionally blue, although the latter color should be regarded with suspicion. Skin lines may or may not be present. Nevi frequently contain hair. The junctional nevus is a light to dark brown macule. Compound and intradermal nevi are flesh-colored or brown, smooth- or rough-surfaced papules that occur in older children and adults (Fig. 7–5).

Differential Diagnosis. The most important task is to differentiate a nevus from a *malignant melanoma*. Regular brown color, surface, and border are characteristic features of a nevus that differentiate it from melanoma. A junctional nevus may appear similar to other pigmented macules such as a *lentigo* or *freckle*. Compound and intradermal nevi, when flesh colored, can be confused with a *skin tag*, *basal cell carcinoma*, and *neurofibroma*. The presence of telangiectasia and central depression as well as recent acquisition in an adult are characteristic of a nodular basal cell carcinoma. When pigmented, these nevi can resemble *seborrheic keratoses* and *dermatofibromas*. The presence of scale and pasted-on appearance is typical of seborrheic keratosis. Dermatofibromas are hard dermal papules that dimple when pinched, whereas nevi are soft.

The *Spitz nevus (benign juvenile melanoma)* is composed of spindle and epithelioid nevus cells. It is a smooth, round, slightly scaling, pink nodule that occurs most frequently in children. The most important aspect of dealing with this lesion is to recognize that it is a nevus and not a melanoma and to avoid extensive surgical intervention.

Blue nevi are small, steel-blue nodules that usually begin early in life. Their importance in diagnosis is their similar appearance to nodular melanoma. If any doubt exists, a biopsy should be performed.

The *dysplastic nevus*, or *atypical mole*, is both controversial and confusing (Fig. 7–6). Controversy exists about its propensity to develop into a malignant melanoma. The confusion stems from differing histologic criteria for diagnosis. Clinically, the atypical mole is larger than 5 mm, is variegated in color with an erythematous background, and has an irregular, indistinct border. Atypical moles were initially recognized as markers for increased risk of melanoma in family members with a familial form of malignant melanoma, the *familial atypical mole and melanoma syndrome* or *dysplastic nevus syndrome*. In these families, virtually all members with atypical moles developed a melanoma in their lifetime, whereas family members without atypical moles did not. Subsequently, investigators discovered that approximately 5% of the healthy Caucasian population in the United States has atypical moles. The risk of developing a melanoma in these individuals, many of whom have only one or a few atypical moles and no personal or familial history of melanoma, is unclear, but for most, a melanoma never develops.

Congenital nevi are present at birth or shortly thereafter and are usually elevated and have uniform, dark brown pigmentation with discrete borders. One percent of newborns have congenital nevi. Large congenital nevi (greater than 20

Uniform color, surface, and border are characteristics of nevi.

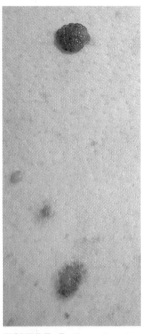

FIGURE 7–5. Several nevi showing variation in appearance.

Special nevi
1. **Spitz**
2. **Blue**
3. **Dysplastic**
4. **Congenital**

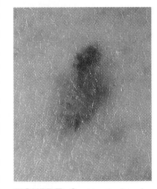

FIGURE 7–6. Atypical mole.

cm across or covering 5% of body area) have a 6% to 12% chance of developing into a malignant melanoma. Small congenital nevi have little to no increased risk of transformation into melanoma and therefore do not need to be removed prophylactically.

Laboratory and Biopsy. Nevus cells vary in morphology, depending on their location in the skin. They are arranged in nests in the basal layer of the epidermis and upper dermis. When they extend deeper, cord-like or sheet-like formations occur. In the upper dermis and epidermis, the individual cells are epithelioid in appearance with a cuboidal or oval shape, indistinct cytoplasm, and a round or oval nucleus and are pigmented. In the middle dermis, nevus cells are smaller, do not contain pigment, and have a lymphoid appearance. In the lower dermis, they have a spindle cell appearance, resembling fibroblasts. Atypical moles histologically have (1) abnormal architecture of melanocytes within the epidermis, (2) dermal fibrotic response, and (3) depending on the pathologist, variable cytologic atypia. Investigators have suggested that the pathologic diagnosis of atypical moles be changed to *nevus with architectural disorder*.

Therapy. The prophylactic removal of nevi is not required. Worrisome lesions are those that have changed in color, shape, or size; have been acquired in adulthood; bleed; or are itching. An excisional biopsy with narrow margins (2 to 3 mm) is recommended for suspicious lesions. Clinically benign and cosmetically unsightly nevi may be removed by shaving off the lesion with a scalpel (shave excision). However, a shave biopsy leaves some residual nevus cells at the biopsy site that may become darkly pigmented.

All nevi that are removed should be examined by a pathologist.

The management of *congenital nevi* is difficult when these lesions are large (diameter greater than 20 cm or covering 5% of body area) and controversial when they are small. Large congenital nevi, such as the bathing-suit nevus, cover extensive areas of the trunk in a garment-like fashion and are generally associated with many satellite lesions. They are rare but have a significant potential for developing into malignant melanoma (6% to 12%). The optimal treatment is excision of these lesions, but the technical difficulty of removing such wide areas of skin may preclude this therapy. At the least, patients should be carefully followed, with excision of nodules that develop within the nevus. Large congenital nevi covering the head and neck are sometimes associated with underlying meningeal melanosis, seizures, mental retardation, and development of meningeal malignant melanoma. Opinion differs concerning removal of small congenital nevi. Some clinicians recommend that all these lesions be excised because of a possible increased potential for the development of melanoma. Others disagree with this opinion and recommend no excision unless the lesion changes clinically. Data from recent studies support the latter opinion.

The recommended advice to the healthy person with (multiple) atypical moles but no personal or familial history of malignant melanoma is patient edu-

---

THERAPY OF NEVUS

- Elliptical excision
- Shave excision

TABLE 7–2 ■ GUIDELINES FOR MANAGEMENT AND FOLLOW-UP OF PATIENTS WITH ATYPICAL MOLES

Baseline Evaluation
Excisional biopsy of at least two lesions to confirm diagnosis
Total skin photographs, including close-ups of suspicious lesions
Sun protection
Patient self-examination monthly
Screen blood relatives for atypical nevi and melanoma

Follow-up Frequency
In patients with no personal or family history of melanoma, every 12 months
In patients with personal or family history of melanoma, every 3 months for 2 years; if no change, then every 6 months for 3 years.
Then, reevaluate yearly.

cation about sun exposure, self-examination, and yearly full skin examination by a physician (Table 7–2).

Course and Complications. Approximately 50% of malignant melanomas have associated nevi. The relative risk of melanoma increases as the number of nevi increases; that is, persons with large numbers of nevi have a greater risk of melanoma than do persons with a few nevi. No evidence indicates that mild irritation or rubbing results in transformation of a nevus into a melanoma.

Some nevi develop a surrounding depigmented zone and are referred to as *halo nevi* (Fig. 7–7). They occur singularly or multiply, usually on the trunk in teenagers. The development of a halo around the nevus is a harbinger of its disappearance. Both humoral and cellular immunities appear to be involved with the development of halo nevi, a process that results in destruction of nevus cells. On rare occasions, a depigmented halo develops around a malignant melanoma. If the central lesion has a uniform brown color typical of a nevus, an excisional biopsy is not necessary.

Pathogenesis. Nevus cells are derived from the neural crest. Morphologically, one can recognize the nevus cell because it has no dendritic processes and groups together in nests within the epidermis and dermis.

Halo nevi are rarely a malignant melanoma.

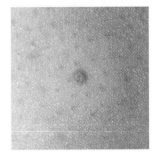

FIGURE 7–7. Halo nevus.

■ MALIGNANT MELANOMA

Definition. Malignant melanoma is a cancerous neoplasm of pigment-forming cells, melanocytes, and nevus cells. Clinically, its hallmarks are an irregularly shaped and colored papule or plaque. Four types of melanoma are recognized (Table 7–3): (1) superficial spreading (Fig. 7–8), (2) lentigo maligna (Fig. 7–9), (3) nodular, and (4) acral lentiginous (Fig. 7–10).

Incidence. The occurrence of malignant melanoma has rapidly increased over the past several decades and is increasing faster than any other cancer in the United States. The reason for this rapid rise is not certain. Increased sunlight exposure, however, has been implicated as one possible factor. More than 40,000 new cases of melanoma are diagnosed yearly in the United States, with the majority occurring in the 15- to 50-year-old age group. The estimated lifetime risk of developing

The incidence of malignant melanoma is increasing.

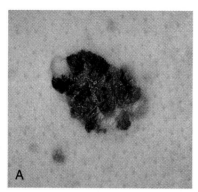

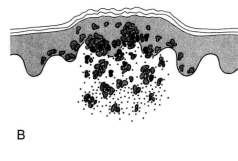

FIGURE 7–8. Superficial spreading melanoma. **A,** Epidermis—irregular brown-black color, irregular border. Dermis—papule; red, white, blue. **B,** Epidermis—atypical pigmented melanoma cells. Dermis—variously sized nests of atypical melanoma cells, inflammation.

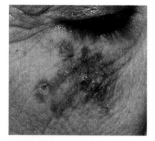

FIGURE 7–9. Lentigo maligna melanoma.

Melanoma signs (ABCDs):
1. **Asymmetry**
2. **Border irregularity—notched border**
3. **Color variegation—red, white, blue**
4. **Diameter greater than 6 mm**

a malignant melanoma is approaching 1 in 90. Excluding other skin cancers, melanoma represents 2% of all cancers and 1% of all cancer deaths in the United States.

History. An increase in the lesion's size or a change in its color is noted in at least 70% of patients who have melanoma. Development of a new growth, bleeding, and itching are other symptoms that may accompany a melanoma. Occasionally, patients have a family history of malignant melanoma.

Physical Examination. Lentigo maligna melanoma (see Fig. 7–9), superficial spreading melanoma, and acral lentiginous melanoma (see Fig. 7–10) are characterized by a horizontal growth phase that allows for clinical identification before deeper invasion and metastasis occurs. The ABCDs of identifying characteristics for these three types of melanoma are *a*symmetry, *b*order irregularity, *c*olor variegation, and *d*iameter greater than 6 mm. The suspicious lesion is red, white, and blue, has a notched border, and has a papule or nodule within it. However, in approximately 10% of melanomas, the ABCD rule does not apply. Therefore, any pigmented lesion or "nevus" that looks significantly different from an individual's

TABLE 7–3 ▪ CLINICAL FEATURES OF MELANOMA

Type	Location	Median Age (Years)	Premetastatic	Frequency (%)*	Race
Lentigo maligna	Sun-exposed surfaces (head, neck)	70	5–15 years	10	Caucasian
Superficial spreading	All surfaces (back, legs)	47	1–7 years	27	Caucasian
Nodular	All surfaces	50	Months–2 years	9	Caucasian
Acral lentiginous	Palms, soles, nail beds	61	Months–8 years	1	Black, Asian

*53% of melanomas are unclassified.

other nevi—the "ugly duckling" mole—should be viewed suspiciously and should probably be examined by biopsy.

Lentigo maligna melanoma occurs on sun-exposed skin, especially the head and neck. It is multicolored, with dark brown, black, red, white, and blue hues, and it is elevated in areas. It is preceded by lentigo maligna (in situ melanoma), which extends peripherally and is an unevenly pigmented, dark brown and black macule. Lentigo maligna often reaches a diameter of 5 to 7 cm before showing signs of invasion. The change in size and darkening is insidious, occurring over a period of years.

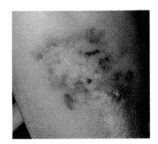

FIGURE 7–10. Acral lentiginous melanoma on the sole of the foot. (Courtesy of Mary Maloney, M.D.)

The most common type of melanoma is the *superficial spreading melanoma*. This lesion is irregular in color (red, white, and blue), surface (papular or nodular), and border (notched) and may occur anywhere on the body. It is most frequently found on the upper back in males and the upper back and lower legs in females. During the horizontal growth phase, the lesion is flat, extending to approximately 2.5 cm in diameter before invasion develops.

Nodular melanoma is a rapidly growing, blue-black, smooth or eroded nodule. It occurs anywhere on the body. It begins in the vertical growth phase, so it is less likely to be diagnosed in a premetastatic stage.

Acral lentiginous melanoma occurs on the palms, soles, and distal portion of the toes or fingers. It is an irregular, enlarging, black growth similar to a lentigo maligna melanoma. The vertical growth phase in this type of melanoma can be deceptive, showing only a small degree of papular elevation associated with a deep invasion. In contrast to the other melanomas, acral lentiginous melanoma is most frequent in blacks and Asians.

Differential Diagnosis. Although the clinical criteria outlined previously allow for the early diagnosis of malignant melanoma, other pigmented lesions must be considered before definitive therapy is undertaken. In one study, two thirds of the pigmented lesions that were clinically thought to be malignant melanoma were not by histopathologic criteria.

The differential diagnosis of lentigo maligna melanoma includes *actinic lentigo* and *seborrheic keratosis*. The brown color of these latter lesions is a reassuring sign of their benignity.

Pigmented basal cell carcinoma, seborrheic keratosis, nevus, and *angioma* can look like superficial spreading malignant melanoma.

Nodular melanoma can resemble *pyogenic granuloma, angioma, blue nevus,* and *dermatofibroma*. A pyogenic granuloma is an easily bleeding nodule composed of numerous benign blood vessels. It often occurs after minor trauma and can be viewed as excessive granulation tissue.

Tinea nigra palmaris, a rare superficial fungal infection, and nevus should be considered in the differential diagnosis of acral lentiginous melanoma. Tinea nigra palmaris can easily be diagnosed with a potassium hydroxide scraping that reveals fungal hyphae.

Biopsy. *All suspicious pigmented lesions must undergo biopsy*, preferably by excision with narrow 2- to 3-mm margins of normal skin. Definitive treatment by wide surgical excision should not be undertaken until confirmation of malignant melanoma is made histologically. In extensive lesions such as lentigo maligna melanoma, it is acceptable to do an incisional biopsy before definitive therapy. The histologic features vary with the type of melanoma and require a skilled pathologist for interpretation.

All suspicious pigmented lesions that could be melanoma should undergo biopsy.

THERAPY OF MALIGNANT MELANOMA

- Excisional biopsy
- Sentinel lymph node biopsy
- Wider excision down to the fascia with margins of normal skin based on thickness of melanoma

Thickness	Margin
<1 mm	1 cm
1–4 mm	2 cm
>4 mm	3 cm

- Chemotherapy—DTIC (dacarbazine)
- Radiation
- Immunotherapy—interferon alfa-2b

Cure of malignant melanoma rests in the hands of the surgeon, if the lesion is treated early enough.

Therapy. The survival of patients with malignant melanoma depends on early diagnosis, when surgical excision is often curative. A more conservative attitude toward the surgical treatment of melanoma has evolved in the past 10 years, with narrower margins advocated. In thin melanomas less than 1.0 mm, a 1.0-cm margin of normal skin around the melanoma is adequate. Thicker malignant melanomas are usually excised with more than 1.0-cm margins of normal skin, although no scientific evidence indicates that this approach improves survival, and no uniform standard exists.

Radiolymphatic sentinel node mapping and biopsy have been used for melanomas greater than 1 mm thick in patients with clinically negative lymph nodes. A radioactive tracer is injected at the site of the primary melanoma before wider excision is performed. The first draining or sentinel lymph node can be identified by lymphoscintigraphy and can be examined by biopsy for the presence of metastatic melanoma. In this way, the clinician can identify patients who may benefit from regional lymphadenectomy and adjuvant immunotherapy. Prognostic information is also garnered. The surgical management of regional lymph nodes remains controversial. Patients with stage I and II (American Joint Commission on Cancer Staging System) nonmetastatic and intermediate-thickness melanoma (1.0 to 4.00 mm) may have improved survival rates after elective lymphadenectomy. Those with thin (less than 1.0 mm) and thick (more than 4.0 mm) melanomas do not appear to benefit from elective lymph node dissection. Stage III patients (nodal metastasis) have a poor survival rate, despite regional lymph node dissection. Stage IV patients (systemic metastasis) have a grave prognosis.

Once a malignant melanoma has metastasized, therapy is with dimethyltriazenyl imidazolecarboxamide alone or in combination with other chemotherapeutic agents. The response rate is 20% to 30%. Radiation therapy is used for palliation of bone and brain metastasis and when lentigo maligna is so large that surgical removal is technically difficult.

Immunotherapeutic approaches for the treatment of disseminated melanoma include cytokines (interferons and interleukins), monoclonal antibodies, autologous lymphocytes, and specific immunization. Interferon alfa-2b (Intron A) is approved as an adjuvant to surgical treatment in patients at high risk of systemic recurrence of the disease. These patients have melanomas greater than 4 mm thick or they have nodal involvement. Median overall survival was increased by 12 months with interferon alfa-2b compared with no treatment.

Course and Complications. Lentigo maligna melanoma, superficial spreading melanoma, and acral lentiginous melanoma initially have a horizontal growth phase manifested as a macular or slightly raised pigmented lesion. During the horizontal growth phase, malignant melanoma is totally curable. Nodular melanoma has only a vertical growth phase. Certain principles are important concerning malignant melanoma:

1. A horizontal growth phase makes surgical cure possible for superficial melanoma.
2. The prognosis is related to tumor thickness (Fig. 7–11).
3. Clinical criteria allow for an early diagnosis of malignant melanoma.

Clark and Breslow correlated survival with tumor thickness. Clark and coworkers devised a system of microstaging melanoma based on level of invasion in the dermis. The difficulty with this system is variability in differentiating between level 3 and level 4 melanomas. Breslow, using an ocular micrometer, measured tumor thickness from the stratum granulosum to the depth of invasion. These measurements are reproducible and are the preferred method of calculating tumor thickness and, thus, of predicting 5-year survival. Recommended follow-up of patients with melanoma is presented in Table 7–4. Extensive laboratory tests such as brain, bone, or liver and spleen scans are not indicated unless the history or physical examination suggests possible metastasis to these organs.

Pathogenesis. The pathogenesis of malignant melanoma is unknown. However, sunlight and heredity have been implicated as risk factors. Other risk factors for melanoma include a large number of small nevi, large nevi, and dysplastic nevi. The production of melanoma by ultraviolet radiation is suggested both epidemiologically and experimentally. The cause-and-effect relationship, however, is less

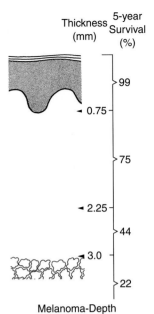

FIGURE 7–11. Prognosis is related to depth of invasion.

TABLE 7–4 ■ GUIDELINES FOR FOLLOW-UP OF MALIGNANT MELANOMA PATIENTS

SUBJECTIVE
Date of Diagnosis _____
Location _____
Breslow thickness _____
Review of Systems _____

OBJECTIVE

	Breslow Thickness of Melanoma		
	In-situ	<1.0 mm	>1.0 mm
Total skin exam	Done	Done	Done
Lymph node exam		Done	Done
Liver/Spleen exam			Done
Annual CBC, LFT's, CXR			Done

PLAN
Melanoma in-situ   Annual skin exam
Melanoma <1.0 mm: Exam Q 6 months for 2 years, then Q 12 months
Melanoma >1.0 mm: Exam Q 3 months for 2 years, then Q 6 months
                                     for 3 years, then Q 12 months

Patients should perform total skin and lymph node self-exam monthly

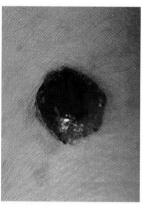

FIGURE 7–12. Unknown.

well proven than with other skin cancers. Familial occurrence of malignant melanoma is rare but well established. The *familial atypical mole and melanoma syndrome (dysplastic nevus syndrome* or B-K mole syndrome) occurs in family members with numerous atypical-appearing, haphazardly colored and bordered nevi *(atypical moles)* who have one or several malignant melanomas. Biopsy of these atypical moles reveals disordered melanocytic proliferation. These atypical moles are markers for an increased risk of developing malignant melanoma and, in some cases, precursors of melanoma. This syndrome also occurs sporadically as well as in a familial pattern. Close clinical follow-up and excision of suspicious nevi are mandatory (see Table 7–2).

■ UNKNOWN (Fig. 7–12)

This 29-year-old white woman was seen in the dermatology clinic because of a bleeding growth. It had been present for 6 months and had grown rapidly. Her medical history was otherwise unremarkable.

What is your differential diagnosis of this lesion?

This 6-mm nodule has the blue-black color and eroded surface typical of a nodular malignant melanoma. The differential diagnosis includes a blue nevus, nodular pyogenic granuloma, and hemangioma.

What would you do now?

An excisional biopsy revealed histopathologic changes typical of a nodular melanoma invading to a depth of 3.7 cm. The remainder of the skin examination and a general physical examination were normal. A sentinel lymph node biopsy was free of tumor. A 3.0-cm margin of normal skin was excised around the biopsy scar.

How would you determine the prognosis of this patient?

The prognosis of malignant melanoma is related to tumor thickness. Because this is a thick melanoma, the patient's prognosis is poor. Staging studies, including a complete blood count, liver function tests, and a chest radiograph, were negative.

Important Points

1. All bleeding pigmented lesions should be examined by biopsy, not merely watched.
2. Patients with thick melanomas have a poor prognosis.
3. Most melanomas can be removed (and cured) when they are thin—if physicians and the public are alert to these diagnostic signs.

R E F E R E N C E S
Freckle

Breathnach AS, Wyllie LM: Electron microscopy of melanocytes and melanosomes in freckled human epidermis. J Invest Dermatol 42:389–394, 1964.

Lentigo

Bolognia JL: Reticulated black solar lentigo ("ink spot" lentigo). Arch Dermatol 128:934–940, 1992.

Giardiello FM, Welsh SB, Hamilton SR, et al.: Increased risk of cancer in the Peutz-Jeghers syndrome. N Engl J Med 316:1511–1514, 1987.

Griffiths CEM, Goldfarb MT, Finkel LJ, et al.: Topical tretinoin (retinoic acid) treatment of hyperpigmented lesions associated with photoaging in Chinese and Japanese patients: a vehicle-controlled trial. J Am Acad Dermatol 30:76–84, 1994.

Rafal ES, Griffiths CEM, Ditre CM, et al.: Topical tretinoin (retinoic acid) treatment for liver spots associated with photodamage. N Engl J Med 326:368–374, 1992.

Voron DA, Hatfield HH, Kalkhoff RK: Multiple lentigines syndrome: case report and review of the literature. Am J Med 60:447–454, 1976.

Melasma

Grimes PE: Melasma: etiologic and therapeutic considerations. Arch Dermatol 131:1453–1457, 1995.

Kimbrough-Green CK, Griffiths CEM, Finkel LJ, et al.: Topical retinoic acid (tretinoin) for melasma in black patients. Arch Dermatol 130:727–733, 1994.

Sanchez JL, Pathak M, Sato S, et al.: Melasma: a clinical, light microscopic, ultrastructural, and immunofluorescence study. J Am Acad Dermatol 4:698–710, 1981.

Smith AG, Shuster S, Thody AJ, et al.: Chloasma, oral contraceptives, and plasma immunoreactive beta-melanocyte-stimulating hormone. J Invest Dermatol 68:169–170, 1977.

Vazquez M, Sanchez JL: The efficacy of a broad-spectrum sunscreen in the treatment of melasma. Cutis 32:92–96, 1983.

Nevus

Elder DE: The dysplastic nevus. Pathology 17:291–297, 1985.

Halpern AC, Du Pont G, Elder DE, et al.: Dysplastic nevi as risk markers of sporadic (nonfamilial) melanoma: a case-control study. Arch Dermatol 127:995–999, 1991.

Klein LJ, Barr RJ: Histologic atypia in clinically benign nevi: a prospective study. J Am Acad Dermatol 22:275–282, 1990.

Murphy GF, Halprin A: Dysplastic melanocytic nevi: normal variants or melanoma precursors? Arch Dermatol 126:519–522, 1990.

Rhodes AR, Melski JW: Small congenital nevocellular nevi and the risk of cutaneous melanoma. J Pediatr 100:219–224, 1982.

Swerdlow AJ, English JSC, Qiao Z: The risk of melanoma in patients with congenital nevi: a cohort study. J Am Acad Dermatol 32:595–599, 1995.

Tucker MA, Halpern A, Holly EA, et al.: Clinically recognized dysplastic nevi: a central risk factor for cutaneous melanoma. JAMA 277:1439–1444, 1997.

Walton RG, Jacobs AH, Cox AJ: Pigmented lesions in newborn infants. Br J Dermatol 95:389–396, 1976.

Malignant Melanoma

Balch CM: Surgical management of regional lymph nodes in cutaneous melanoma. J Am Acad Dermatol 3:511–524, 1980.

Brady MS, Coit DG: Sentinel lymph node evaluation in melanoma. Arch Dermatol 133:1014–1020, 1997.

Chang AE, Karnell LH, Menck HR: The National Cancer Data Base report on cutaneous and noncutaneous melanoma. Cancer 83:1664–1678, 1998.

Consensus Conference: Precursors to malignant melanoma. JAMA 251:1864–1866, 1984.

Day CL, Mihm MC, Sober AJ, et al.: Narrower margins for clinical stage I malignant melanoma. N Engl J Med 306:479–482, 1982.

Drake LA, Ceilley RI, Cornelison RL, et al.: Guidelines of care for malignant melanoma. J Am Acad Dermatol 28:638–641, 1993.

Epstein DS, Lange JR, Gruber SB, et al.: Is physician detection associated with thinner melanomas? JAMA 281:640–643, 1999.

Glass FL, Cottam JA, Reintgen DS, et al.: Lymphatic mapping and sentinel node biopsy in the management of high-risk melanoma. J Am Acad Dermatol 39:603–610, 1998.

Grin-Jorgensen C, Kopf AW, Maize JC: Cutaneous malignant melanoma. J Am Acad Dermatol 25:714–716, 1991.

Ho VC, Sober AJ: Therapy for cutaneous melanoma: an update. J Am Acad Dermatol 22:
    159–176, 1990.
Johnson TM, Smith JW, Nelson BR, et al.: Current therapy for cutaneous melanoma. J Am
    Acad Dermatol 32:689–707, 1995.
Johnson TM, Yahanda AM, Chang AE, et al.: Advances in melanoma therapy. J Am Acad
    Dermatol 38:731–741, 1998.
NIH Consensus Development Panel on early melanoma: Diagnosis and treatment of early
    melanoma. JAMA 268:1314–1319, 1992.
Piepkorn M, Odland PB: Quality of care in the diagnosis of melanoma and related melan-
    ocytic lesions. Arch Dermatol 133:1393–1396, 1997.
Rigel D: Malignant melanoma: incidence issues and their effect on diagnosis and treatment
    in the 1990s. Mayo Clin Proc 72:367–371, 1997.
Rigel D, Kopf AW, Friedman RJ: The rate of malignant melanoma in the United States: are
    we making an impact? J Am Acad Dermatol 17:1050–1053, 1987.
Sahin S, Levin L, Kopf AW, et al.: Risk of melanoma in medium-sized congenital melano-
    cytic nevi: a follow-up study. J Am Acad Dermatol 39:428–433, 1998.
Sober AJ, Fitzpatrick TB, Mihm MC: Primary melanoma of the skin: recognition and man-
    agement. J Am Acad Dermatol 2:179–197, 1980.
Stevens G, Cockerell CJ: Avoiding sampling error in the biopsy of pigmented lesions. Arch
    Dermatol 132:1380–1382, 1996.
Tucker MA, Halpern A, Holly EA, et al.: Clinically recognized dysplastic nevi: a central
    risk factor for cutaneous melanoma. JAMA 277:1439–1444, 1997.
Veronesi UV, Cascinelli N, Adamus J, et al.: Thin stage I primary cutaneous malignant
    melanoma: comparison of excision with margins of 1 or 3 cm. N Engl J Med 318:1159–
    1162, 1988.
Weiss M, Loprinzi CL, Creagan ET, et al.: Utility of follow-up tests for detecting recurrent
    disease in patients with malignant melanomas. JAMA 274:1703–1705, 1995.
Whited JD, Grichnik JM: Does this patient have a mole or a melanoma? JAMA 279:696–
    701, 1998.

DERMAL AND SUBCUTANEOUS GROWTHS

EPIDERMAL INCLUSION CYST
HEMANGIOMA
DERMATOFIBROMA
KELOID
LIPOMA
NEUROFIBROMA
XANTHOMA
KAPOSI'S SARCOMA
OTHER MALIGNANT DERMAL TUMORS

This chapter deals with nodular and cystic "lumps" in the skin. With the exception of lipomas, the lesions are located in the dermis, often with no alteration in the overlying epidermis. For many patients, common lesions such as epidermal inclusion cysts, small hemangiomas, dermatofibromas, and lipomas are not troubling and are not brought to the attention of a physician. However, these lesions are often found in routine physical examinations, and it is important to be able to distinguish them from malignant dermal growths. In patients for whom a "lump" in the skin is the presenting complaint, their usual question is, "Is it malignant?" This concern is appropriate and must always be addressed.

Color and consistency are helpful distinguishing clinical features (Table 8–1). The color of the lesions sometimes reflects the nature of the proliferating elements. Vascular lesions, for example, have hues ranging from red to purple. Consistency often distinguishes a nodule from a cyst; a cyst is usually fluctuant or malleable. For nodules, a soft consistency lends reassurance that the lesion is benign, a firm consistency is of intermediate concern, and a hard consistency should lead one to be more suspicious of a possible malignant process.

Color and consistency are helpful distinguishing features.

Sometimes, the diagnosis can be made only with biopsy. This is particularly important for firm-to-hard nodules in which the clinical diagnosis is uncertain. A general and important rule, then, is that for any skin nodule of uncertain origin, a biopsy is indicated to rule out malignancy.

For dermal nodules, if the clinical diagnosis is uncertain, a biopsy must be done to rule out malignancy; hard nodules are particularly suspect.

■ EPIDERMAL INCLUSION CYST

Definition. An epidermal inclusion cyst (Fig. 8–1) is derived from the upper portion (infundibulum) of the epithelial lining of a hair follicle and is located in the dermis. It is also called a *follicular cyst.*

TABLE 8–1 ■ DERMAL AND SUBCUTANEOUS GROWTHS

	Frequency*	Physical Examination	Differential Diagnosis†	Laboratory Test (Biopsy)	
				Diagnostic but Usually Not Necessary	Diagnostic and Necessary
Epidermal inclusion (follicular) cyst	0.5	Flesh-colored, firm, but malleable nodule	Pilar cyst Lipoma	X‡	
Hemangioma	0.8	Red or purple (often *blanchable*) soft-to-firm macule, papule, or nodule	Blue nevus Melanoma Kaposi's sarcoma	X	
Dermatofibroma	0.2	Tan-to-brown, firm, flat to slightly elevated papule *"dimples"* with lateral pressure	Nevus Melanoma Dermatofibrosarcoma protuberans (rare)	X	
Keloid	0.2	Pink, firm, elevated scar	Hypertrophic scar Dermatofibrosarcoma protuberans (rare)	X	
Lipoma	0.2	Flesh-colored, rubbery, *subcutaneous* nodule	Epidermal inclusion cyst Angiolipoma Metastatic tumor	X	
Neurofibroma	0.1	Flesh-to-brown, soft, and often compressible *("buttonhole" sign)* papule or nodule	Skin tag Nevus	X	
Xanthoma	<0.1	*Yellow* papules and nodules Hard subcutaneous tendon nodules	Sebaceous gland tumor Juvenile xanthogranuloma Rheumatoid nodules	X	
Kaposi's sarcoma	<0.1	*Purple* macules, plaques, or nodules	Bruise Hemangioma Bacillary angiomatosis		X
Other malignant tumors	<0.1	Flesh, red, or purple, *hard* nodules	Any of the above		X

* Percentage of new dermatology patients with this diagnosis seen in the Hershey Medical Center Dermatology Clinic, Hershey, PA.

† A malignant tumor should be in the differential diagnosis for all dermal growths.

‡ Incision and drainage reveals cheesy, foul-smelling material.

Epidermal inclusion cysts are common and benign; they often are mislabeled as sebaceous cysts.

This lesion is often misnamed a sebaceous cyst, but the contents are keratin, not sebum. It clinically appears as a flesh-colored, firm, but often malleable nodule in the skin.

Incidence. These lesions are common, but they usually are not brought to the attention of a physician, so the exact incidence is not known. They may occur at

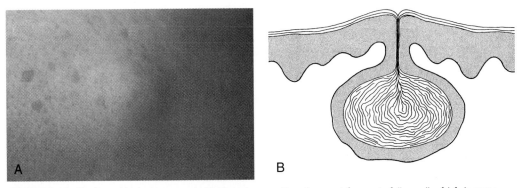

FIGURE 8–1. Epidermal inclusion cyst. **A,** Epidermis—unaltered, except for central "pore," which is sometimes visible. Dermis—firm, malleable nodule. **B,** Epidermis—invaginates into dermis. Dermis—keratin-filled, epidermal-line cyst.

any age. Epidermal inclusion cysts accounted for 59% of excised nodules in one large pediatric series (Knight and Reiner, 1983).

History. Epidermal inclusion cysts usually are asymptomatic and most frequently are found incidentally by either the patient or the examining physician. Occasionally, they are the primary complaint in a patient concerned about the possibility of malignancy. Another cause for medical attention is rupture of the cyst or secondary infection, either of which causes inflammation, pain, and drainage of foul-smelling material.

Physical Examination. Characteristically, the lesion is a flesh-colored, dome-shaped nodule that feels firm (but not hard). On palpation, it often feels slightly malleable, a finding suggesting that the contents are semisolid. This is a helpful diagnostic aid, as is the finding of a *central pore*, which represents the opening of the follicle from which the cyst originated. Lesions range in size from 0.5 to 5 cm. They may be located anywhere but occur most frequently on the head and trunk. If the central pore is patent, the diagnosis sometimes is confirmed by squeezing the lesion and expressing some of the whitish, cheesy, foul-smelling material that is trapped within. This material represents macerated keratin.

> A central pore is characteristic of a cyst.

Differential Diagnosis. *Pilar cysts* (also mistakenly termed sebaceous cysts) arise from the middle third (isthmus) of the follicular canal. They occur most frequently on the scalp, where they are the most common type of cyst. In other locations, they are less common than epidermal inclusion cysts, but the two may be clinically indistinguishable, and histologically some cysts may have elements of both. The difference is not critical; both are benign. A *lipoma* usually is deeper than an epidermal inclusion cyst, and although a lipoma may feel rubbery, it usually is not malleable. If the diagnosis is uncertain, particularly if the lesion feels firm, a *malignant tumor* must be considered.

Laboratory and Biopsy. Usually, the diagnosis can be made clinically. If desired, confirmation can be obtained by incising and draining the lesion, which reveals the cheesy, foul-smelling keratinous contents. A biopsy is equally confirmatory but usually is not necessary.

> The cheesy, foul-smelling material in the cyst represents macerated keratin; expression of this material is diagnostic.

Therapy. Frequently, no therapy is requested or needed. If removal is desired, one should remove the entire cyst with its lining, to prevent recurrence. This is accomplished by incising the skin overlying the cyst without disrupting the cyst wall

THERAPY OF EPIDERMAL CYSTS

- None
- Incision and Drainage
- Excision

To prevent recurrence, the entire cyst, with its lining, should be removed.

and then bluntly dissecting the entire cyst, along with its wall. If the cyst breaks, a curette can be used to remove the remaining contents and cyst wall. Elliptical excision is usually required for removal of cysts that have previously ruptured and scarred.

Course and Complications. Untreated, most epidermal inclusion cysts reach a stable size, often in the range of 1 to 3 cm, rarely larger.

Complications are rare and usually are limited to occasional rupture or infection. Rupture or infection results in redness and tenderness of the cyst and, on examination, increased fluctuance. If this occurs, the lesion should be treated as an abscess with incision and drainage and, occasionally, oral antibiotics.

Multiple epidermal inclusion cysts are a feature of *Gardner's syndrome*, an uncommon, autosomal dominant, heritable disorder manifested by multiple epidermal cysts, fibromas, osteomas, and intestinal polyps. The intestinal polyps often undergo malignant degeneration.

Pathogenesis. Epidermal inclusion cysts arise from the upper portion (infundibulum) of a hair follicle. The epidermal lining of the cyst is identical to that of the surface epidermis and produces keratin, which, having no place to shed, accumulates and forms the cystic mass.

■ HEMANGIOMA

Categories of hemangiomas:
1. **Capillary**
   a. **Nevus flammeus**
   b. **Strawberry**
   c. **Cherry**
2. **Cavernous**

Definition. A hemangioma is a benign proliferation of blood vessels in the dermis. The vascularity imparts a red, blue, or purple color to these lesions. Their clinical appearance further depends on the number, size, and depth of the proliferative vessels. Capillary hemangiomas are composed of small and superficial vessels. Nevus flammeus, strawberry hemangiomas (Fig. 8–2), and cherry angiomas fall into this category. In cavernous hemangiomas, the vessels are larger and deeper.

Incidence. Faint nevus flammeus lesions occur in the eyelid areas in as many as one third of newborns and the back of the neck in an additional 30%. Darker nevus flammeus lesions (port-wine stains) and strawberry and cavernous hemangiomas are much less common but are more likely to be brought to the attention of a physician because of cosmetic concerns. Strawberry and cavernous hemangiomas each occur in fewer than 1% of newborns. Cherry or "senile" (a term that, in general, is best avoided in describing skin lesions) angiomas appear in middle to late adulthood and are extremely common. Most older adults have at least several of these but are appropriately unconcerned about them.

History. Port-wine stains are usually present at birth. Strawberry and cavernous hemangiomas usually are not noted at birth or may be detected as only a faint bluish macule. They rapidly enlarge over the ensuing weeks. Cherry angiomas

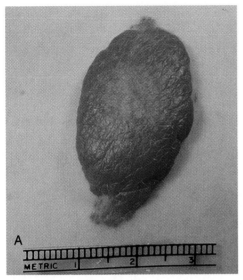

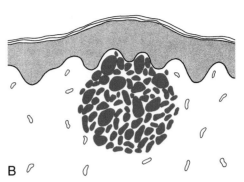

FIGURE 8-2. "Strawberry" hemangioma. **A,** Epidermis—normal, although surface may be irregular, as seen here. Dermis—red nodule. **B,** Epidermis—normal. Dermis—focal proliferation of blood vessels and endothelial cells.

usually are multiple and are acquired later in life. Hemangiomas are asymptomatic, except when they are large and cause local obstruction, a fortunately rare occurrence.

Physical Examination. The four types of hemangiomas listed previously differ in their physical appearance, as their names suggest:

Nevus flammeus is flat and occurs most often as a transient pink mark over the eyelids or as a persistent lesion on the back of the neck (erythema nuchae). The latter is colloquially called a "stork bite" because it is present at birth in the location where the "stork" would carry the baby. A *port-wine stain* is a nevus flammeus that is dark red to purple; it usually is located on the face.

A *strawberry hemangioma*, as implied by its name, has a protruding, roughened surface and a bright red color. These lesions may be single or multiple and can be located anywhere.

Cherry angiomas are small (2 to 5 mm), smooth, dome-shaped papules superficially protruding from the skin (Fig. 8–3). They usually are multiple lesions located on the trunk, and they range in color from red to purple.

Cavernous hemangiomas are dome-shaped, deep, soft, bluish nodules. Fortunately, they are rare. Some cavernous hemangiomas also have a superficial capillary component.

Differential Diagnosis. The diagnosis of childhood hemangiomas is usually made clinically without difficulty. In an adult, sometimes erythema nuchae is confused with *seborrheic dermatitis* or some other inflammatory rash.

Occasionally, a cherry angioma, particularly when it is purplish, may be confused with a *blue nevus* or even a *melanoma*. If the lesion is partly blanchable, this supports a vascular origin. Hemangiomas, however, are not always blanchable; when the diagnosis is in doubt, a biopsy should be performed. Rarely, lesions of *Kaposi's sarcoma* may be confused with hemangiomas. Clinically, Kaposi's sarcoma lesions appear as purple macules, papules, or nodules. A biopsy is diagnostic.

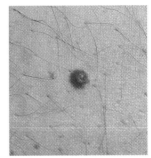

FIGURE 8-3. Cherry angioma.

Blanchability is a diagnostic feature found in many (but not all) hemangiomas.

Laboratory and Biopsy. A biopsy, if done, reveals a marked increase in blood vessels, many of which are dilated. A nevus flammeus early in life may show no histologic abnormality. Later, persistent lesions show dilated capillaries (telangiectasia). In the other hemangiomas, endothelial cell proliferation is found in association with the increased number of vessels.

Therapy. Skillful neglect is the most appropriate therapy for most childhood hemangiomas of the strawberry and cavernous types. Although these lesions may grow over the first 1 to 2 years of life (and during this time, the parents will need repeated reassurance), they usually spontaneously involute over the ensuing years with a cosmetic result that is superior to any that can be obtained by therapeutic intervention. Accordingly, skillful neglect frequently is the best option for these hemangiomas.

Port-wine stains are persistent. Laser therapy has been used with moderate success. As this technology continues to improve, so do the clinical results. Patients with evolving strawberry hemangiomas have also been treated with laser therapy, and the best results are obtained if laser therapy is administered early, within the first months of life. For many patients with port-wine stains, covering the lesions provides an inexpensive, and cosmetically acceptable result. Covermark and Dermablend are cosmetic products specifically designed for covering port-wine stains and other macular marks in the skin.

Course and Complications. Faint nevus flammeus eyelid lesions resolve within the first year of life. Port-wine stain lesions are persistent and occasionally are associated with angiomatosis in the brain and eye—the *Sturge-Weber syndrome*. This syndrome is manifested by one or more of the following: early-onset epilepsy, hemiparesis, intracranial calcifications, cerebral atrophy, and choroidal vascular lesions in the eye with glaucoma. Patients at risk for the Sturge-Weber syndrome are limited to those in whom the port-wine stain involves the V1 ophthalmic area of the trigeminal nerve. If Sturge-Weber syndrome is suspected, a computer assisted tomography scan of the head should be obtained to search for central nervous system involvement, and an eye examination should be performed to check for increased intraocular pressure.

Strawberry hemangiomas often increase in size over the first year but then subside spontaneously, so by the age of 5 years, 50% are involuted; 90% are involuted by age 9. Strawberry hemangiomas occasionally ulcerate and may be further complicated by infection. In infants with numerous strawberry hemangiomas, internal organ involvement should be suspected; this rare syndrome occasionally leads to death from high-output cardiac failure or compromise of an affected vital organ.

Cavernous hemangiomas may involute, but less often and less completely than strawberry hemangiomas. Depending on their location, large cavernous or mixed cavernous-capillary hemangiomas may cause functional compromise of

Most strawberry hemangiomas involute spontaneously during childhood.

THERAPY OF HEMANGIOMAS

- None
- Laser therapy
- Covering cosmetics

neighboring and underlying structures (e.g., the eye or oral pharynx). Systemic steroid therapy may ameliorate this rare complication. Platelet consumption may also occur within the tortuous vessels in patients with large hemangiomas (Kasabach-Merritt syndrome), but fortunately, this also is rare.

Once acquired, cherry angiomas persist but without complications.

Pathogenesis. With the exception of cherry angiomas, hemangiomas represent congenital malformations. Transient nevus flammeus lesions probably are the result of a localized congenital weakness of capillary walls that leads to vessel dilatation. With the other congenital capillary and cavernous hemangiomas, patients have a localized proliferation of endothelial cells and the supporting stroma, resulting in a cellular mass containing increased vascular channels.

■ DERMATOFIBROMA

Definition. A dermatofibroma is an area of focal dermal fibrosis, often accompanied by overlying epidermal thickening and hyperpigmentation (Fig. 8–4). It clinically appears as a small brown papule, often more indurated than elevated. The origin is unknown.

Incidence. Dermatofibromas are common and are often found incidentally in cutaneous examinations. Occasionally, they cause a patient to seek medical advice. They are seen most often in young adults.

History. Dermatofibromas usually are asymptomatic. The patient's concern, if any, is over the possibility of malignancy.

Physical Examination. Typical dermatofibromas are approximately 5 mm in size and are slightly elevated. They vary in color from light tan to dark brown. The fibrotic nature of the lesion is best appreciated by palpation, which reveals a firm consistency. A helpful diagnostic test is the "dimple sign," in which pinching results in central dimpling. Most dermatofibromas exhibit this sign; it is rarely seen with any other skin lesion. Dermatofibromas may occur anywhere, but the thighs and legs are the most common locations. One or several lesions may be present.

The "dimple sign" is characteristic of dermatofibroma.

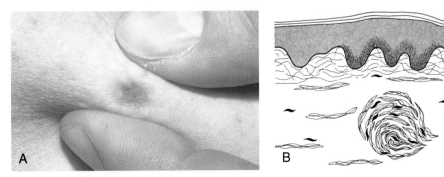

FIGURE 8–4. Dermatofibroma. **A,** Dermatofibroma with "dimple sign." Epidermis—increased pigment ranging from tan to brown; accentuated skin markings. Dermis—slightly elevated nodule, more palpable than elevated. **B,** Epidermis—slightly thickened and hyperpigmented. Dermis—nodular aggregate of fibroblasts and densely packed collagen.

Differential Diagnosis. With its brown color, a dermatofibroma may be confused with a *nevus*. Nevi, however, usually are softer and do not exhibit the "dimple sign." Darker dermatofibromas may raise a clinical suspicion of a *melanoma*. Dermatofibromas are usually purely brown (a benign color), whereas a nodular melanoma usually has shades of dark gray or blue. If any doubt exists, however, a biopsy should be performed.

Dermatofibrosarcoma protuberans is a low-grade malignant fibrous tumor that grows slowly but persistently and rarely metastasizes. It is a rare tumor and is distinguished clinically from a dermatofibroma by its larger size, irregular shape, and continued growth.

Laboratory and Biopsy. The diagnosis usually is made clinically. If any doubt exists, a biopsy should be performed to rule out malignancy. The histologic picture is diagnostic and shows a focal proliferation of densely packed collagen bands that are twisting and intertwining. Fibroblasts are interspersed and increased in number. Increased pigmentation of the slightly thickened overlying epidermis accounts for the frequent brown color of these lesions.

Therapy. Therapy usually is not indicated. If desired, a simple excision is sufficient for removal and histologic examination.

Course and Complications. Dermatofibromas are chronic and usually stable in size. They have no complications.

Pathogenesis. Although the origin is unknown, trauma (e.g., an insect bite) may be an initiating factor for some of these lesions. The proliferation of fibroblasts and subsequent fibrosis may represent an exuberant healing response to injury. However, most patients do not recollect a history of trauma in the area.

Two other lesions are considered within the spectrum of a dermatofibroma. A *histiocytoma* (an aggregate of histiocytes in a focal area within the dermis) probably represents an early phase in the formation of a dermatofibroma. A *sclerosing hemangioma,* as the name suggests, shows more of a vascular component, but the end result is that of dermal fibrosis as well.

■ KELOID

Definition. A keloid represents excessive proliferation of collagen (scar tissue) after trauma to the skin (Fig. 8–5). Clinically, a keloid appears as an elevated, firm, protuberant nodule or plaque.

Incidence. Keloids are relatively common. The incidence is highest in persons 10 to 30 years old. Blacks are particularly prone to keloids; in African populations, the prevalence is approximately 6%.

History. The trauma responsible for inducing the keloid almost always is remembered by the patient. Often, the trauma is obvious, such as ear piercing, surgical incisions, or other wounds. Keloids develop over weeks to months after the trauma. New and actively growing keloids often itch, whereas stable, long-standing ones are asymptomatic.

Physical Examination. A keloid looks like an overgrown scar, which is what it is. It is protuberant and firm and usually conforms roughly to a pattern of the original

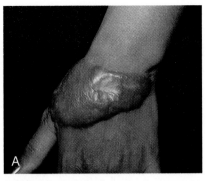 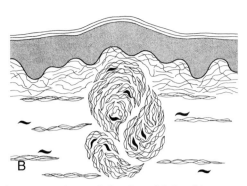

FIGURE 8–5. Keloid. **A,** Epidermis—smooth. Dermis—firm nodule, often pink in white patients, dark brown in black patients. **B,** Epidermis—may be atrophic. Dermis—highly compacted whorls of collagen.

trauma, although it is more extensive. Keloids are often pink or dark brown and have an irregular border with claw-like extensions. They may occur anywhere but they are more common on the earlobes (secondary to ear piercing), shoulders, upper chest, and back.

Differential Diagnosis. The difference between a keloid and a *hypertrophic scar* is mainly quantitative, with a keloid expanding beyond the limits of the original trauma.

A *dermatofibrosarcoma protuberans* is a rare, malignant fibrous tumor that may clinically look like a keloid, but the patient usually has no history of prior trauma, and the lesion continues to enlarge. If malignancy is suspected, a biopsy should be performed.

Laboratory and Biopsy. The diagnosis can usually be made on clinical grounds. If doubt remains, a biopsy can be performed for confirmation. The histologic examination shows whorls and nodules of highly compacted hyalinized bands of collagen. Fibroblasts may be increased in number but not markedly so in mature keloids. Mast cells are prominent, and release of their histamine content may be the cause of the often associated pruritus. The overlying epidermis may be atrophic.

Therapy. Surgical removal alone, although tempting, is contraindicated because it often is followed by a recurrence that is larger than the original lesion. Repeated intralesional injections of steroids (triamcinolone [Kenalog-40]) at monthly intervals may cause keloids to flatten, which is a goal desired by some patients. Surgery may be used if it is combined with another modality such as intralesional steroids or low-dose radiotherapy. Pressure dressings are also helpful when applied after surgery or injections. Silicone (Silastic) gel dressings applied daily for 2 months have been shown to help flatten hypertrophic scars by mechanisms that are unknown. Experimental cytokine therapies have been used: intralesional injections with interferon-α or with anti–transforming growth factor-β have been reportedly useful.

Surgery should never be used alone in treating keloids.

Course and Complications. Untreated, the usual course of a keloid is that of gradual enlargement to a steady-state size. Keloids are much less likely to regress than are hypertrophic scars, but in either case, the time course for regression (if it occurs at all) is measured in years. The major complication is cosmetic disfigurement, which may be profound.

THERAPY OF KELOIDS

- None
- Intralesional steroids
- Surgery with intralesional steroids

Pathogenesis. Increased fibroblast activity, initiated by tissue injury, results in a marked increase in collagen synthesis. Dermal ground substance (primarily the chondroitin 4-sulfate component) is also increased; investigators have suggested that this change may inhibit collagen degradation. Collagen production may also be affected by imbalance in, or altered fibroblastic responsiveness to, tissue cytokines. For example, collagen synthesis by fibroblasts is stimulated by transforming growth factor-β and is inhibited by interferons. These observations form the basis for the cytokine-directed therapies mentioned earlier.

■ LIPOMA

Definition. A lipoma represents a benign tumor of subcutaneous fat (Fig. 8–6). Clinically, it is a rubbery nodule that appears only slightly elevated above the skin's surface but is easily palpable deep in the skin. The origin is unknown.

Incidence. Most lipomas are never brought to a physician's attention. When they are, it is because of the patient's concern that the lesions may be malignant. They are most common in midlife.

History. Lipomas usually are asymptomatic. They may grow slowly, but most patients are not aware of any change in size.

Physical Examination. A typical lipoma is flesh colored and imparts a slight elevation to the normal-appearing overlying skin. It feels rubbery but not hard and usually is freely movable. Lipomas range in size from 1 to 10 cm, rarely larger. They may occur anywhere but are found most often on the trunk, neck, and upper extremities.

Differential Diagnosis. A lipoma usually is deeper, more freely movable, and more rubbery than an *epidermal* inclusion cyst.

Angiolipomas are uncommon tumors that often are painful and sometimes are locally invasive. Histologically, they have a prominent vascular component.

Metastatic *malignant tumors* of the skin can be deep but usually are firm (if not hard) and also involve the dermis, so the skin cannot be freely moved over them. A lipoma may also be mistaken for a soft tissue sarcoma, which is harder.

Laboratory and Biopsy. The diagnosis can usually be made clinically. If any doubt exists, particularly if a malignant tumor is even remotely suspected, a biopsy should be performed. One needs to be sure to extend the biopsy deep enough to sample the tumor. A deep elliptical excision is preferred. Histologically, a lipoma is an encapsulated collection of normal fat cells.

Therapy: None required

Therapy. Therapy usually is not required.

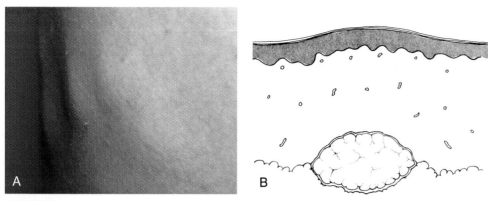

FIGURE 8–6. Lipoma. **A,** Multiple lipomas. Epidermis—normal. Dermis—deep, soft, rubbery nodule. **B,** Epidermis—normal. Dermis—impinged on by encapsulated tumor of normal-appearing fat cells.

Course and Complications. Lipomas found incidentally by the physician are usually reported by the patient to have been present without change in size for a number of years. For lesions recently detected or those that appear to be growing, a biopsy should be considered to confirm the diagnosis. These lesions have no complications.

■ NEUROFIBROMA

Definition. A neurofibroma represents a focal proliferation of neural tissue within the dermis (Fig. 8–7). Clinically, neurofibromas may appear in two ways: (1) most often, as soft, protruding papules and nodules; and (2) less often, as deep, firm, subcutaneous nodules. Multiple neurofibromas are a cutaneous expression of neurofibromatosis 1 (von Recklinghausen's disease), a dominantly inherited neurocutaneous disorder with prominent skin, skeletal, and nervous system abnormalities. Neurofibromatosis 2 is characterized primarily by bilateral acoustic neuromas and usually lacks the cutaneous findings of neurofibromatosis 1.

Incidence. Solitary neurofibromas are infrequent and inconsequential. Neurofibromatosis 1 is one of the more common genetic disorders, with an overall prevalence of approximately 3 in 10,000.

> Solitary neurofibromas are inconsequential; multiple ones are a sign of neurofibromatosis.

History. In von Recklinghausen's disease, the onset of skin tumors usually occurs in late childhood, with more rapid growth occurring in adolescence and pregnancy. Inheritance is determined by an autosomal dominant mechanism, but the expressivity is variable. A family history is important and should be followed by a cutaneous examination of both parents. However, spontaneous mutations are common and account for approximately 50% of patients with neurofibromatosis 1. Patients with neurofibromatosis may have signs and symptoms relative to other organ involvement, most often, the skeletal and central nervous systems.

Physical Examination. A typical neurofibroma appears as a soft, flesh-colored, protruding papule or nodule that characteristically, on compression, can be invaginated into what feels like a defect in the skin. This is the so-called *buttonhole sign.* These soft lesions sometimes attain nodule size. Less often, neurofibromas appear as deep, firm, dermal or subcutaneous nodules, which sometimes become extremely large (plexiform neurofibromas) and occasionally are tender. Neurofibro-

> Soft papules and nodules can often be invaginated into an apparent defect in the skin; this "buttonhole" sign is characteristic of neurofibromas.

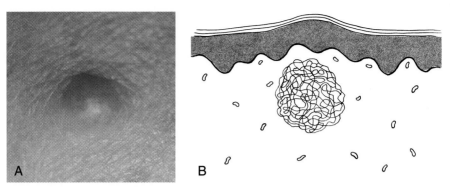

FIGURE 8–7. Neurofibroma. **A,** Epidermis—normal. Dermis—soft papule or nodule that invaginates into skin with applied pressure. **B,** Epidermis—normal. Dermis—circumscribed collection of loosely packed neural fibers.

mas in von Recklinghausen's disease are multiple, occasionally numbering in the thousands in a given patient. In the extreme ease, particularly when combined with bony abnormalities, the condition can be remarkably disfiguring.

Café-au-lait spots are light brown macules and are another cutaneous finding in neurofibromatosis. They are present early in life. Six or more café-au-lait spots, each more than 1.5 cm in diameter, are diagnostic for neurofibromatosis. Axillary freckling is another characteristic sign.

Ophthalmologic examination for Lisch nodules is useful in diagnosing neurofibromatosis 1.

The diagnostic criteria for neurofibromatosis 1 are given in Table 8–2. Ophthalmologic evaluation is extremely helpful. In neurofibromatosis 1, iris hamartomas (Lisch nodules) are invariably found.

Differential Diagnosis. *Skin tags* are also soft but more superficial, are narrower at the base (pedunculated), and lack the buttonhole sign.

A *dermal nevus* can appear as a soft, flesh-colored papule in the skin that clinically is similar to a small neurofibroma. Sometimes, only a biopsy differentiates the two with certainty. Biopsies are more often done for solitary neurofibromas than for multiple neurofibromas, in which the diagnosis is more clinically evident.

Laboratory and Biopsy. The diagnosis of neurofibromatosis can usually be made clinically. Magnetic resonance imaging is helpful in detecting brain hamartomas in children affected with neurofibromatosis 1 and in revealing acoustic neuromas in patients with neurofibromatosis 2. For solitary neurofibromas or when histologic confirmation is needed for neurofibromatosis, a biopsy specimen provides the diagnosis. The histologic picture shows a well-circumscribed collection of fine, wavy fibers loosely packed in the dermis. Special stains for nerve fibers are positive.

**Therapy:
Genetic counseling**

Therapy. Individual lesions can be removed surgically, but if excision is incomplete, recurrence is common. No known medical therapy is available to treat, prevent, or retard the progression of either the cutaneous features or the systemic disease in neurofibromatosis. Patients who are diagnosed with neurofibromatosis should have genetic counseling, preferably performed by a clinical geneticist.

Course and Complications. Solitary neurofibromas are of little consequence. They are usually asymptomatic, have no complications, and are stable. In von Recklinghausen's disease, the cutaneous condition usually is progressive. Lesions continue to form and grow, sometimes to the point of resulting in marked cosmetic

TABLE 8-2 ■ DIAGNOSTIC CRITERIA FOR NEUROFIBROMATOSIS 1

The diagnostic criteria are met if a person has two or more of the following:
Six or more café-au-lait macules more than 5 mm in greatest diameter in prepubertal persons and more than 15 mm in greatest diameter in postpubertal persons
Two or more neurofibromas of any type or one plexiform neurofibroma
Freckling in the axillary or inguinal regions
Optic glioma
Two or more Lisch nodules (iris hamartomas)
A distinctive osseous lesion
A first-degree relative with neurofibromatosis 1 by the above criteria

Modified from Mulvihill JJ, Parry DM, Sherman JL, et al.: Neurofibromatosis 1 (Recklinghausen disease) and neurofibromatosis 2 (bilateral acoustic neurofibromatosis). Ann Intern Med *113*:39–52, 1990.

disfigurement. With the variable expressivity of the disease, some patients are only mildly affected. Deep nodular lesions (plexiform neurofibromas) can rarely degenerate into malignant neurofibrosarcoma. Clinical clues that this is occurring include lesion enlargement and the development of tenderness. In most patients, the skin lesions remain histologically benign, although, as mentioned, they can become a source of cosmetic disfigurement and social stigmatization. Systemic complications of von Recklinghausen's disease are potentially numerous and include the following: central nervous system involvement with tumors, mental retardation, and seizures; skeletal abnormalities, including kyphoscoliosis, pseudarthrosis, and localized gigantism; and endocrine disorders such as precocious puberty and pheochromocytoma. Patients with neurofibromatosis and hypertension should be screened for pheochromocytoma.

Pathogenesis. Neurofibromatosis is caused by an abnormal gene transmitted in an autosomal dominant manner. The gene locations are on chromosome 17 for neurofibromatosis 1 and on chromosome 22 for neurofibromatosis 2. The gene on chromosome 17 encodes for a protein named *neurofibromin*, which appears to possess tumor-suppressor activity. Accordingly, inherited abnormalities of this gene may lead to tumor development, for example, neurofibromas and possibly other tumors found in patients with neurofibromatosis. The increased mast cells associated with neurofibromas may also promote tumor growth by release of growth factors such as histamine and tumor necrosis factor.

■ XANTHOMA

Definition. A xanthoma represents a focal collection of lipid-laden dermal histiocytes in the dermis or tendons (Fig. 8–8). Clinically, xanthomas located in the dermis appear as yellowish (*xanthous* is Greek for yellow) papules, plaques, and nodules. Tendon xanthomas are deep, flesh-colored, hard nodules located within peripheral tendons. Xanthomas usually are a manifestation of a hyperlipoproteinemic state.

Xanthomas are yellow tumors in the skin.

Incidence. Flat xanthomas on the eyelids (xanthelasmas) are the most frequently encountered xanthomas but still are not common. Other xanthomas are even less common, both as a presenting complaint in a dermatology clinic and as an incidental finding in the general population. Familial hypertriglyceridemia and familial hypercholesterolemia are both inherited as autosomal dominant traits, each

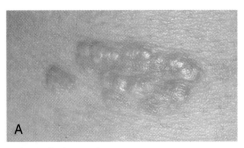
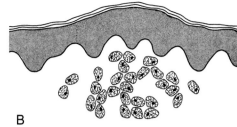

FIGURE 8-8. Xanthomas. **A,** Eruptive xanthomas. Epidermis—normal. Dermis—yellow papules and small nodules. **B,** Epidermis—normal. Dermis—dense infiltrate of lipid-laden histiocytes.

at a frequency of 1 in 500 of the general population. Patients who are homozygous for the disease obviously are much fewer in number but are more severely affected and more likely to have xanthomas.

History. In patients with one of the inherited hyperlipoproteinemias, a positive family history may be elicited. In addition, the patient may have systemic signs and symptoms that accompany the cutaneous xanthomas, including a history of coronary artery disease and diabetes. Patients with eruptive xanthomas have markedly elevated triglyceride levels that usually result from a familial metabolic abnormality combined with a secondary factor such as alcohol, obesity, glucose intolerance, hyperinsulinemia, and drugs, including estrogens, corticosteroids, and isotretinoin. Eruptive xanthomas appear relatively quickly in several weeks— and correspondingly disappear rapidly after reduction of serum triglyceride levels.

Physical Examination. Several types of xanthomas have been characterized. In all except the tendon type, the yellow color of the lesion provides the clue to its lipid nature. The most common types are as follows:

Xanthelasmas are yellowish plaques on the eyelids (Fig. 8–9). This is the only type that is not invariably accompanied by an elevation in either plasma cholesterol or triglycerides.

Eruptive xanthomas are reddish-yellowish papules and plaques that occur in patients with markedly elevated triglycerides. They occur most frequently on extensor surfaces but may appear anywhere.

Tuberous xanthomas are "potato-like" papules and nodules, which are yellowish and are most often found on the elbows and buttocks. Tuberous xanthomas are associated with increased serum triglycerides or cholesterol.

Tendon xanthomas are stony hard nodules occurring on tendons, most often the Achilles tendon and the extensor tendons of the fingers (Fig. 8–10). Because of their depth, the yellow color cannot be appreciated clinically. Tendon xanthomas are usually associated with severe hypercholesterolemia.

Differential Diagnosis. Sebaceous glands and lipids are the two major causes of the yellow color in skin papules. The lesions of *sebaceous gland hyperplasia* usually occur on the face as small superficial papules, often with a central umbilication.

The yellowish papules and plaques of *juvenile xanthogranuloma* also contain lipid, which is responsible for their color. As the name suggests, these lesions occur in childhood and usually involute spontaneously. Histologically, they have a distinctive appearance. They are not associated with elevated plasma lipids. Both *rheumatoid nodules* and *tendon xanthomas* are subcutaneous, but only tendon xanthomas are affixed to the tendon structures.

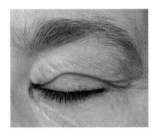

FIGURE 8-9. Xanthelasma.

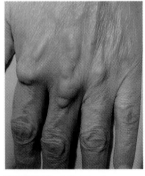

FIGURE 8-10. Tendon xanthomas on extensor tendons of the hand.

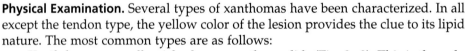

Xanthoma Type	Elevated Plasma Lipids
Xanthelasma	Often none
Eruptive	Triglycerides
Tendon	Cholesterol
Tuberous	Both or either of the above

Laboratory and Biopsy. Diagnosis is usually made clinically. All patients with xanthomas should have a screening fasting lipid profile. In patients with xanthelasma, results are normal in approximately 50%. For the other types of xanthoma, lipid abnormalities are to be expected. Biopsy reveals an infiltrate of numerous lipid-laden histiocytes.

Therapy. Therapy is aimed at lowering the abnormal lipid levels with diet and, for patients with marked lipid elevations, drugs. Xanthelasma lesions may be removed surgically for cosmetic reasons.

Therapy:
Lower lipid level with diet and drugs

Course and Complications. Eruptive xanthomas involute spontaneously after the lowering of the serum triglycerides. The other types of xanthomas are more persistent but may slowly regress if the lipids are lowered.

Eruptive xanthomas usually resolve when triglyceride levels are lowered; other xanthomas are more persistent.

The cutaneous lesions usually have no complications, but the lipid abnormality may have significant systemic complications such as premature myocardial infarction in patients with elevated cholesterol and pancreatitis in patients with marked elevations of serum triglycerides.

Pathogenesis. Xanthomas represent accumulations of lipid-laden histiocytes. The lipid is thought to be extracted from plasma, although some evidence suggests that intracellular lipid synthesis may also be operative in some instances.

Patients with familial hypertriglyceridemia have increased endogenous hepatic production of very low-density lipoproteins (VLDL), which are particles with a high triglyceride content. In these patients, VLDL production is further increased with high carbohydrate or alcohol ingestion, obesity, or diabetes, so triglyceride levels of more than 2,000 mg/mL may be attained. Triglyceride deposits are polar and thereby more susceptible to intracellular lysosomal hydrolases; hence, eruptive xanthomas quickly resolve when the triglyceride level is lowered.

Patients with familial hypercholesterolemia have high levels of circulating low-density lipoproteins (LDL), which are particles with a high cholesterol content. In these patients, the gene affected is the one that controls the synthesis of LDL cell-surface receptors. As a result, LDL cannot be adequately removed from the plasma by cellular uptake. In addition, the cells perceive an intracellular deficiency of LDL and hence are stimulated to produce more LDL, a process resulting in even higher serum levels. Individuals who are heterozygous for this disease have plasma LDL levels that are twice to three times normal levels and develop tendon xanthomas and premature atherosclerotic cardiovascular disease in midlife. Homozygotic patients have plasma LDL levels that are six to eight times normal levels, with cholesterol levels of more than 800 mg/dL, and they develop symptomatic coronary artery disease before the age of 20 years. The nonpolar cholesterol esters are more resistant to degradation and therefore persist both in skin (tendon xanthomas) and in blood vessels (atherosclerosis).

■ KAPOSI'S SARCOMA

Definition. Kaposi's sarcoma is a malignant tumor derived from endothelial cells. It is manifested by multiple vascular tumors that usually first occur in the skin, where they appear as purple macules, plaques, or nodules (Fig. 8–11).

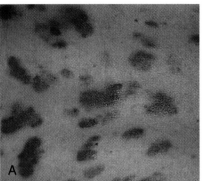
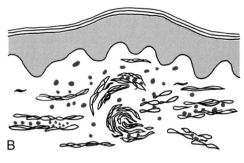

FIGURE 8-11. Kaposi's sarcoma. **A,** Epidermis—normal. Dermis—purple plaque. **B,** Epidermis—normal. Dermis—strands and clusters of spindle cells, hemorrhage, and blood-filled vascular slits.

Types of Kaposi's sarcoma:
1. Classic
2. Lymphadenopathic
3. AIDS-associated

Incidence. The disease occurs in three settings. Classic Kaposi's sarcoma is a chronic cutaneous disorder that occurs primarily in elderly men, usually those of Eastern European descent. This is the type described by Moriz Kaposi in 1872. It remains an uncommon disorder with an annual incidence in the United States of approximately 0.05 per 100,000 population. It affects men 10 to 15 times more often than women and occurs most often in people older than 50 years.

An aggressive lymphadenopathic form primarily occurs in equatorial Africa, where it accounts for approximately 9% of all cancers. This type mainly affects young men and is rapidly fatal.

AIDS-associated Kaposi's sarcoma was first noted in 1979 and represents the most common neoplasm associated with AIDS. Kaposi's sarcoma occurs most frequently in homosexual AIDS patients. In AIDS patients, Kaposi's sarcoma disseminates and is frequently fatal. In the United States, the incidence of Kaposi's sarcoma has been decreasing in AIDS patients in recent years.

Test for HIV in patients newly diagnosed with Kaposi's sarcoma.

History. The skin lesions in Kaposi's sarcoma are usually asymptomatic, so patients seek advice because of concern over appearance or uncertainty about the nature of newly appearing skin lesions. In some patients, Kaposi's sarcoma may be an incidental physical finding. In this setting, it often is the first sign of AIDS, so the physician should obtain a blood test for HIV. Kaposi's sarcoma can also develop in patients receiving immunosuppressive therapy for organ transplantation and other diseases.

Kaposi's sarcoma lesions are purple.

Physical Examination. Lesions in Kaposi's sarcoma may appear as macules, papules, dermal plaques, and nodules. However, in all forms, the lesions are characteristically *purple*. In the classic type of Kaposi's sarcoma, multiple lesions are usually located on the lower legs, where they may be accompanied by edema. In AIDS-associated Kaposi's sarcoma, lesions may occur anywhere on the skin and range in number from one to innumerable. Lymphadenopathy frequently is also present in patients with AIDS. Kaposi's sarcoma may also involve the mucous membranes. When examining the mouth, one should also look for oral hairy leukoplakia (see Chapter 23) as another sign of AIDS. Additional skin manifestations of AIDS are listed in Chapter 25.

Differential Diagnosis. A solitary macule of Kaposi's sarcoma may be subtle and may resemble a *bruise*. Papules and nodules may be confused with benign *hemangiomas*, but hemangiomas usually are redder. *Bacillary angiomatosis* is a condition that also occurs in AIDS patients. It is manifested by red or purple papules that may resemble Kaposi's sarcoma. Biopsy of bacillary angiomatosis, however, shows a benign process, and a Warthin-Starry stain reveals clusters of *Bartonella* bacteria, the same microorganisms that cause cat-scratch disease. Distinguishing bacillary angiomatosis from Kaposi's sarcoma is important because the former is benign and responds to erythromycin therapy.

Biopsy is diagnostic for Kaposi's sarcoma.

Laboratory and Biopsy. The diagnosis of Kaposi's sarcoma is confirmed with a biopsy that shows a proliferation in the dermis of spindle cells arranged in strands and small nodular aggregates. The spindle cells also attempt to form small blood vessels, resulting in slit-like spaces filled with red blood cells. Hemorrhage is common; lymphocytes and histiocytes also may be present. As previously mentioned, patients suspected to have AIDS-associated Kaposi's sarcoma should have an HIV serologic test.

Therapy. Early classic Kaposi's sarcoma may require no therapy or only occasional excision of a papule or nodule. With more advanced cutaneous disease, local radiation therapy is highly effective. Patients with disseminated disease are treated with one or more chemotherapeutic agents.

AIDS-associated Kaposi's sarcoma has been treated with local radiation therapy, cryosurgery, intralesional interferon-α, or intralesional chemotherapy (e.g., vinblastine). Disseminated disease is treated with a combination of zidovudine (AZT) and systemic interferon-α or with systemic chemotherapy using agents such as vincristine, vinblastine, bleomycin, and etoposide, either alone or in combination.

Course and Complications. Classic Kaposi's sarcoma progresses slowly, and because it primarily affects elderly patients, many die of other causes. In the United States, the average survival time for patients with classic Kaposi's sarcoma has been reported to be 8 to 13 years, but much longer times have been noted, and spontaneous remissions have occurred. Patients have an increased frequency of second malignant diseases, especially lymphoma and leukemia.

Lymphadenopathic Kaposi's sarcoma rapidly disseminates to internal organs and results in early death. AIDS-associated Kaposi's sarcoma also disseminates early in its course, but some patients respond to therapy, and many die of other causes, such as opportunistic infections.

Pathogenesis. Kaposi's sarcoma is a malignant disease in which endothelial cells proliferate to form tumors. Multiple tumors apparently result from a multifocal rather than a metastatic process. Immunosuppression may play a permissive role because, in the United States, the disease occurs most frequently in patients who are immunosuppressed by drugs or by AIDS. The findings of Kaposi's sarcoma in several homosexual patients who are HIV negative and the epidemic occur-

---

THERAPY OF KAPOSI'S SARCOMA

- Excision
- Radiation therapy
- Interferon-α (intralesional or systemic)
- Chemotherapy (intralesional or systemic)

rences of lymphadenopathic Kaposi's sarcoma in Africa also suggest an etiologic role for an infectious, transmittable organism. In this regard, human herpesvirus type 8 has now been detected in all forms of Kaposi's sarcoma and so is strongly implicated in the pathogenetic process.

■ OTHER MALIGNANT DERMAL TUMORS

Definition. These tumors result from deposition or proliferation of malignant cells in the dermis. They usually manifest clinically as hard nodules in the skin (Fig. 8–12).

Malignant tumors from endogenous dermal elements are rare. Metastatic tumors are more common.

Incidence. Malignant dermal tumors can be primary or metastatic. Kaposi's sarcoma, as discussed previously, is an example of a primary (albeit multifocal) malignant tumor derived from endothelial cells in the skin. Tumors from other endogenous elements such as collagen (dermatofibrosarcoma protuberans), neural tissue (neurofibrosarcoma), vascular tissue (angiosarcoma), appendageal structures (sweat gland and sebaceous gland carcinomas), and subcutaneous fat (liposarcoma) are all extremely rare and are not discussed except with the usual admonition that for undiagnosed nodules in the skin, a skin biopsy is necessary.

The more common cause of malignant dermal tumors is metastatic disease. We performed a tumor registry survey of 4,020 patients with metastatic carcinoma and found that 420 (10%) had cutaneous metastases. The incidence of metastatic nodules in the skin depends on the type of malignancy. For example, skin involvement is relatively common in acute myelomonocytic leukemia (occurring in 10% to 20% of cases) but uncommon in acute lymphocytic leukemia. Moreover, skin nodules are common in metastatic breast carcinoma but extremely rare in prostatic carcinoma. Table 8–3 lists the tumor types that we found most likely to metastasize to skin.

Skin metastases occasionally are the first sign of internal cancer.

Cutaneous metastases occasionally serve as the *first sign* of an internal malignancy. In a retrospective survey of 7,316 patients with cancer, we found 37 (0.5%) who presented with local (9 cases) or distant (17 cases) metastases as the first manifestation of their cancer. Most had breast cancer.

History. In patients with a known history of internal malignant disease, one should be particularly suspicious of a possible malignant origin of any new skin nodule. The nodules are usually asymptomatic, but the patient may have other signs and

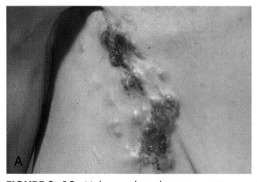
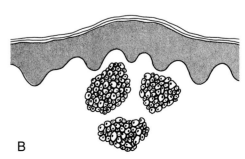

FIGURE 8–12. Malignant dermal tumors. **A,** Metastatic breast carcinoma. Epidermis—normal (occasionally ulcerated). Dermis—firm or hard nodules. **B,** Epidermis—normal. Dermis—dense aggregates of malignant cells.

TABLE 8–3 ■ FREQUENCY OF SKIN METASTASES IN INTERNAL MALIGNANCIES

	Frequency (%)
Malignancy	
Leukemia	
Acute myelomonocytic	10–20
Chronic lymphocytic	5–10
Acute lymphocytic	Rare
Lymphoma (not including mycosis fungoides)	
Non-Hodgkin's	3–20
Hodgkin's	0.5
Multiple myeloma	4
Metastatic carcinoma	10
Type of Carcinoma Responsible for Skin Metastases	
Women	
Breast	73
Melanoma	11
Ovary	3
Oral cavity	2
Lung	2
Men	
Melanoma	34
Lung	12
Large intestine	12
Oral cavity	10

symptoms of malignancy, including weight loss, lymphadenopathy, or symptoms related to the location of the primary tumor.

Physical Examination. Malignant tumors in the dermis are characteristically hard, or at least extremely firm. They vary in color from flesh tones to pink, red, and purple. Skin nodules of lymphoma and myeloma frequently are plum colored (Fig. 8–13). Large nodules sometimes ulcerate. Lymphadenopathy or hepatosplenomegaly may also be present in patients with metastatic disease.

Differential Diagnosis. A malignant tumor in the skin may be confused with any of the benign dermal growths. As is repeatedly emphasized, if any doubt exists, a biopsy is required.

Laboratory and Biopsy. The biopsy is diagnostic, showing an infiltrate of malignant cells, often in nodular aggregates. Occasionally, the histologic features are tumor specific, that is, the likely primary source can sometimes (but by no means always) be suggested by the histology of the skin involvement. Special histochemical stains for cellular components (e.g., keratin) or tumor markers (e.g., carcinoembryonic antigen) may be helpful.

Therapy. For a primary malignant process in the skin, the preferred therapy is surgical excision. Therapy of metastatic disease is that of the primary tumor. The effect of systemic therapy often can be evaluated by measuring the metastatic skin lesion, an easily assessable marker. Troublesome skin metastases sometimes are also treated with palliative radiation or surgery.

Malignant tumors are hard.

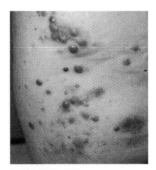

FIGURE 8–13. Cutaneous plasmacytomas: plum-colored papules in a patient with myeloma metastatic to the skin.

Initial therapy:
1. **Excision for primary tumors**
2. **Chemotherapy for metastases**

Course and Complications. For metastatic disease, the course is similar to that of the primary process. For many diseases, the development of skin metastasis indicates a particularly poor prognosis. Acute myelomonocytic leukemia is an example.

The skin nodules of metastatic disease may ulcerate and may become secondarily infected. This condition can lead to sepsis and death. The major complications, however, usually do not result from the skin but from the systemic disease.

Pathogenesis. Spread to the skin from an internal malignant disease usually occurs by a hematogenous route. Some tumors may also reach the skin through lymphatic pathways. Once lodged in the skin, the malignant cells proliferate in a three-dimensional fashion, which is clinically expressed as a nodule. Why some tumors have a greater propensity for the skin than others is not known.

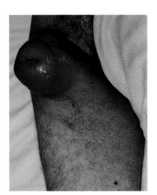

FIGURE 8–14. Unknown.

■ UNKNOWN (Fig. 8–14)

This 50-year-old man sought medical attention because of the large nodule on his right hip. Otherwise, he felt well. On examination, the nodule felt extremely firm. A healing excision from a recent biopsy was present.

What is the most likely diagnosis?

Malignancy must be suspected for all firm dermal nodules. A benign process would be particularly unlikely in this patient because of the size and firmness of the nodule.

What should be done next?

All suspicious nodules must be examined by biopsy. Biopsy of this nodule was initially interpreted as undifferentiated metastatic malignancy, not further classifiable.

Do you see any other skin lesions of note?

The patient was hospitalized to search for the primary tumor. On admission, the housestaff noted on the patient's midthigh a small, darkly pigmented plaque with bluish color, irregular border, and white halo (see Fig. 8–14). Excision and histologic examination of this lesion revealed a primary malignant melanoma. Retrospective review of the original biopsy from the nodule showed it to be metastatic melanoma.

Important Points

1. For firm nodules in the skin, malignancy must be suspected, and biopsy must be performed.

2. A complete skin examination is an important part of every physical examination. In this case, it revealed the source of the primary malignant disease.

REFERENCES

Epidermal Inclusion Cyst

Baldwin HE, Berck CM, Lynfield YL: Subcutaneous nodules of the scalp: preoperative management. J Am Acad Dermatol 25:819–830, 1991.

Knight PJ, Reiner CB: Superficial lumps in children: what, when, and why? Pediatrics 72: 147–153, 1983.

Hemangioma

Alper JC, Holmes LB: The incidence and significance of birthmarks in a cohort of 4,641 newborns. Pediatr Dermatol 1:58–68, 1983.

Ashinoff R, Geronemus RG: Capillary hemangiomas and treatment with the flash lamp-pumped pulsed dye laser. Arch Dermatol 127:202–205, 1991.

Bowers RE, Graham EA, Tomlinson KM: The natural history of the strawberry nevus. Arch Dermatol 82:667–680, 1960.

Enjolras O, Riche MC, Merland JJ: Facial port-wine stains and Sturge-Weber syndrome. Pediatrics 76:48–51, 1985.

Goldman L, Dreffer R: Laser treatment of extensive mixed cavernous and port-wine stains. Arch Dermatol 113:504–505, 1977.

Osburn K, Schosser RH, Everett MA: Congenital pigmented and vascular lesions in newborn infants. J Am Acad Dermatol 16:788–792, 1987.

Dermatofibroma

Fitzpatrick TB, Gilchrest BA: Dimple sign to differentiate benign from malignant pigmented cutaneous lesions. N Engl J Med 296:1518, 1977.

Taylor HB, Helwig EB: Dermatofibrosarcoma protuberans: a study of 115 cases. Cancer 15: 717–725, 1962.

Keloid

Alster TS, West TB: Treatment of scars: a review. Ann Plast Surg 39:418–432, 1997.

Berman B, Bieley H: Adjunct therapies to surgical management of keloids. Dermatol Surg 22:126–130, 1996.

Tredget EE, Nedelec B, Scott PG, et al.: Hypertrophic scars, keloids, and contractures: the cellular and molecular basis for therapy. Surg Clin North Am 77:701–730,1997.

Lipoma

Lin JJ, Lin F: Two entities in angiolipoma: a study of 459 cases of lipoma with review of the literature on infiltrating angiolipoma. Cancer 34:720–727, 1974.

Neurofibroma

Crowe FW, Schull WJ: Diagnostic importance of the café-au-lait spot in neurofibromatosis. Arch Intern Med 91:758–766, 1963.

Gutmann DH, Aylsworth A, Carey JC, et al.: The diagnostic evaluation and multidisciplinary management of neurofibromatosis 1 and neurofibromatosis 2. JAMA 278:51–57, 1997.

Lubs MLE, Bauer MS, Formas ME, Djokic B: Lisch nodules in neurofibromatosis type 1. N Engl J Med 324:1264–1266, 1991.

Mulvihill JJ, Parry DM, Sherman JL, et al.: Neurofibromatosis 1 (Recklinghausen disease) and neurofibromatosis 2 (bilateral acoustic neurofibromatosis). Ann Intern Med 113: 39–52, 1990.

Sorensen SA, Mulvihill JJ, Niwlawn A: Long-term follow-up of Von Recklinghausen neurofibromatosis: survival and malignant neoplasms. N Engl J Med 314:1010–1015, 1986.

Xanthoma

Bergman R: Xanthelasma palpebrum and risk of atherosclerosis. Int J Dermatol 37:343–345, 1998.

Hu C, Ellefson RD, Winkelmann RK: Lipid synthesis in cutaneous xanthoma. J Invest Dermatol 79:80–85, 1982.

Parker F: Xanthomas and hyperlipidemias. J Am Acad Dermatol 13:1–30, 1985.

Kaposi's Sarcoma

Krown SE, Gold JWM, Niedzwiecki D, et al.: Interferon-α with zidovudine: Safety, tolerance, and clinical and virologic effects in patients with Kaposi sarcoma associated with the acquired immunodeficiency syndrome (AIDS). Ann Intern Med 112:812–821,1990.

Martin JN, Ganem DE, Osmond DH, et al.: Sexual transmission and the natural history of human herpesvirus 8 infection. N Engl J Med 338:948–954, 1998.

Serfling U, Hood AF: Local therapies for cutaneous Kaposi's sarcoma in patients with acquired immunodeficiency syndrome. Arch Dermatol 127:1479–1481, 1991.

Tappero JW, Conant MA, Wolfe SF, et al.: Kaposi's sarcoma: epidemiology, pathogenesis, histology, clinical spectrum, staging criteria, and therapy. J Am Acad Dermatol 28:371–395, 1993.

Other Malignant Dermal Tumors

Brownstein MH, Helwig EB: Metastatic tumors of the skin. Cancer 29:1298–1307, 1972.

Kois JM, Sexton FM, Lookingbill DP: Cutaneous manifestations of multiple myeloma. Arch Dermatol 127:69–74, 1991.

Lookingbill DP, Spangler N, Helm KF: Cutaneous metastases in patients with metastatic carcinoma: a retrospective study of 4020 patients. J Am Acad Dermatol 29:228–236,1993.

Lookingbill DP, Spangler N, Sexton FM: Skin involvement as the presenting sign of internal carcinoma: a retrospective study of 7316 cancer patients. J Am Acad Dermatol 22:19–26, 1990.

Shaikh BS, Frantz E, Lookingbill DP: Histologically proven leukemia cutis carries a poor prognosis in acute nonlymphocytic leukemia. Cutis 39:58–60, 1987.

3

RASHES WITH

EPIDERMAL

INVOLVEMENT

∎

ECZEMATOUS RASHES

9

NONSPECIFIC DERMATITIS
CONTACT DERMATITIS
ATOPIC DERMATITIS
SEBORRHEIC DERMATITIS
STASIS DERMATITIS
LICHEN SIMPLEX CHRONICUS

The term *eczema* is derived from a Greek word that means "to boil out or over." It is a convenient "wastebasket" for many undiagnosed rashes but is best applied to epidermal eruptions that are characterized histologically by intercellular edema, called *spongiosis* (Table 9–1). *Eczema and dermatitis* are synonyms. Acute dermatitis has a marked amount of spongiosis causing vesiculation. Subacute dermatitis has less spongiosis, resulting in "juicy papules." Chronic dermatitis has a markedly thickened epidermis *(lichenification)* with only slight spongiosis.

The hallmarks of dermatitis are marked pruritus, indistinct borders (except for contact dermatitis), and epidermal changes characterized by vesicles, juicy papules, or lichenification. Dermatitis may be localized or diffuse; it may be idiopathic or may have a specific cause. Contact allergy is the best-understood cause of an eczematous reaction and potentially is the most correctable. For any eczematous rash, the first question to be asked is, "Could it be contact dermatitis?"

> **Types of dermatitis:**
> 1. **Acute—vesicles**
> 2. **Subacute—juicy papules**
> 3. **Chronic—lichenification**

> **If it does not itch, reconsider the diagnosis of dermatitis.**

■ NONSPECIFIC DERMATITIS

Definition. Nonspecific dermatitis is an epidermal eruption that may be acute (Fig. 9–1) or chronic (Fig. 9–2) and localized or generalized. It is a diagnosis that is made by exclusion when an underlying cause such as an allergen or an irritant cannot be found, and its distribution is not typical of defined eczematous eruptions such as atopic or seborrheic dermatitis.

Incidence. Nonspecific dermatitis is one of the eruptions most frequently seen by the clinician. Eleven percent of our patients had this diagnosis.

History. Itching is the chief complaint prompting patients to seek medical attention. It is often severe enough to interfere with normal daily activities and to interrupt sleep. The itching may be episodic or constant. The patient frequently

TABLE 9–1 ■ ECZEMATOUS ERUPTIONS

	Frequency*	History	Physical Examination	Differential Diagnosis	Laboratory Test
Nonspecific dermatitis	11.4	Pruritus	Acute: vesicles, weeping, crusted patches Subacute: juicy papules Chronic: lichenified, scaling plaques	Contact dermatitis Atopic dermatitis Seborrheic dermatitis Fungal infection Psoriasis Drug rash	—
Contact dermatitis	2.8	Irritant: contact precedes rash by hours to days Allergic: contact precedes rash by 1–4 days	Vesicles, juicy papules, lichenified plaques Sharp margins Geometric or linear configuration Conforms to area of contact	Eczematous dermatitis Fungal infection Cellulitis	Patch test
Atopic dermatitis	2.6	Allergic rhinitis Asthma	Vesicles, juicy papules—infants Lichenified plaques—adults and older children Head, neck, antecubital and popliteal fossa	Contact dermatitis Scabies	IgE
Seborrheic dermatitis	3.7	Dandruff	Scaling papules and patches Scalp, eyebrows, nose, sternum	Atopic dermatitis Psoriasis Fungal infection Histiocytosis X Lupus erythematosus	—
Stasis dermatitis	0.4	Varicose veins Leg swelling Thrombophlebitis	Juicy papules Lichenified plaques Brown pigmentation Lower legs	Cellulitis Contact dermatitis Arterial disease Fungal infection	—
Lichen simplex chronicus	0.8	Rash subsequent to pruritus	Lichenified plaque within reach of fingers	Psoriasis	—

*Percentage of new dermatology patients with this diagnosis seen in the Hershey Medical Center Dermatology Clinic, Hershey, PA.

has a history of "sensitive skin" that is intolerant to topical preparations such as moisturizers, soaps, and detergents.

Physical Examination. The varied appearance of nonspecific dermatitis occurs because of its evolution from an acute to a chronic process. Acutely, intercellular edema leads to vesiculation. Chronically, lichenification occurs. The polymorphism is manifested by vesicles, juicy papules, and plaques. Secondary changes

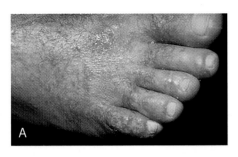
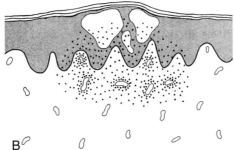

FIGURE 9–1. Nonspecific dermatitis (acute). **A,** Epidermis—vesicles. Dermis—erythema. **B,** Epidermis—vesicles, spongiosis. Dermis—perivascular inflammation.

include oozing, crusting, scaling, and fissuring. Characteristic of nonspecific dermatitis is the indistinct border between normal and abnormal skin.

Depending on the morphology and location, various types of dermatitis have been classified. *Dyshidrotic eczema* is characterized by deep-seated vesicles (which resemble the pearls in tapioca pudding) involving the palms, soles, and sides of the digits. It occurs bilaterally and symmetrically. *Autosensitization* or *id eruption* is a generalized subacute dermatitis that follows a localized acute dermatitis, usually of the feet or hands. It is thought to be a hypersensitivity reaction to a substance produced by the acute dermatitis. *Xerotic eczema* (Fig. 9–3) is the result of low humidity and dry skin. It occurs in the winter and is manifested by dry fissured skin of the trunk and extremities. It particularly affects the elderly and the lower legs of all age groups. *Nummular eczema* is characterized by oval, weeping, patches with crusted papulovesicles. It occurs on the trunk and extremities.

Types of idiopathic eczemas:
1. **Dyshidrotic**
2. **Autosensitization**
3. **Xerotic**
4. **Nummular**

Differential Diagnosis. The differential diagnosis of an acute vesiculopapular dermatitis includes, first, *contact dermatitis*. Also to be considered are infectious processes by a *dermatophyte, herpes simplex virus, varicella-zoster virus,* or *bacteria,* as in impetigo. The appearance of rectangular or linear areas of dermatitis would lead one to suspect contact dermatitis. Removal of the top of the vesicle or scales from the edge of the patch for potassium hydroxide (KOH) examination reveals the typical hyphae of a fungal infection. Scraping the base of the vesicle for a Tzanck preparation reveals the multinucleated giant cells of herpesvirus, which clinically

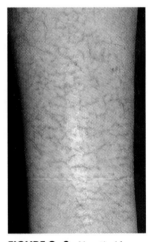

FIGURE 9–3. Xerotic (dry skin) eczema.

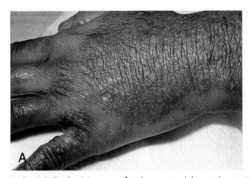
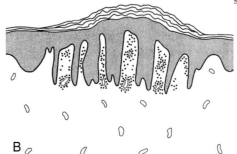

FIGURE 9–2. Nonspecific dermatitis (chronic). **A,** Epidermis—lichenified, scale. Dermis—erythema. **B,** Epidermis—thickened, hyperkeratosis. Dermis—perivascular inflammation.

appear as grouped vesicles on an erythematous base. Impetigo can be ruled out by a Gram stain or culture of the yellow crusts typical of this infectious process.

The differential diagnosis of chronic nonspecific dermatitis includes chronic *contact dermatitis*, *psoriasis*, *drug eruption*, and *fungal infection*. The history and patch tests differentiate chronic nonspecific dermatitis from contact dermatitis. Clinically, psoriasis is usually easy to distinguish by its sharply demarcated, silvery scaling plaques that affect but are not limited to the scalp, elbows, and knees. In any nonspecific dermatitis, one should consider drugs as the cause. Discontinuation of medication with subsequent clearing is the only reliable way to rule out a drug eruption. Fungal infections of the skin can mimic dermatitis, especially if lesions are treated with topical steroids. Any scaling patch, particularly if it has an annular inflammatory border, should be scraped and the scale should be examined for fungal hyphae (KOH preparation).

Spongiosis is the histologic hallmark of eczema.

Biopsy. The histologic hallmark of dermatitis is intercellular edema of the epidermis leading to widening of intercellular spaces with a sponge-like appearance of the epidermis (spongiosis). When the process is acute and severe, it results in intraepidermal vesicle formation. When it is chronic, the epidermis becomes hyperkeratotic and thickened (acanthotic). The dermis is characterized by a lymphocytic infiltrate.

Avoid the use of long-term systemic steroids because of systemic side effects.

Therapy. Corticosteroids are the cornerstone of dermatitis treatment. They may be applied topically, injected intralesionally, or administered systemically. Steroid creams are used for acute papulovesicular eczema, whereas ointments are better for chronic lichenified dermatitis. Therapy with topical steroids such as hydrocortisone 1% (Hytone), triamcinolone 0.1% (Kenalog), and fluocinonide 0.05% (Lidex) are discussed in detail in Chapter 5. Thick, hyperkeratotic plaques that are unresponsive to topical steroids may be injected with intralesional steroids (Kenalog 10). This should be done cautiously because skin atrophy may occur. Severe, widespread acute or subacute dermatitis is most effectively treated with prednisone, but long-term use must be avoided if possible. In adults, prednisone, starting at a dosage of 40 to 60 mg daily and tapered over 2 to 4 weeks, is usually effective. Topical steroids may be added during the tapering period for recurrence of small areas of dermatitis. An alternative to prednisone is triamcinolone at a dose of 40 mg intramuscularly (Kenalog-40), which has an effect for 2 to 4 weeks. Again, long-term administration should be avoided.

Astringent dressings (Domeboro) applied for 15 minutes twice daily are helpful in treating acute weeping dermatitis. For widespread dermatitis, baths have a soothing effect on the skin by reducing inflammation and oozing and by removing crust and scaling. Colloidal oatmeal (Aveeno) or tar (Cūtar) may be added to the bath water. Patients should soak in the bath for 15 to 20 minutes once or twice daily and should apply a steroid to the dermatitis *immediately* after towel drying.

Itching is a prominent component of dermatitis and must be reduced to prevent scratching. Antihistamines such as hydroxyzine (Atarax) or diphenhydramine (Benadryl) can be used three or four times daily, particularly at bedtime. The nonsedating antihistamines, unfortunately, are not effective in reducing pruritus.

Secondary bacterial infections with *Staphylococcus aureus* often complicate dermatitis, in which case a course of erythromycin, dicloxacillin, or cephalexin for 7 days is indicated. Penicillin is *not* prescribed because *S. aureus* is usually resistant to this antibiotic. Impetiginized eczema has yellow crusting, purulent weeping, and pustules.

THERAPY OF NONSPECIFIC DERMATITIS

- Steroids
    - Topical
        - Hydrocortisone 1% (lowest potency)
        - Triamcinolone 0.1% (medium potency)
        - Fluocinonide 0.05% (high potency)
    - Intralesional
        - Triamcinolone suspension (Kenalog-10)
    - Systemic
        - Prednisone: 1 mg/kg/day or 40–60 mg/day in adults
        - Triamcinolone suspension (Kenalog-40): 1 mL, IM
- Antihistamines
    - Hydroxyzine: 10–25 mg QID; syrup, 10 mg/5 mL–2 mg/kg/day in 4 divided doses
    - Diphenhydramine: 25–50 mg QID; elixir, 12.5 mg/5 mL–5 mg/kg/day in 4 divided doses
- Baths and compresses
    - Oatmeal
    - Tar
    - Aluminum acetate
- Antibiotics if secondary infection
    - Dicloxacillin: 500 mg BID
    - Erythromycin: 500 mg BID
    - Cephalexin: 500 mg BID; suspension, 250 mg/5 mL–25–50 mg/kg/day in divided doses

Pathogenesis. The cause of nonspecific dermatitis is unknown. Scratching results in histamine release, which causes more itching, more dermatitis, and a chronic, self-perpetuating eruption.

■ CONTACT DERMATITIS

Definition. Contact dermatitis (Fig. 9–4) is an inflammatory reaction of the skin precipitated by an exogenous chemical. The two types of contact dermatitis are irritant and allergic. *Irritant contact dermatitis* is produced by a substance that has a direct toxic effect on the skin. *Allergic contact dermatitis* triggers an immunologic reaction that causes tissue inflammation. Examples of irritants include acids, alkalis, solvents, and detergents. Innumerable chemicals cause allergic contact dermatitis, including metals, plants, medicines, cosmetics, and rubber compounds. Clinical appearance can range from acute (vesicles) to chronic (lichenification) eczematous reactions.

Types of contact dermatitis:
1. Irritant
2. Allergic

Incidence. Contact dermatitis is a frequent problem that most people experience during their lifetime. Statistics from industry indicate that it accounts for more

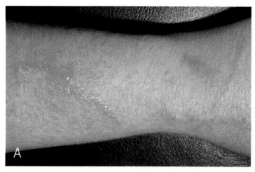
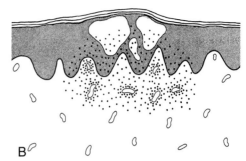

FIGURE 9–4. Contact dermatitis. **A,** Epidermis—vesicles. Dermis—erythema. **B,** Epidermis—vesicles, spongiosis. Dermis—perivascular inflammation.

than 40% of all occupational illness (excluding injury) and one fourth of all time lost from work. One of every 1,000 workers is affected by contact dermatitis, and the total cost of this condition is millions of dollars per year. In occupational contact dermatitis, approximately 70% is irritant and 30% is allergic.

Causes of allergic contact dermatitis:
1. **Poison ivy or oak**
2. **Cosmetics**
3. **Nickel**
4. **Rubber compounds**
5. **Medications**

History. One should first determine whether the contact dermatitis is an allergic or an irritant phenomenon. Skin damage is usually evident within several hours after contact with a strong irritant. Weaker irritants, however, may require multiple applications and days before the development of dermatitis. Allergic contact dermatitis usually requires 24 to 48 hours after exposure before the development of clinical disease. Occasionally, the dermatitis may develop as soon as 8 to 12 hours after contact or may be delayed as long as 4 to 7 days. The history of a precipitating contactant may be either obvious or obscure. Detailed history of occupation, hygienic habits, and hobbies is frequently necessary to find the contactant.

The most common sensitizers are poison ivy or oak, cosmetics, nickel, rubber compounds, and medications.

Poison ivy or *oak* is a frequent cause of allergic contact dermatitis in the summer (Fig. 9–5). The sensitizing allergens are pentadecylcatechol and heptadecylcatechol, chemicals located in the sap (oleoresin-urushiol) of the plant. Another familiar member of this family of poisonous plants is poison sumac. Less frequently recognized family members are cashew, mango, lacquer, and ginkgo trees. Sensitization to poison ivy results in sensitivity to the other poisonous plants in this family. The characteristic eruption resulting from contact with poison ivy or oak is manifested by linear streaks of papules and vesicles. Contact with the smoke of burning plants can result in confluent severe dermatitis of the exposed skin.

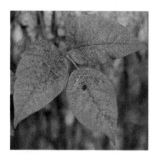

FIGURE 9–5. Poison ivy plant.

Cosmetics contain fragrances and preservatives that cause allergic contact dermatitis, particularly affecting the faces of women from the use of make-up and moisturizers, for example. Paraphenylenediamine is a dye found in permanent hair coloring. Sensitization to paraphenylenediamine occurs in hairdressers and in clients who have their hair colored. When completely oxidized, as the dye on a fur coat, paraphenylenediamine is not allergenic.

Nickel sensitivity is most often seen in women as a result of wearing "cheap" pierced earrings. It is found in many metal alloys (Fig. 9–6). One cannot be certain that the commonly advertised "hypoallergenic" earrings are nickel free. Although stainless steel contains nickel, it is bound so tightly that it usually does not allow an allergic reaction to occur.

Rubber compounds are ubiquitous. Shoes and gloves are the most common sources of allergic contact dermatitis caused by these chemicals. An eczematous reaction limited to the feet or hands is typical of shoe and glove dermatitis, respectively. The most frequent rubber allergens are *mercaptobenzothiazole* and *thiuram*.

In sleuthing the causes of contact dermatitis, one must not overlook the possibility of a topical medication perpetuating or exacerbating a pre-existing dermatitis. *Neomycin* and *bacitracin*, found in topical antibiotic preparations, cause allergic contact dermatitis when these agents are used to treat cuts and abrasions, chronic ulcers, and surgical wounds. *Ethylenediamine* is the preservative contained in the original Mycolog cream. The frequent use of this topical agent resulted in sensitization to ethylenediamine in many individuals. Mycolog-II does not contain ethylenediamine, but generic nystatin creams still contain this allergen. Other sources of ethylenediamine are widespread. Industrial exposure can occur through dyes, insecticides, rubber accelerators, synthetic waxes, and resins. Of importance to physicians, ethylenediamine is the preservative used in aminophylline. An ethylenediamine-sensitive patient who is given aminophylline may develop generalized eczematous dermatitis.

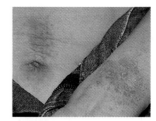

FIGURE 9–6. Allergic contact dermatitis in response to nickel found in a metal snap and a watch band.

Physical Examination. Contact dermatitis may be acute or chronic. The configuration of the lesions depends on the nature of the exposure, which may result in patches or plaques with angular corners, geometric outlines, and sharp margins. Poison ivy or oak characteristically causes linear streaks of papulovesicles.

The location of the dermatitis is helpful in predicting the causative irritant or allergen. The head and neck are frequent sites of contact dermatitis from fragrances and preservatives found in cosmetics. Hair dyes, permanent wave solutions, and shampoos produce dermatitis on the scalp. Eczema of the eyelids is caused by eye cosmetics or allergens that have been transferred from the hands, such as nail polish. Photoallergic contact dermatitis from sunscreens and fragrances is produced by a photoreaction between sunlight and an allergen in exposed areas of the skin, such as the head, neck, V-shaped area of the chest, and arms. The hands are the most common area of contact dermatitis from industrial chemicals, particularly an irritant reaction from petroleum products and solvents. Dermatitis of the feet is produced by allergens in shoes, such as rubber chemicals and leather tanning agents. The groin and buttocks in infants are frequently affected by diaper dermatitis (Fig. 9–7). This condition is an irritant contact dermatitis from moisture and feces. Diaper dermatitis is often complicated by secondary infection with bacteria and yeast.

Streaks of vesicles are characteristic of contact dermatitis to poison ivy or oak.

The location of the dermatitis often provides a clue to the nature of the contactant.

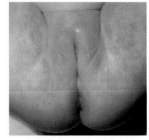

FIGURE 9–7. Irritant contact dermatitis (diaper dermatitis).

Differential Diagnosis. Morphologically, contact dermatitis is identical to other *eczematous eruptions* and may complicate atopic or stasis dermatitis if the patient becomes sensitized to the topical preparation used to treat these dermatoses. Other causes of eczematous-appearing dermatoses that may need to be ruled out include superficial *fungal infections* and *bacterial cellulitis*. In bacterial cellulitis, the skin is painful (rather than pruritic), and the patient is often febrile.

For any dermatitis, ask, "Could it be contact dermatitis?"

Laboratory and Biopsy. No standard testing method is available for diagnosing irritant contact dermatitis. For allergic contact dermatitis, the causative agent can be identified by patch tests, but these tests must be properly performed and interpreted (see Chapter 4). Patch testing is done with a screening patch test series

Patch tests help in identifying the responsible allergen or allergens.

(T.R.U.E. test). This series is composed of medications, fragrances, preservatives, metals, rubber compounds, and miscellaneous chemicals. Individual chemicals and special trays (e.g., allergens found in plants) supplement the screening series. The chemicals are applied to patches that are taped on the back of the test subject. After 48 hours, the patches are removed, and the test site is examined for an eczematous reaction that is graded according to a standard interpretation key: a +1 reaction indicates palpable erythema, a +2 reaction indicates papules and vesicles, and a +3 reaction indicates bullae. Another delayed reading 1 to 2 days after patch test removal is mandatory. Although the patch testing procedure is simple, its interpretation is often difficult. A positive patch test must be relevant to the eruption to be meaningful. Unknown chemicals and potential irritants must be patch tested cautiously and are best left to trained personnel who have experience in patch testing.

Biopsy of contact dermatitis cannot differentiate between irritant and allergic causes. Contact dermatitis also cannot be histologically differentiated from other causes of eczematous eruptions such as atopic or seborrheic dermatitis.

Therapy. Prevention of contact dermatitis is the most logical, but often most difficult, solution. Avoidance of an irritant or allergen may require a change in lifestyle or occupation. Sometimes, protective clothing is curative. Allergens that have high sensitizing potential are best used in closed systems in which workers have virtually no contact with the offending chemicals. Protective or barrier creams (Ivy Block, Pro Q) are of benefit when matched to the contactant they block. Sometimes, the offending material can be substituted with another, less toxic or allergenic chemical. Predictive testing for contact irritancy or sensitivity is standard procedure before introducing new cosmetics or chemicals. Immunization is a promising mode of therapy, although no *scientifically proven* preparations are available to hyposensitize persons who are sensitive to poison ivy or poison oak. Application of IvyBlock before exposure, however, reduces the development of poison ivy or oak dermatitis.

Acute severe, generalized contact dermatitis is treated with a short course of systemic steroids: 40 to 60 mg prednisone daily for a *minimum* of 5 days and then tapered over the next 5 days or 1 mL triamcinolone suspension (Kenalog-40) intramuscularly. Astringent dressings (Domeboro) or soothing baths (Aveeno) reduce weeping and itching. Milder dermatitis responds to topical steroids (see Table 5–1). Systemic antihistamines such as 10 to 25 mg hydroxyzine (Atarax) or 25 to 50 mg diphenhydramine (Benadryl) four times daily are helpful for pruritus.

THERAPY OF CONTACT DERMATITIS

- Avoidance of irritant or allergen
- Protective clothing—gloves, etc.
- Barrier creams
    - IvyBlock—poison ivy and oak
    - Pro Q—detergents
- Steroids, antihistamines, baths, and compresses
    - (See Therapy of Nonspecific Dermatitis)

Course and Complications. Acute allergic contact dermatitis subsides within 3 to 4 weeks. If the patient has repeated exposure to the contactant, chronic dermatitis will develop. With the breakdown of the epidermal barrier, secondary bacterial infection may complicate contact dermatitis. Although contact dermatitis may start locally, generalized hypersensitivity of the skin can occur, with resultant generalized dermatitis autosensitization.

Pathogenesis. Irritant contact dermatitis is a nonspecific inflammatory reaction resulting from toxic injury of the skin. Allergic contact dermatitis is a cell-mediated, delayed type IV immunologic reaction. It is divided into a sensitization phase and an elicitation phase. The sensitization phase occurs when a chemical (hapten) is applied to the skin of a nonsensitized individual. This chemical in itself is unable to induce an allergic reaction because of its small molecular size, which is usually less than 500 daltons. It must combine with an epidermal protein thought to be on the surface of the Langerhans cell (epidermal macrophage). After the formation of the hapten-protein complex, the Langerhans cell presents the allergen to T-lymphocytes in the lymph node, where effector, memory, and suppressor lymphocytes are produced. The period of sensitization requires approximately 7 to 10 days. The elicitation phase occurs in sensitized individuals 1 to 2 days after reexposure to the antigen. After presentation of the antigen by Langerhans cells to memory T-cells in the skin, effector T-cells produce lymphokines, which recruit other inflammatory cells and produce allergic contact dermatitis. The dermatitis usually appears clinically 1 to 2 days after the elicitation exposure. The reaction is thought to be ultimately extinguished by suppressor T-cells.

> **Allergic contact dermatitis is a cell-mediated, delayed type IV immunologic reaction.**

■ ATOPIC DERMATITIS

Definition. Atopic dermatitis is a chronic, pruritic, eczematous condition of the skin that is associated with a personal or family history of atopic disease (e.g., asthma, allergic rhinitis, or atopic dermatitis). The origin of atopic dermatitis is unknown, but patients appear to have a genetic predisposition that can be exacerbated by numerous factors, including food allergy, skin infections, irritating clothes or chemicals, change in climate, and emotions. Lichenification is the clinical hallmark of chronic atopic dermatitis (Fig. 9–8).

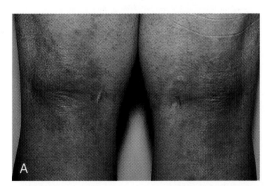
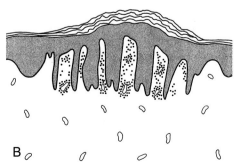

FIGURE 9–8. Atopic dermatitis. **A,** Epidermis—lichenification, scaling. Dermis—erythema. **B,** Epidermis—thickened, hyperkeratosis. Dermis—perivascular inflammation.

Incidence. Atopic dermatitis is predominantly a disease of childhood, with 5% of children affected. It usually starts after 2 months of age, and by 5 years of age, 90% of the patients who will develop atopic dermatitis have manifested the disease. It is uncommon for adults to develop atopic dermatitis without a history of eczema in childhood.

History. A history of allergic respiratory disease is found in one third of patients with atopic dermatitis and in two thirds of their family members. Pruritus is the most distressing and prominent symptom (Table 9–2).

> **Lichenification is the clinical hallmark of chronic atopic dermatitis.**

Physical Examination. The morphology and distribution of atopic dermatitis are age dependent (Fig. 9–9). Infantile atopic dermatitis is characterized by acute-to-subacute eczema with papules, vesicles, oozing, and crusting. It is distributed over the head, diaper area, and extensor surfaces of the extremities. In children and adults, the eruption is a chronic dermatitis with lichenification and scaling. The distribution includes the neck, face, upper chest, and, characteristically, antecubital and popliteal fossae (see Fig. 9–8).

Atopic individuals have a characteristic expression. The face has mild-to-moderate erythema, perioral pallor, and infraorbital folds (Dennie-Morgan lines) associated with dermatitis and hyperpigmentation. The skin generally is dry and may have generalized fine, whitish scaling. The palms often have increased linear markings.

> **Atopic dermatitis in infants is papular or vesicular; in children and adults, it is lichenified, especially affecting the antecubital and popliteal fossae.**

Differential Diagnosis. The differential diagnosis of atopic dermatitis includes other eczematous eruptions and *scabies*. The history of other family members with pruritus and a thorough skin examination that reveals burrows, particularly on the hands, are diagnostic of scabies. Infants with *histiocytosis X* and immunodeficiency syndromes such as *Wiskott-Aldrich syndrome, ataxia-telangiectasia,* and *Swiss-type agammaglobulinemia* have dermatitis that resembles atopic dermatitis, but these conditions are rare, and the infants have systemic symptoms that distinguish their conditions from atopic dermatitis.

Laboratory and Biopsy. The diagnosis of atopic dermatitis is made clinically. The skin biopsy (rarely required) reveals an eczematous change that is not specific for atopic dermatitis. Serum immunoglobulin (Ig) E frequently is elevated but usually is not necessary to make the diagnosis.

> **To be successful, treatment must eliminate pruritus.**

Therapy. The treatment of atopic dermatitis is the same as for other eczematous eruptions and includes topical steroids and systemic antihistamines. These should be given in appropriate strength and frequency to reduce inflammation and itching significantly. A common error is undertreatment. Occasionally, a short course of systemic steroids is necessary to bring the disease under control. Wet dressings (plain water) and baths (Aveeno) are helpful in treating acute atopic dermatitis. Avoidance of environmental factors that enhance itching, such as wool clothes,

---

TABLE 9–2 ■ DIAGNOSTIC CRITERIA FOR ATOPIC DERMATITIS

Pruritus
Typical morphology and distribution
    Flexural lichenification in adults and older children
    Facial and extensor papulovesicles in infancy
Chronic—relapsing course
Personal or family history of atopic disease

emotional stress, and uncomfortable climatic conditions, is important. Moisturizers reduce dry skin and itching. Tacrolimus ointment, ultraviolet radiation B (UVB), or psoralen plus ultraviolet radiation A (PUVA) may be considered if satisfactory control is not achieved with initial treatment.

In some children, food allergy can cause atopic dermatitis. Skin testing or radioallergosorbent tests may help to identify foods that are responsible. Positive tests must be confirmed with controlled food challenges and elimination diets. Eggs, peanuts, milk, and wheat appear to be the most frequent offending foods. Investigators have suggested that atopic dermatitis can be prevented by avoiding cow's milk, wheat, and eggs for the first 6 months of life. However, this approach is controversial and not generally recommended. Patients with atopic dermatitis have a higher frequency of immediate skin test reactivity in general, but hyposensitization is rarely of value in atopic dermatitis. As a last resort, severe atopic dermatitis is treated with azathioprine or cyclosporine.

Course and Complications. Atopic dermatitis is a chronic disease punctuated by repeated acute flare-ups followed by longer periods of slow resolution. The cause of these flare-ups is frequently unknown, a feature that adds to the frustration of this disease. Most children (90%) outgrow their disease by adolescence, although as adults, some continue to have localized forms of atopic dermatitis such as chronic hand or foot dermatitis, patches of lichen simplex chronicus, or eyelid dermatitis.

Atopic dermatitis is frequently complicated by skin infections. Atopic skin has a higher rate of colonization with *S. aureus*. The most serious cutaneous infection is *Kaposi's varicelliform eruption*. This widespread vesiculopustular eruption is caused by herpes simplex, variola, or vaccinia virus. Patients with this infection are acutely ill and may die; for this reason, smallpox immunization was contraindicated in these patients. The *hyper-IgE syndrome* refers to a syndrome of atopic dermatitis characterized by recurrent pyoderma (skin infections), elevated serum IgE, and decreased chemotaxis of mononuclear cells.

Pathogenesis. Disturbed immunology and abnormal vascular response have been implicated in the etiology of atopic dermatitis. Neither of these mechanisms alone or in combination can completely account for the clinical findings.

The immunologic changes are most notable and frequent in patients with severe atopic dermatitis. These changes include elevation of serum IgE, defective cell-mediated immunity, decreased chemotaxis of mononuclear cells, elevated T-lymphocyte activation, and hyperstimulatory Langerhans cells. The elevation of IgE is thought to reflect decreased T-suppressor cells and uninhibited production of IgE. Depressed cell-mediated immunity is manifested by increased susceptibility to cutaneous viral and bacterial infections. In addition, in vitro tests of cell-mediated immunity such as lymphocyte blastogenesis to mitogens and antigens are blunted. Food allergy in atopic individuals is thought to occur during the first months of life, when a transient deficiency of IgA in the bowel exists. This situation allows antigens (e.g., cow's milk) to gain access to the immune system, with the production of specific IgE antibodies and dermatitis. This is the rationale for breast feeding and dietary discretion for the first 6 months of life.

The vascular abnormalities are explained by disturbances in the autonomic nervous system in the skin. Nicotinic acid and cholinergic agents, when applied or injected into the skin of patients with atopic dermatitis, result in a white blanch rather than a red flare. However, this result is not specific for atopic dermatitis because it also occurs in allergic contact dermatitis. Blockade of the autonomic

Bacterial and viral skin infections are common in atopic dermatitis.

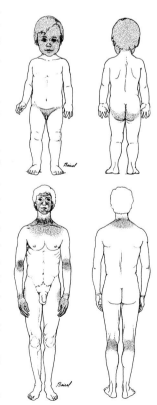

FIGURE 9–9. Distribution of atopic dermatitis.

THERAPY OF ATOPIC DERMATITIS

- Steroids, antihistamines, baths, compresses, and antibiotics
  (See Therapy of Nonspecific Dermatitis)
- Avoidance of irritants—wool clothes, harsh soaps, uncomfortable climate
- Moisturizers
- Avoidance of food allergens—(eggs, peanuts, milk, wheat) in selected patients
- Tacrolimus ointment
- Ultraviolet light—UVB, PUVA
- Immunomodulants—azathioprine, cyclosporine

nervous system has been the explanation for these vascular changes, but the actual mechanism and pathogenic importance are unknown.

■ SEBORRHEIC DERMATITIS

Definition. Seborrheic dermatitis is a chronic, superficial, inflammatory process affecting the hairy regions of the body, especially the scalp, eyebrows, and face (Fig. 9–10). Its cause is thought to be an inflammatory reaction to the yeast *Pityrosporum ovale*. Dandruff is scaling of the scalp without inflammation.

***Pityrosporum ovale* may contribute to the cause of seborrheic dermatitis.**

Incidence. Seborrheic dermatitis is a common problem affecting 3% to 5% of the healthy population.

History. The occurrence of seborrheic dermatitis parallels the increased sebaceous gland activity occurring in infancy and after puberty. It has a waxing and waning course with a variable amount of pruritus. It has been associated with Parkinson's disease and AIDS. Approximately one third of patients with AIDS and AIDS-related complex have seborrheic dermatitis.

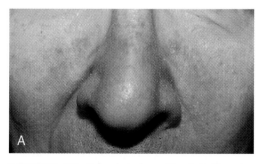
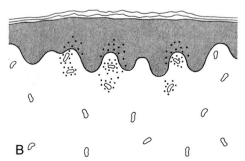

FIGURE 9–10. Seborrheic dermatitis. **A,** Epidermis—scaling. Dermis—erythema. **B,** Epidermis—hyperkeratosis. Dermis—perivascular inflammation.

Physical Examination. Seborrheic dermatitis has a predilection for the hairy regions of the skin, where sebaceous glands are numerous (Fig. 9–11). These regions are the scalp, eyebrows, eyelids, nasolabial creases, ears, chest, intertriginous areas, axilla, groin, buttocks, and inframammary folds. The rash is bilateral and symmetrically distributed. In its mildest form, dandruff, one sees fine, white scale without erythema. The patches and plaques of seborrheic dermatitis are characterized by indistinct margins, mild-to-moderate erythema, and yellowish, greasy scaling. It is uncommon for hair loss to result from seborrheic dermatitis.

Differential Diagnosis. The differential diagnosis of seborrheic dermatitis includes atopic dermatitis, psoriasis, tinea capitis, histiocytosis X, lupus erythematosus, and rosacea. The distinction between *seborrheic dermatitis* and *atopic dermatitis* in infancy is often difficult, so many clinicians use the term "infantile eczema." When the dermatitis involves solely the diaper area and axillae, a diagnosis of seborrheic dermatitis is favored. Lesions on the forearms and shins favor the diagnosis of atopic dermatitis. *Psoriasis* may also enter into the differential diagnosis. Psoriasis limited to the scalp may be impossible to differentiate from seborrheic dermatitis. Involvement of nails, knees, and elbows favors the diagnosis of psoriasis. *Tinea capitis* should be considered in the differential diagnosis of seborrheic dermatitis, especially when the usual antiseborrheic agents have failed, when the patient has hair loss, and when the patient is a black person living in an urban area. *Otitis externa* usually is not due to a fungal infection but rather is a manifestation of seborrheic dermatitis. *Histiocytosis X*, an uncommon Langerhans cell neoplasm, may appear as a seborrheic dermatitis–like eruption. The occurrence of petechiae and the failure of standard therapy should make one suspect this cancer and obtain a skin biopsy. Facial involvement with seborrheic dermatitis may mimic lupus erythematosus or rosacea. *Lupus erythematosus* lacks yellowish, greasy scales and generally does not involve the eyebrows, as does seborrheic dermatitis. If in doubt, the history, physical examination, laboratory tests, and skin biopsy will rule out lupus. *Rosacea* has inflammatory papules and pustules not seen in seborrheic dermatitis.

Laboratory and Biopsy. Seborrheic dermatitis usually is not examined by biopsy unless concern exists about the possibility of another disease such as histiocytosis X. The histopathologic changes in seborrheic dermatitis are those of dermatitis and therefore are nondiagnostic with reference to other eczematous conditions.

Therapy. Antiseborrheic shampoos containing zinc pyrithione, selenium sulfide, or ketoconazole are the mainstay of treatment. Some over-the-counter shampoos are available. Some examples are 1% selenium sulfide (Selsun Blue, Head & Shoulders Intensive Treatment) and 1% zinc pyrithione (Head & Shoulders). We prefer either the over-the-counter zinc pyrithione products or the prescription shampoos containing 2.5% selenium sulfide (Selsun, Exsel) or 2% ketoconazole (Nizoral). The shampoo must be rubbed into the wet scalp, rinsed, and then reapplied for 3 to 5 minutes before the final rinse. Patients with inflammatory seborrheic dermatitis that has not responded to shampoos benefit from a topical steroid lotion or gel in hairy areas and hydrocortisone cream or ketoconazole cream for nonhairy skin. High-potency steroids are contraindicated, particularly on the face.

Course and Complications. In infants, seborrheic dermatitis can be expected to remit after 6 to 8 months. In adults, the course is chronic and unpredictable. However, it is usually easily controlled with shampoos and topical hydrocortisone preparations. Rarely, it can cause widespread exfoliative dermatitis. In infants, the

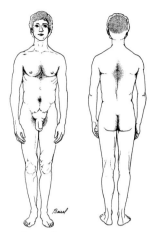

FIGURE 9–11. Distribution of seborrheic dermatitis.

Seborrheic dermatitis is the most common cause of a "butterfly" rash.

High-potency steroid creams should be avoided in the treatment of seborrheic dermatitis.

THERAPY OF SEBORRHEIC DERMATITIS

- Shampoos—2 or 3 times/week
  Zinc pyrithione 1%
  Selenium sulfide 1% or 2.5%
  Ketoconazole 1% or 2%
- Hydrocortisone cream 1% or 2.5%—BID as needed
- Ketoconazole cream 2%—BID as needed

---

association of a seborrhea-like dermatitis with failure to thrive and diarrhea is called *Leiner's disease.*

Pathogenesis. The pathogenesis of seborrheic dermatitis is thought to be an inflammatory reaction to the resident skin yeast *Pityrosporum ovale.* This lipophilic yeast is normally found on the seborrheic regions of skin, and proliferation is believed to play a role in this disease. The most effective antiseborrheic shampoos have antifungal activity against these yeast organisms.

■ STASIS DERMATITIS

Characteristics of stasis dermatitis:
1. **Edema**
2. **Brown pigmentation**
3. **Petechiae**
4. **Subacute and chronic dermatitis**

Definition. Stasis dermatitis is an eczematous eruption of the lower legs secondary to peripheral venous disease (Fig. 9–12). Venous incompetence causes increased hydrostatic pressure and capillary damage with extravasation of red blood cells and serum. In some patients, this condition causes an inflammatory eczematous process.

Incidence. Stasis dermatitis is a disease of adults, predominantly of middle and old age.

History. Patients have a history of a chronic, pruritic eruption of the lower legs preceded by edema and swelling. Patients with stasis dermatitis often have had thrombophlebitis.

Physical Examination. Varicose veins are often prominent, as is pitting edema of the lower leg. The peripheral pulses are intact. The involved skin has brownish hyperpigmentation, dull erythema, petechiae, thickened skin, scaling, or weeping. Any portion of the lower leg may be affected, but the predominant site is above the medial malleolus.

Differential Diagnosis. *Contact dermatitis, superficial fungal infection,* and *bacterial cellulitis* must be considered in the differential diagnosis of stasis dermatitis. The history of application of a topical preparation to the skin and KOH testing will help to differentiate the first two conditions from stasis dermatitis. Gram stains and bacterial cultures from bacterial cellulitis may be helpful but often are negative. An acute onset with fever particularly favors bacterial cellulitis.

Laboratory and Biopsy. The diagnosis of stasis dermatitis is usually made clinically. The biopsy shows a subacute or chronic dermatitis with hemosiderin, fibrosis, and dilated capillaries in the dermis. Vascular laboratory studies may be used to assess for peripheral vascular disease (see Chapter 20).

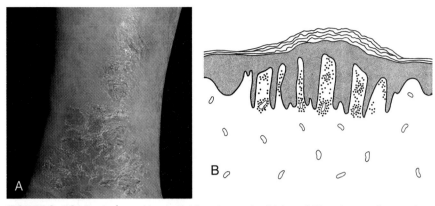

FIGURE 9–12. Stasis dermatitis. **A,** Epidermis—scale, thickened. Dermis—erythema, pigmentation. **B,** Epidermis—hyperkeratosis, thickened. Dermis—perivascular inflammation.

Therapy. The cornerstone of stasis dermatitis management is the prevention of venous stasis and edema. This is done by use of supportive hose (Jobst) while the patient is ambulatory. Standing should be restricted, and patients who are obese should be placed on weight-reduction programs. If this approach fails, bed rest with elevation of the legs is required. The dermatitic skin is treated with topical steroids (Kenalog, Lidex) and wet compresses (Domeboro) if oozing or crusting is present.

Course and Complications. Stasis dermatitis is a chronic and slowly progressive disease unless treated. Dusky erythema in areas of stasis dermatitis is the harbinger of leg ulceration.

Allergy to topical preparations occurs in 60% of patients with stasis dermatitis. The compromised epidermal barrier from stasis allows sensitization to occur more easily than in normal skin. Contact dermatitis can easily be misdiagnosed as a flare-up of stasis dermatitis. Topical antibiotics are particularly prone to cause allergic contact dermatitis.

> **Of patients with stasis dermatitis, 60% develop allergies to topical medications.**

Pathogenesis. Venous incompetence results in increased venous pressure of the lower legs. This increased hydrostatic pressure results in swelling and edema. Capillary proliferation and leakage of red blood cells and vascular fluids result in inflammation. If the condition is unchecked, fibrin deposition will occur around the capillaries, resulting in tissue hypoxia, sclerosis, and necrosis with ulceration.

■ LICHEN SIMPLEX CHRONICUS

Definition. Lichen simplex chronicus (also called "neurodermatitis") is a chronic eczematous eruption of the skin that is the result of scratching (Fig. 9–13). Pruritus precedes the scratching and is precipitated by frustration, depression, and stress. The scratching then causes the lichenification and further itching, resulting in an "itch-scratch-itch" cycle that perpetuates the process.

> **Itching typically precedes the rash of lichen simplex chronicus.**

Incidence. Of all new patients seen in our clinic, 0.8% have presented with lichen simplex chronicus.

THERAPY OF STASIS DERMATITIS

- Reduction of leg edema
    Support stocking (custom-fitted, knee high, medium pressure)
    Leg elevation
- Topical steroids
    Triamcinolone 0.1%
    Fluocinonide 0.05%
- Compresses
    Aluminum acetate
- Avoidance of prolonged use of topical antibiotics

History. Some patients with lichen simplex chronicus have a history of emotional or psychiatric problems. However, for most, it is simply a nervous habit. Preceding the eruption, the patient has a pruritic area of skin that is scratched, producing a plaque of chronic dermatitis.

Physical Examination. The patient may appear anxious and may talk with pressured speech. There usually is little insight into the cause of the eruption. The lichenified plaque always occurs within reach of scratching fingers.

Types of "psychodermatoses":
1. **Lichen simplex chronicus**
2. **Neurotic excoriations**
3. **Factitious dermatitis**
4. **Delusions of parasitosis**

Differential Diagnosis. The diagnosis of lichen simplex chronicus is usually obvious in patients who have a localized itching plaque of chronic dermatitis. Several more serious "psychodermatoses" are neurotic excoriations, factitious dermatitis, and delusions of parasitosis.

Neurotic excoriations (Fig. 9–14) are characterized by linear, "dug-out" lesions that typically spare the upper midback, where scratching fingers cannot reach. Patients usually are neurotic women.

Factitious dermatitis is a self-inflicted injury of the skin that presents as a bizarre eruption (often ulcerated) with linear and geometric outlines. The patient's history is vague and unclear. The diagnosis is made when the clinician has a high

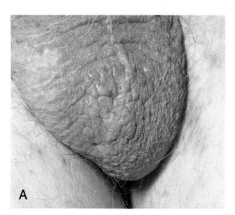
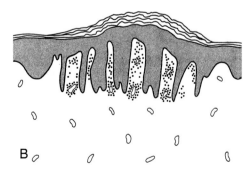

FIGURE 9–13. Lichen simplex chronicus. **A,** Epidermis—lichenification. Dermis—erythema. **B,** Epidermis—thickened. Dermis—perivascular inflammation.

THERAPY OF LICHEN SIMPLEX CHRONICUS

- Steroids
  - Topical under occlusion
  - Intralesional — triamcinolone suspension: 10 mg/mL
- Buspirone: 5–10 mg TID
- Emotional support

---

index of suspicion in a patient who has apparent secondary gain from perpetuating the condition.

Delusions of parasitosis occur in disturbed or anxious eccentric individuals. This disorder begins as intractable pruritus with a crawling sensation in the skin. The patients are convinced that they are harboring parasites and usually bring "specimens" to prove infestation. These bits of material or skin must be examined to rule out a true infestation and to assure the patient of your interest in the problem. More than half these patients have no visible skin lesions. Those with active lesions have excoriated, crusted papules secondary to picking.

Laboratory and Biopsy. The biopsy in lichen simplex chronicus is nonspecific, showing only chronic dermatitis.

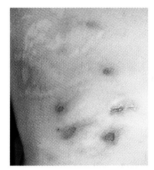

FIGURE 9–14. Neurotic excoriations.

Therapy. Treatment may be difficult, particularly if the patient has poor insight concerning the nature and cause of the eruption. Topical steroids under occlusion (Cordran tape) and intralesional steroids (triamcinolone [Kenalog-10]) are helpful. Cordran tape, a plastic tape with the steroid incorporated into its adhesive, is beneficial because the tape protects the area from scratching fingers as well as providing a topical steroid. Tranquilizers (buspirone [BuSpar]) and antidepressants have a role in treating underlying emotional difficulties if such conditions are present.

Course and Complications. Lichen simplex chronicus is a chronic, waxing and waning problem that accompanies the mood changes of the patient.

■ UNKNOWN

This 40-year-old man was using povidone-iodine ointment dressings on a non-healing wound. Two weeks after starting this therapy, he developed a markedly pruritic eruption under the dressing. The physical examination revealed a 3-cm necrotic ulcer with a surrounding erythematous, papulovesicular rash conforming to the rectangular area covered by the povidone-iodine dressing (Fig. 9–15).

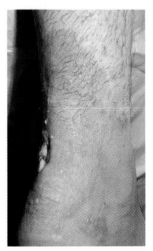

FIGURE 9–15. Unknown.

What is your differential diagnosis?

This eczematous eruption confined to the area underneath the dressing is typical of contact dermatitis. A less likely cause would be a fungal or bacterial infection.

How would you treat the patient?

The dermatitis cleared when the povidone-iodine dressings were replaced with saline compresses and a topical steroid cream.

How would you prove your diagnosis?

The patient had no history of iodine sensitivity. However, he had been applying the povidone-iodine dressing for 2 weeks, which is sufficient time to develop sensitivity to this compound. A patch test to 10% povidone-iodine solution was positive, confirming the diagnosis of allergic contact dermatitis.

Important Points

1. Topical medicaments are an important cause of allergic contact dermatitis and should be suspected when an eczematous eruption occurs in areas that conform to application of the medication.
2. Avoidance of the allergen is the treatment of choice. Topical steroids hasten resolution of allergic contact dermatitis.
3. Patch testing confirms the diagnosis of allergic contact dermatitis.

REFERENCES

Contact Dermatitis

Drake LA, Dorner W, Goltz RW, et al.: Guidelines of care for contact dermatitis. J Am Acad Dermatol. 32:109–113, 1995.
Kalish RS: Recent developments in the pathogenesis of allergic contact dermatitis. Arch Dermatol. 127:1558–1563, 1991.
Marks JG, DeLeo VA: Contact and Occupational Dermatology. 2nd ed. St. Louis, Mosby–Year Book, 1997.
Marks JG, Martini MC: Contact dermatitis and contact urticaria. In Sams WM, Lynch PJ (eds.): Principles and Practice of Dermatology. 2nd ed. New York, Churchill Livingstone, 1996, pp. 419–430.

Atopic Dermatitis

Drake LA, Ceilley, RI, Cornelison RL, et al.: Guidelines of care for atopic dermatitis. J Am Acad Dermatol 26:485–488, 1992.
Hanifin JM: Atopic dermatitis: new therapeutic considerations. J Am Acad Dermatol 24:1097–1101, 1991.
Hanifin JM, Cooper KD, Roth HL: Atopy and atopic dermatitis. J Am Acad Dermatol 15:703–706, 1986.
Morren MA, Przybilla B, Bamelis M, et al.: Atopic dermatitis: triggering factors. J Am Acad Dermatol 31:467–473, 1994.
Rajka G: Atopic Dermatitis. Philadelphia, WB Saunders, 1975.
Rasmussen JE: Advances in nondietary management of children with atopic dermatitis. Pediatr Dermatol 6:210–215, 1989.
Rothe MJ, Grant-Kels JM: Atopic dermatitis: an update. J Am Acad Dermatol 35:1–13, 1996.
Ruzicka T, Bieber T, Schöpf E, et al.: A short-term trial of tacrolimus ointment for atopic dermatitis. N Engl J Med 337:816–821, 1997.

Seborrheic Dermatitis

Danby FW, Maddin WS, Margesson LJ, et al.: A randomized, double-blind, placebo-controlled trial of ketoconazole 2% shampoo versus selenium sulfide 2.5% shampoo in the treatment of moderate to severe dandruff. J Am Acad Dermatol 29:1008–1012, 1993.

Heng MCY, Henderson CL, Barker DC, Haberfelde G: Correlation of *Pityrosporum* ovale density with clinical severity of seborrheic dermatitis as assessed by a simplified technique. J Am Acad Dermatol 23:82–86, 1990.

VanCutsem J, Van Gerven F, Fransen J, Schrooten P, Janssen PAJ: The *in vitro* antifungal activity of ketoconazole, zinc pyrithione, and selenium sulfide against *Pityrosporum* and their efficacy as a shampoo in the treatment of experimental pityrosporosis in guinea pigs. J Am Acad Dermatol 22:993–998, 1990.

Stasis Dermatitis

Browse NL, Burnand KG: Hypothesis: the cause of venous ulceration. Lancet 2:243–245, 1982.

Fraki JE, Peltonen L, Hopsu-Havu VK: Allergy to various components of topical preparations in stasis dermatitis and leg ulcer. Contact Dermatitis 5:97–100, 1979.

Kitahama A, Elliott LF, Kerstein MD, et al.: Leg ulcer: conservative management or surgical treatment? JAMA 247:197–199, 1982.

Lichen Simplex Chronicus

Cotterill JA (ed.): Psychodermatology. J Semin Dermatol 2:171–226, 1983.

Driscoll MS, Rothe MJ, Grant-Kels JM, et al.: Delusional parasitosis: a dermatologic, psychiatric, and pharmacologic approach. J Am Acad Dermatol 29:1023–1033, 1993.

Zomer SF, DeWit RFE, Van Bronswijk JEHM, et al.: Delusions of parasitosis: a psychiatric disorder to be treated by dermatologists? An analysis of 33 patients. Br J Dermatol 138:1030–1032, 1998.

10

SCALING PAPULES, PLAQUES, AND PATCHES

■

PSORIASIS
FUNGAL INFECTIONS
    Tinea Corporis
    Tinea Cruris
    Tinea Pedis
    Tinea Manuum
    Tinea Faciale
PITYRIASIS ROSEA
SECONDARY SYPHILIS
MYCOSIS FUNGOIDES
DISCOID LUPUS ERYTHEMATOSUS

In papulosquamous lesions, the borders are sharply demarcated; in eczematous lesions, they are not.

Scale is the common characteristic of the diseases discussed in this chapter. Scaling disorders have also been called the papulosquamous (squamous means scaly) diseases. As previously emphasized, *scale* represents thickened stratum corneum and is to be distinguished from *crust*, which represents dried surface fluid, as is found in the vesicular and pustular disorders. The elevation of scaling papules and plaques results from thickening of the epidermis (acanthosis) or underlying dermal inflammation. A *patch* is a scaling macule. It is flat because it has no epidermal thickening (the epidermis may even be atrophic) and little dermal inflammation.

The papulosquamous disorders have diverse causes, as seen in Table 10–1. The lesions, in addition to being scaly, are sharply demarcated. The latter feature helps to distinguish them from scaling lesions of eczematous dermatitis, in which the borders usually are indistinct. Exceptions are *nummular (coin-shaped) eczema*, which can resemble tinea corporis, and *seborrheic dermatitis*, which in the scalp can be confused with psoriasis and on the chest can be confused with tinea corporis. *Lichen planus* often is also included in the papulosquamous disorders, but usually the scale is not readily evident, so we have designated this disease as a papular disorder (see Chapter 12). *Tinea versicolor* can appear as finely scaling patches, but patients more often present because the lesions appear as white spots; hence, this disease is discussed in Chapter 14.

The diagnostic approach to sealing diseases should include consideration of the distribution of the lesions and sometimes also the presence or absence of nail and mucous membrane involvement. Of the laboratory tests that are listed, the

TABLE 10–1 ■ SCALING PAPULES, PLAQUES, AND PATCHES*

	Frequency†	Etiology	Physical Examination — Appearance of Lesions	Physical Examination — Characteristic Distribution	Differential Diagnosis	Laboratory Test
Psoriasis	5.2	Unknown	Erythematous plaques with *silvery scales*	Anywhere: Scalp, elbows, knees, and *intergluteal cleft* are favored locations. Nails often involved	Seborrheic dermatitis (scalp) Fungal infection (nails)	
Fungus	2.5	Infection (dermatophyte)	*Annular* patches with elevated borders surmounted by scale	Anywhere	(See Table 10–2)	Potassium hydroxide preparation Fungal culture
Pityriasis rosea	1.1	Unknown	Tannish-pink *oval* papules and plaques with delicate *collarette of scale*; rash preceded by *herald patch*	"Christmas tree" pattern on trunk, spares face and distal extremities	Secondary syphilis Tinea corporis	
Secondary syphilis	<0.1	Infection (spirochete)	*Red-brown* or *copper-colored* scaling papules and plaques sometimes annular in shape	Generalized, *palms* and *soles* often included Mucous membranes sometimes involved	Pityriasis rosea Lichen planus Drug eruption	Serologic test for syphilis
Mycosis fungoides	0.2	Neoplastic (lymphoma)	*Yellowish-red* or *violaceous*, irregularly shaped patches and plaques with only slight scale	*Asymmetric:* Girdle area often the first area involved	Psoriasis Eczematous dermatitis	Biopsy
Lupus, discoid	0.2	"Autoimmune"	Red to *purplish* papules and plaques with adherent scale and *follicular plugging*, older lesions atrophic	Sun-exposed areas favored	Psoriasis	Biopsy with immunofluorescence Antinuclear antibodies

*See also discussions of seborrheic dermatitis (Chapter 9), lichen planus (Chapter 12), and tinea versicolor (Chapter 14).
†Percentage of new dermatology patients with this diagnosis seen in the Hershey Medical Center Dermatology Clinic, Hershey, PA.

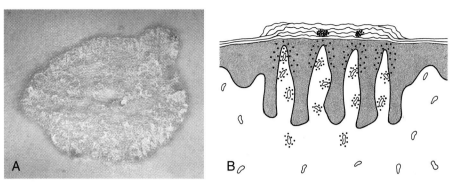

FIGURE 10–1. **A,** Epidermis—plaque with silvery scales. Dermis—erythema. **B,** Epidermis—hyperkeratosis, acanthosis with elongated rete pegs, and infiltration by neutrophils, forming microabscesses in the stratum corneum. Dermis—capillary proliferation with perivascular inflammation.

For scaling rashes of uncertain etiology, "If it scales, scrape it!"

one that should be done most frequently is a potassium hydroxide (KOH) preparation of the scale to look for fungal elements. The general rule for scaling rashes of uncertain etiology is "If it scales, scrape it!"

■ PSORIASIS

Definition. Psoriasis is an inflammatory rash with increased epidermal proliferation resulting in an accumulation of stratum corneum (Fig. 10–1). The etiology is unknown. The clinical appearance is that of sharply demarcated, erythematous papules and plaques, surmounted by silvery scales.

Incidence. The prevalence in the general population is 0.6%. Psoriasis may begin at any age but is most common in adults, with an average onset at age 35 years.

History. The disease usually starts gradually, although occasionally it is explosive in onset or exacerbation. The sudden appearance of multiple small (guttate) lesions of psoriasis in a generalized distribution is often preceded by a streptococcal throat infection. In patients with severe sudden onset or rapidly worsening large-plaque psoriasis, a predisposing HIV infection should be considered: 1% of patients with AIDS develop severe psoriasis, and sometimes the psoriasis is the presenting manifestation of AIDS. Other aggravating factors that have been implicated in psoriasis include trauma to the skin that precipitates a psoriatic lesion (Koebner phenomenon) and emotional stress, which, although difficult to document scientifically, is believed by many patients to be a contributing factor. A few drugs have been found to aggravate psoriasis. Lithium is the best proven culprit, but β-blockers and nonsteroidal anti-inflammatory drugs have also been implicated. Itching (psoriasis is derived from the Greek word for itching) ranges from mild to severe. A family history of psoriasis can be elicited from approximately one third of patients.

Physical Examination. The lesions are sharply demarcated, erythematous papules and plaques surmounted by scale, which characteristically is silvery. In intertriginous areas, maceration prevents scales from accumulating, but the lesions remain red and sharply defined. Psoriasis is classically distributed on the scalp, elbows,

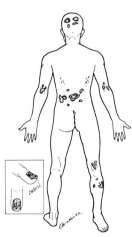

FIGURE 10–2. Typical distribution of psoriasis. The intergluteal cleft is a common location.

and knees (Fig. 10–2). The intergluteal cleft is also a common site that is frequently overlooked (Fig. 10–3). Although these are typical sites, psoriatic lesions can occur anywhere and can cover the entire skin surface.

The intergluteal cleft is often involved in psoriasis.

Nail involvement is present in as many as 50% of patients with psoriasis. The nails can be pitted with small, ice pick–like depressions in the nail plate. Onycholysis (separation of nail plate from the nail bed) can also occur. This condition is caused by a plaque of psoriasis in the distal nail bed with accumulation of scale that lifts the plate from the nail bed.

Pustular psoriasis is an uncommon variant. In this form of the disease, superficial pustules occur in one of three presentations: (1) pustules studding more typical plaques, (2) pustules confined to the palms and soles, and (3) a rare generalized eruption in which the pustules erupt abruptly on large areas of erythematous skin and are accompanied by fever and leukocytosis.

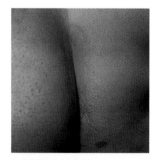

FIGURE 10–3. Psoriasis of the intergluteal cleft. Scales are not seen in intertriginous skin.

Differential Diagnosis. Diagnosis usually is not difficult, especially when the lesions have the characteristic silvery scale and involve the typical locations. It may be more difficult when scale is not present, as in extremely early lesions or in lesions in the intertriginous areas. Intertriginous lesions may be confused with *tinea cruris, candidiasis,* and *intertrigo* (see the discussion of tinea cruris later in this chapter). Psoriasis of the scalp (Fig. 10–4) is most often confused with *seborrheic dermatitis,* in which the scaling is usually finer, yellower, and more diffuse. Guttate psoriasis on the trunk is sometimes confused with *pityriasis rosea.* Nail involvement may be clinically indistinguishable from a *fungal infection;* a positive KOH preparation or fungal culture enables one to diagnose the latter.

Laboratory and Biopsy. A biopsy usually is not necessary; in fact, the clinical picture often is more characteristic than the histologic findings. If a biopsy is performed, the pathologic examination shows hyperkeratosis, parakeratosis, decreased granular layer with an acanthotic epidermis, and inflammatory infiltrate in the dermis that includes neutrophils, some of which may migrate into and through the epidermis, forming small collections within the stratum corneum (Munro's abscesses).

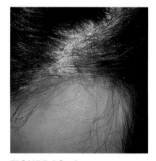

FIGURE 10–4. Psoriasis of the scalp.

Therapy. The goal of therapy is to decrease the epidermal proliferation and the underlying dermal inflammation. Five types of topical agents are used: steroids, tar and anthralin preparations, calcipotriene (a vitamin D derivative), tazarotene (a vitamin A derivative), and ultraviolet (UV) light.

Topical steroids are both antimitotic and anti-inflammatory. Over-the-counter hydrocortisone preparations are ineffective, and the stronger, "fluorinated" preparations are required (see Chapter 5). These agents are expensive but are useful in patients with limited areas of involvement. A good response is usually noted within several weeks, but tachyphylaxis (loss of effect with continued use of a drug) often develops. Therefore, for long-term use of topical steroids, we instruct patients to use an intermittent regimen—for example, use the agent only 2 of every 3 weeks. This practice may also reduce the potential for developing steroid atrophy of the skin. Psoriasis also responds to systemic steroids, but these should be avoided because of their well-known long-term side effects and because psoriasis often rebounds badly after the drug is discontinued.

Initial therapy:
1. Topical steroids
2. Tars

Topical tars and *anthralin* are hydrocarbons with antimitotic activity; tars can also be anti-inflammatory. These products can stain skin (temporarily) and fabrics (permanently) and are slow to produce a response, but the responses that are achieved tend to last longer, and tachyphylaxis is less likely to develop than with topical steroids. Tar oil (Balnetar, Cūtar) added to a bath is a convenient way to

THERAPY OF PSORIASIS

Topical
- Steroids—midpotency to strong potency (e.g., triamcinolone cream 0.1% BID)
- Tars and anthralin
    5% LCD in Aquaphor daily or Micanol 1% cream daily
- Vitamin D derivative
    Calcipotriene ointment 0.005% daily
- Retinoid
    Tazarotene gel 0.05% or 0.1% daily
- Ultraviolet B light

Systemic
- Psoralens with ultraviolet A (PUVA)
- Methotrexate
- Retinoid (acitretin)
- Cyclosporine

apply tar to the total skin surface. The patient should be advised, however, that these tar oils stain plastic (but not porcelain) bathtubs. Tar preparations applied directly to the skin may be more effective than tar baths but are messier to use. Hence, we instruct patients to apply tar at bedtime. Commercial tar preparations are available, but we more often prescribe a compounded preparation containing a tar liquid—5% liquor carbonis detergens—contained in Aquaphor. To this, 3% salicylic acid may be added as a keratolytic to help remove thick scales if they are present. Anthralin is commercially available in a cream (Drithocreme) preparation ranging in concentrations from 0.1% to 1.0%. Because of potential irritancy, this therapy is initiated with the low concentrations and is advanced as tolerated. A 30-minute, short-contact regimen can be used, but we usually suggest an overnight application. Skin irritation and staining are the main disadvantages of anthralin therapy. Micanol cream is a newer anthralin formulation with reduced side effects, but possibly also reduced efficacy.

Calcipotriene (Dovonex ointment, cream, and lotion) is a vitamin D derivative with antimiotic activity. It is applied twice daily and requires several months of use for full effect. Some patients respond well, but many do not. It is expensive and may cause irritation, but it is otherwise safe for long-term use in limited-plaque disease.

Tazarotene (Tazorac gel 0.05% and 0.1%) is a retinoid that is the most recent addition to the list of topical agents available for psoriasis. In general, retinoids promote differentiation and inhibit proliferation—desirable effects for an anti-psoriatic drug. Topical tazarotene is applied at bedtime, often in conjunction with a topical steroid in the morning. It is effective for many patients, but it is also extremely expensive and may cause irritation (that is ameliorated by the morning steroid). Tazaroc gel is also rated category X for pregnancy, so it should not be used in women with childbearing potential.

Short-wave UV light (UVB) therapy can be used alone or in combination with tar therapy. The least expensive source of UVB is the sun. UV light theory therapy also can be provided in the offices of many dermatologists and hospital physical therapy departments. Some patients find it convenient to purchase a UVB unit for their use at home during the winter months. Commercial units designed for this purpose are available but should be used only with a physician's guidance.

Four systemic agents are approved for use in psoriasis. All are reserved for patients with severe widespread disease that is poorly responsive to topical measures.

Psoralen in combination with long-wave UV light (PUVA) is the least toxic systemic approach, but it requires frequent office visits. The psoralen drug intercalates between the DNA strands and binds to them during irradiation with UVA. Therefore, although when the drug is taken by mouth it reaches all the body's tissues, only those tissues that receive the UV radiation (i.e., the skin and the eyes, unless shielded) are affected. This treatment could result in cataracts, so the eyes must be protected with special glasses. The major long-term concerns involve premature aging of the skin and the development of skin cancers, including melanoma.

Methotrexate, a folate antagonist, inhibits cellular proliferation and is highly effective in many patients with psoriasis. It is administered on a weekly schedule. Complete blood cell counts need to be monitored at frequent intervals. The major long-term concern is liver toxicity, so regular liver function blood tests and intermittent liver biopsies are required. Familiarity with methotrexate and careful follow-up of patients are necessary to avoid serious side effects of this drug.

Acitretin (Soriatane) is a retinoid with profound effects on keratinization. It is administered orally on a daily basis and is particularly effective for pustular psoriasis. Acitretin often improves but seldom clears the more common plaque-type psoriasis. It can be used in conjunction with PUVA for additive effect. Acitretin is a *teratogen*, and it is not safe for use in women with childbearing potential. Additional common side effects include drying of skin and mucous membranes, hair loss, peeling of palms and soles, bony hyperostoses, and numerous other less common problems including effects on bones, eyes, liver, and blood lipids. In addition, the medication is expensive.

Systemic *cyclosporine* (Neoral) is a drug used to prevent rejection of transplanted organs. It is also approved for treating psoriasis and is effective in this role. It is, however, expensive and potentially nephrotoxic.

Course and Complications. Psoriasis is a chronic condition that waxes and wanes, frequently without obvious cause. Perhaps because of the favorable influence of sunlight, many patients note that their psoriasis is better in summer and worse in winter. With the foregoing therapies, the disease can usually be controlled, although not cured. This skin disease, like many others, can be socially stigmatizing and, in some individuals, physically disabling.

Psoriatic skin is often colonized with *Staphylococcus aureus*. With scratching, secondary infection occasionally occurs. Uncommonly, psoriasis affects the total body surface, resulting in erythroderma with its associated complications, which include loss of heat, fluid, and protein; hospitalization may be required.

Arthritis accompanies psoriasis in approximately 5% of patients. It classically affects the distal interphalangeal joints, but more often it occurs as asymmetric arthritis involving small and medium-sized joints. Ankylosing spondylitis can also occur in psoriatic arthritis. Psoriatic arthritis is usually treated with nonsteroidal anti-inflammatory drugs, although these sometimes aggravate the skin lesions. Methotrexate is often useful for psoriatic arthritis and is particularly indicated in the rapidly destructive type—arthritis mutilans.

Systemic agents for psoriasis are reserved for patients with severe disease.

Arthritis accompanies psoriasis in approximately 5% of patients. Five clinical types are recognized:
1. **Asymmetric small and medium-sized joint involvement**
2. **Distal interphalangeal joint disease**
3. **Rheumatoid arthritis–like**
4. **Ankylosing spondylitis**
5. **Mutilating**

Pathogenesis. Many patients with psoriasis are genetically predisposed. Thirty-five percent have a family history of psoriasis, and in identical twins the disease occurs concurrently in 80%. The precipitating factors responsible for unmasking this genetic predisposition, however, are largely unknown. Whether the initiating event in psoriasis occurs in the epidermis or in the dermis is debated. Some investigators have proposed that mediators such as proteases are released in the epidermis, and these provoke epidermal proliferation and the underlying inflammatory response. The clinical Koebner phenomenon has been used to support this hypothesis. Others have implicated the dermal inflammatory process as being primary in the evolution of a psoriatic lesion. Investigators have noted that neutrophils extravasated from the superficial dermal capillaries invade the epidermis, and this appears to be followed by the epidermal proliferation. Elevated levels of leukotrienes (one of the products of arachidonic acid metabolism) have been found in psoriatic skin, where, as mediators of inflammation, they may attract neutrophils and may provoke epidermal proliferation. Autoantibodies directed against stratum corneum have also been implicated as playing a possible role in the pathogenesis of psoriasis.

T-cell mechanisms have been strongly implicated. Many experimental data now suggest that psoriasis may be a T-cell–mediated autoimmune disease. The therapeutic effectiveness of cyclosporine, a T-cell–targeted drug, supports this theory.

Whatever the provocation, the end result for the epidermis is an accelerated cell cycle or an increased number of cycling cells recruited from the normal resting cell population. This leads to an increased number of dividing cells, culminating in an orgy of epidermal proliferation. Cellular turnover is increased sevenfold, and the transit time from the basal layer to the top of the stratum corneum is decreased from the normal 28 days to 3 or 4 days. This process is too fast for the cells to be shed, so they accumulate, resulting in the characteristic scale.

> **In a psoriatic plaque, epidermal cell production is increased sevenfold.**

■ FUNGAL INFECTIONS

> **Synonyms for a fungal infection of the skin:**
> 1. **Dermatophytosis**
> 2. **Tinea**
> 3. **"Ringworm"**

Definition. These disorders result from infection of the skin by fungal organisms collectively called dermatophytes (*phyte* is the Greek word for plant). Various clinical lesions can result, but the most common are scaling, erythematous papules, plaques, and patches, which often have a serpiginous or worm-like border. The word *tinea* (Latin for worm) is used for these superficial fungal infections. It is followed by a qualifying term that denotes the location of the infection on the body. For example, tinea capitis is a fungal infection of the scalp, and tinea pedis is a dermatophyte infection of the feet. Tinea versicolor is the only exception; its name derives from the several shades of color that lesions may have in this disease.

Incidence. Dermatophytic infections are common, in aggregate representing 2.5% of our new patients. The incidence is higher in warmer, more humid climates. Table 10–2 gives the prevalence of four of the more common skin and fungal infections in the general population in the United States.

History. In most dermatophytic infections, the patient presents with a scaling rash. Pruritus is common and often the chief complaint. A history of exposure to infected persons or other mammals (e.g., dogs, cats, cattle) may be elicited.

TABLE 10–2 ■ FUNGAL INFECTIONS

Name	Prevalence in General Population* (rate/1,000)	Location	Clinical Appearance (Types 1, 2, and 3)	Differential Diagnosis (Types 1, 2, and 3)
Tinea capitis†		Scalp	1. Round, scaling area of alopecia 2. Diffuse scaling 3. Red, boggy, swollen area with pustules (kerion)	1. Alopecia areata 2. Seborrheic dermatitis 3. Bacterial infection
Tinea corporis		Body	Annular, "ringworm"	Nummular eczema Pityriasis rosea (herald patch)
Tinea cruris	7	Groin	Sharply demarcated area with elevated, scaling, serpiginous borders	Psoriasis Impetigo Intertrigo Candidiasis
Tinea pedis	39	Feet	1. Interdigital maceration 2. Diffuse scaling on soles and sides of feet ("moccasin") 3. Vesicles and pustules on instep	1. Hyperhidrosis 2. Dry skin 3. Contact dermatitis Dyshidrotic eczema
Tinea manuum		Hand	Diffuse dry scaling, usually on only one palm	Contact dermatitis Psoriasis
Tinea faciale		Face	Slightly scaling, erythematous patches and plaques; border may not be well demarcated in all areas	Photodermatitis Lupus erythematosus Seborrheic dermatitis
Tinea unguium (onychomycosis)‡	22	Nails	Subungual debris with separation from the nail bed	Psoriasis Trauma
Tinea versicolor§	8	Trunk	White, tan, or pink patches with fine desquamating scale	Vitiligo (white) Seborrheic dermatitis (tan or pink)

*Data from the United States National Health Survey, 1978.
†See Chapter 21.
‡See Chapter 22.
§See Chapter 14.

Physical Examination. The physical findings and differential diagnosis vary with the different tineas. The findings in tinea capitis are discussed in Chapter 21 and in tinea unguium in Chapter 22. Because tinea versicolor most often presents as white spots, it is discussed in Chapter 14. The physical findings and differential diagnosis of the remaining dermatophyte infections are now discussed.

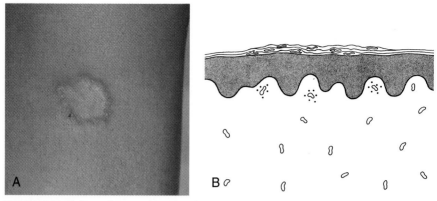

FIGURE 10–5. Tinea Corporis (ringworm). **A,** Epidermis—elevated, scaling border. Dermis—erythema. **B,** Epidermis—thickened stratum corneum infiltrated with fungal hyphae. Dermis—inflammation.

Tinea Corporis

Tinea corporis (Fig. 10–5) is the classic "ringworm." It occurs most often in children. Often, patients have a history of exposure to an infected animal such as a pet dog or cat.

Physical Examination. The typical lesion is annular, with an elevated, scaling border and tendency for central clearing. One or several lesions may be present. In patients predisposed to chronic infection, the eruption may be widespread, and not all the lesions may be annular. In these instances, the finding of elevated serpiginous borders in some of the lesions is a helpful clue (Fig. 10–6).

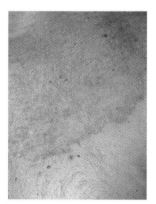

FIGURE 10–6. Tinea Corporis with serpiginous scaling border.

Differential Diagnosis. The coin-shaped lesions of *nummular eczema* are usually multiple and are located on the extremities. They are often mistaken by the patient, and sometimes by the physician, as ringworm. In nummular eczema, one usually sees no central clearing, and the KOH preparation is negative.

Pityriasis rosea starts with a single herald patch, which is frequently mistaken for tinea. The correct diagnosis usually becomes evident when the generalized eruption develops within a few weeks. Although occasionally annular, lesions of psoriasis are usually thicker and more scaling than those of fungal infections. More typical lesions of psoriasis usually are also found, and, of course, the KOH examination is negative.

Uncommonly, *impetigo* present in an annular configuration. The finding of vesicles, pustules, and crusts in annular lesions should lead one to suspect a bacterial, rather than fungal, cause.

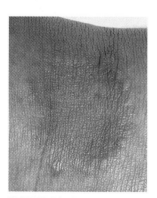

FIGURE 10–7. Granuloma annulare with indurated border and no scale.

Erythema annulare centrificum and *granuloma annulare* (Fig. 10–7) are two uncommon diseases that may be confused with ringworm. Clinically, the differences are that in erythema annulare centrificum, the scale is inside the elevated border and is KOH negative. In granuloma annulare, the border is more indurated and is *not* scaling. A skin biopsy is helpful in confirming the diagnoses of these two disorders. Both conditions are idiopathic and are usually localized but occasionally generalized. The generalized form of erythema annulare centrificum is called *erythema gyratum repens*, a rare condition that is almost always associated with an internal malignant disease (Fig. 10–8). Generalized granuloma annulare is sometimes associated with diabetes mellitus.

Tinea Cruris

A groin rash has several common causes (Fig. 10–9); dermatophytic infection is one. Patients with tinea cruris ("jock itch") frequently also have tinea pedis ("athlete's foot"). The perspiration that occurs with exercise probably is the common predisposing denominator in these "athletic" rashes.

Physical Examination. Dermatophytic infection in the groin may not appear as an annular lesion, but the border is elevated, serpiginous, and scaling. Often, lesions have a tendency for central clearing. The scrotum is seldom involved.

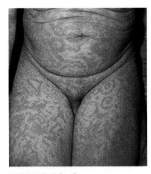

FIGURE 10–8. Erythema gyratum repens.

Differential Diagnosis. In addition to dermatophytic infection are two other common causes of a groin rash. *Candidiasis* appears as a bright, intensely erythematous ("beefy red") eruption with poorly defined borders and satellite papules and pustules. The scrotum is often affected. *Intertrigo* represents simple irritant dermatitis, most often found in obese patients in whom moisture accumulates between skin folds in the inguinal area and, along with friction, causes skin irritation. The eruption is not as erythematous as that of candidiasis and not as sharply demarcated as tinea cruris. The KOH preparation is positive in tinea cruris and candidiasis but negative in intertrigo.

Less often, *psoriasis* and *seborrheic dermatitis* selectively affect the groin. *Erythrasma* is an uncommon disease of intertriginous skin caused by *Corynebacterium minutissimum*. Clinically, it appears as a velvety patch with fine scale that under Wood's light examination fluoresces a diagnostic coral pink.

Three major causes of a groin rash:
1. Tinea cruris
2. Candidiasis
3. Intertrigo

Tinea Pedis

As noted in Table 10–2, the feet are most often involved with dermatophytic infection. Tinea pedis affects approximately 4% of the general population and occurs in three forms, each of which has a different appearance.

Physical Examination. *Interdigital* tinea pedis appears as a macerated scaling process between the toes (Fig. 10–10**A**). It is most common in patients with sweaty feet.

Diffuse plantar scaling is extremely common in older patients. It is usually asymptomatic. The skin of the feet appears dry, with diffuse scaling on the soles extending onto the sides of the feet (see Fig. 10–10**B**). The border may or may not be sharply demarcated. The distribution of this process on the feet has been likened to a "moccasin." Often, patients have accompanying nail involvement.

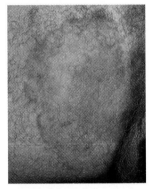

FIGURE 10–9. Tinea Cruris. Sharply marginated scaling border. Scrotum is spared.

The *vesiculopustular* form is the least common type of tinea pedis and the one that is most often misdiagnosed. Vesicles and pustules on the instep of the feet should lead to a suspicion of this type of tinea pedis. A KOH preparation taken from the underside of the roof of the vesicle or pustule reveals fungal hyphae.

Differential Diagnosis. Patients with sweaty feet (hyperhidrosis) may develop *maceration* between the toes, simply as a result of retained moisture in these occluded areas. This then provides a good culture medium for fungus to become secondarily involved. Clinically, simple maceration may be indistinguishable from interdigital tinea pedis. A KOH preparation enables one to diagnose fungus infection, but in both situations measures to decrease sweating also are important.

Diffuse plantar scaling is most often passed off as *dry skin*. *Contact dermatitis* and *dyshidrotic eczema* represent the two diseases that are most often confused with

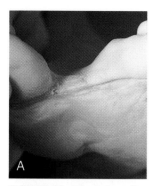

FIGURE 10–10. A, Interdigital tinea pedis: scaling and maceration.

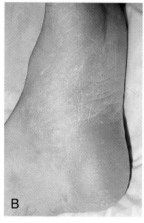

FIGURE 10–10. B, Chronic scaling tinea pedis: diffuse plantar scaling in moccasin distribution.

the vesiculopustular type of tinea pedis. In contact dermatitis and dyshidrotic eczema, however, the vesicles are usually smaller and rarely progress to pustules. *Pustular psoriasis* of the palms and soles is an uncommon disease that can also be confused with vesiculopustular tinea pedis. If doubt exists, a KOH preparation should be performed.

Tinea Manuum

Dermatophytic infection of the palm is uncommon but not rare. It virtually always occurs in a patient who has coexisting tinea pedis.

Physical Examination. Typically, tinea manuum involves only one hand, resulting in the "one hand, two feet" syndrome (Fig. 10–11). It appears as diffuse scaling of the palmar surface, much like the plantar scaling type of tinea pedis. The border on the wrist side is often sharply demarcated.

Differential Diagnosis. *Chronic irritant contact dermatitis,* or "dishpan hands," can also appear as chronic scaling of the palms. However, this condition usually involves both palms, and the border generally is not well demarcated.

Psoriasis can affect the palms with sharply demarcated scaling plaques. Usually, these plaques are bilateral and are more elevated and erythematous than in tinea manuum; often, lesions of psoriasis elsewhere on the body support the diagnosis. KOH preparation is necessary in case of doubt.

Tinea Faciale

This is an uncommon but often missed fungal infection of the skin (Fig. 10–12).

Physical Examination. Tinea faciale appears as an erythematous, usually asymmetric, eruption on the face. An annular pattern is frequently not evident, but usually at least some of the borders are well demarcated and are often serpiginous, providing the clue to the fungal origin. Pustules may be present and may further obscure the clinical diagnosis.

Differential Diagnosis. The lesions in *seborrheic dermatitis* are usually symmetric and are not well demarcated.

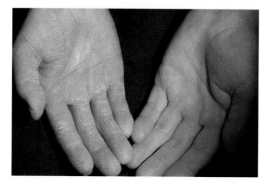

FIGURE 10–11. Tinea Manuum. Diffuse scaling of only one hand in a patient with tinea pedis—the "one hand, two feet" syndrome.

Rashes resulting from sunlight *(photodermatitis)* are distinguished by their distribution, which usually is symmetric, sparing areas that are relatively protected from the sun, such as the eyelids and under the chin.

Occasionally, tinea faciale can appear as a butterfly rash resembling that of *lupus erythematosus.* The finding of sharp serpiginous borders should heighten the suspicion of a fungal origin. However, for any of these conditions, if there is scale and any doubt, scrape it!

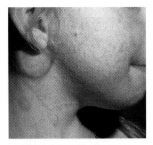

FIGURE 10-12. Tinea Faciale. Sharply demarcated, scaling, serpiginous border is best seen here on neck.

Laboratory Tests

The single most important laboratory test for all of the mentioned fungal infections is the KOH preparation (Fig. 10–13). The details of this procedure are outlined in Chapter 4. The finding of hyphae on a KOH preparation is diagnostic of either dermatophytic or candidal infection. Usually, the clinical presentation distinguishes between the two.

If desired, one can also obtain scales for fungal culture. Cultures distinguish between candidal and dermatophytic infections. Cultures sometimes are also helpful in patients in whom dermatophytic infections are suspected but the KOH examination is negative.

Skin biopsy is not indicated, and contrary to some misconceptions, a Wood's light (black light) is of no help in diagnosing dermatophytic infection of the skin. A Wood's light fluoresces infected scalp hairs in one type of tinea capitis, but infected skin does not show fluorescence.

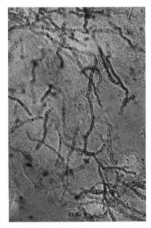

FIGURE 10-13. A positive potassium hydroxide examination showing multiple hyphae.

Therapy

Most dermatophytic infections involve only limited areas and respond well to topical agents. Mycolog cream should never be used because this preparation has

---

THERAPY OF DERMATOPHYTE INFECTIONS

Topical (for limited skin disease)
- Azoles (e.g., miconazole 2% or clotrimazole 1% cream BID)
- Allylamines (e.g., naftifine 1% or terbinafine 1% cream daily)
- Ciclopirox (Loprox cream 1% BID)

Systemic (for scalp, nails, or extensive involvement)
- Griseofulvin—microsize: 20 mg/kg daily
- Terbinafine
    - < 20 kg: 62.5 mg daily
    - 20–40 kg: 125 mg daily
    - > 40 kg: 250 mg daily
- Itraconazole
    - 20 kg: 5 mg/kg daily
    - 20–40 kg: 100 mg daily
    - 40 kg: 200 mg daily

Mycolog cream has no effect on dermatophyte infections.

Initial therapy:
1. **Skin—topical antifungals**
2. **Hair and nails—systemic therapy**

no effect against dermatophytes, despite its misleading name. The only antifungal agent in Mycolog is nystatin, which is effective against only *Candida albicans*. For dermatophyte infections, we usually prescribe one of the many available imidazole creams. Over-the-counter imidazole creams include clotrimazole (Lotrimin) and miconazole (Micatin), either of which is applied twice daily. Non-azole antifungal medications include naftifine (Naftin) and terbinafine (Lamisil), allylamine compounds that are marketed for once-daily use, and ciclopirox olamine (Loprox), a substituted pyridine that exhibits antibacterial as well as antifungal activity. The patient is instructed to apply the topical antifungal to the infected skin until the infection is clinically clear and then to apply it for 1 to 2 weeks longer in hopes of preventing recurrence.

Chronic tinea pedis is notoriously refractory to curative therapy, particularly if the patient has nail involvement. For suppressive therapy, an antifungal powder, such as miconazole powder, should be used daily on an indefinite basis after the skin has been clinically cleared.

For patients with disease that is either widespread or resistant to topical measures, systemic therapy is indicated. Systemic treatment is also most effective for treating scalp and nail infection. The five available oral systemic agents are griseofulvin, ketoconazole (Nizoral), itraconazole (Sporanox), fluconazole (Diflucan), and terbinafine (Lamisil). For dermatophytic infection, griseofulvin had been the standard treatment. Adult patients are treated with either microsized griseofulvin (e.g., Fulvicin U/F), 500 mg twice daily, or ultramicrosized griseofulvin (e.g., Gris-PEG), 250 mg twice daily for 4 to 6 weeks. The newer systemic antifungals, however, can achieve better results with shorter courses of treatment (and fewer side effects). For example, most dermatophyte infections of the skin can be cured with a 1- to 2-week course of itraconazole (200 mg daily) or terbinafine (250 mg daily). Doses for children are adjusted downward according to body weight.

Treatment of tinea capitis requires 2 to 4 weeks of therapy with the newer antifungals. Adjunctive twice-weekly use of a dandruff shampoo containing selenium sulfide (Selsun, Exsel) can shorten the time course of this infection.

Course and Complications

Some acute dermatophytic infections resolve spontaneously. Even in these patients, however, the time course can be shortened by the use of the therapy mentioned previously.

Complications are rare. Secondary bacterial infections are uncommon. Recognizing that fungal infections can produce pustules (particularly when hair follicles are affected), one must be cautious about misdiagnosing such pustules as being bacterial in origin. KOH examinations and cultures clarify the matter if one is in doubt. Intertriginous tinea pedis can allow bacteria to gain access to deeper tissues. This is a common portal of entry in patients with recurrent cellulitis of the lower extremities, so treatment of the dermatophyte infection can prevent subsequent episodes of cellulitis.

Pathogenesis

The three genera of dermatophytes are *Trichophyton*, *Microsporum*, and *Epidermophyton*. Some of these organisms grow only on human hosts (anthropophilic), whereas others can also exist in soil (geophilic) or on animals (zoophilic). All the dermatophytes are keratinophilic, that is, they feed on keratin. They all produce keratinases, a necessary requirement for their keratinophilia. Stratum corneum, hair, and nails are attractive substrates for these fungi, not only because of their keratin composition but perhaps also because of their low density of bacterial inhibitors and competitors. Dermatophytes form hyphae through which nourishment is obtained from the keratin-rich host environment.

The clinical appearance and behavior of a fungal infection of the skin partly depends on the host response. Slow-growing dermatophytes infecting only the outermost layers of the stratum corneum may not elicit an inflammatory response. The diffuse plantar scaling type of tinea pedis is an example. The clinical reaction may also be influenced by the type of dermatophyte; some are more likely than others to elicit an inflammatory reaction. In general, zoophilic dermatophytes provoke more inflammation than anthropophilic ones. Tinea corporis from *Microsporum canis* (*canis* is Latin for canine, or relating to the dog) is an example of an infection from a zoophilic dermatophyte that produces an inflammatory erythematous, scaling annular lesion.

Human dermatophytic infections may resolve spontaneously, probably as a result of cellular immune responses provoked by antigenic material from the organisms. Persistent infections occur in patients who do not mount this immune reaction, either because the fungus has failed to provoke it (e.g., in chronic tinea pedis, in which the fungus growth remains superficial in the thick stratum corneum and does not gain access to the circulation) or because of dermatophyte-specific host immune deficiency. Dermatophytic infections do not invade beyond the epidermis because of their dependence on keratin for nutrition and the fungistatic properties of transferrin and β-globulin in human serum.

■ PITYRIASIS ROSEA

Definition. Pityriasis rosea (*pityriasis* means bran-like scale, and *rosea* means rose colored) is an acute, self-limiting, inflammatory dermatosis of unknown origin. It is clinically characterized by oval, minimally elevated, scaling patches, papules, and plaques that are mainly located on the trunk (Fig. 10–14).

Incidence. The exact incidence is not known, but the disease is relatively common. It is the third most common papulosquamous disease, affecting 1% of the new

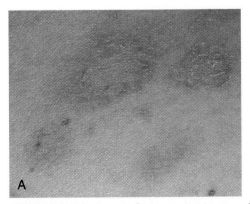
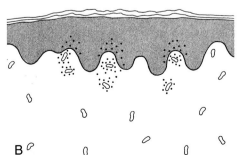

FIGURE 10–14. Pityriasis Rosea. **A,** Epidermis—delicate scale near border of minimally elevated plaque. Dermis—erythema. **B,** Epidermis—slight hyperkeratosis and acanthosis with focal spongiosis and scattered lymphocytes. Dermis—moderate perivascular lymphocytic infiltrate.

patients seen in our dermatology clinic. The disease affects mainly older children and young adults and occurs with some seasonal variation, being least common during the summer months.

History. Characteristically, the generalized eruption is preceded by a single lesion, which is called the "herald patch." This is frequently misdiagnosed as ringworm. The herald patch is followed after several days to weeks by the generalized rash. The patient usually feels well. Itching is often present and ranges in severity from mild to moderate.

Physical Examination. The herald patch is the largest of the lesions and ranges from 2 to 5 cm. The multiple lesions that follow resemble the herald patch but are smaller. They are typically tannish pink or salmon colored, round to oval, and surmounted by a delicate scale that in the mature lesion is located near the border. Typically, oval lesions on the neck and trunk follow the skin cleavage lines in a pattern that, with imagination, has been likened to that of a Christmas tree. The rash is distributed mainly on the trunk and neck and sometimes on the proximal extremities (Fig. 10–15). In children, the face may also be affected. Also in children, papular or vesicular variants of the disease can occur. Oral lesions, although not prominent, have been described and range from erythematous macules to hemorrhagic puncta to small ulcerations.

Differential Diagnosis. Although the diagnosis of pityriasis rosea is usually straightforward, sometimes other disorders must be considered in the differential diagnosis. In *tinea corporis*, patients usually have only a few lesions. If doubt exists, however, a KOH preparation should be done. The explosive onset of the small lesions of *guttate psoriasis*, mainly distributed on the trunk, can be confused with pityriasis rosea. However, the scale in psoriasis is thicker and more silvery, and the course is more prolonged. Uncommonly, generalized *lichen planus* can resemble pityriasis rosea. The purple color of the lesions in lichen planus helps to distinguish the two. *Pityriasis lichenoides chronica* is an uncommon disorder in which the lesions may resemble those of pityriasis rosea but (as the name implies) are chronic rather than transient. Drug eruptions should be considered in any patient with acute generalized dermatosis. Usually, however, a drug eruption is more brightly erythematous, more confluent, less scaling, and more itchy than pityriasis rosea.

The most important diagnosis to consider in the differential is *secondary syphilis*, particularly if the eruption is atypical—for example, if the patient has no herald patch, if the distal extremities (particularly the palms and soles) are involved, or if the patient is systemically ill. In all cases of "atypical" pityriasis rosea, a serologic test for syphilis should be ordered.

Laboratory and Biopsy. The diagnosis is almost always clinical. Skin biopsy is nonspecific and is rarely indicated. If it is performed, the findings will include mild hyperkeratosis with focal parakeratosis, minimal acanthosis with focal spongiosis, and a moderate dermal inflammatory infiltrate, with a few of the cells migrating into the epidermis.

Therapy. Treatment usually is not necessary for this self-limited disease. Occasionally, antihistamines are needed for pruritus, and moisturizing creams are needed for the dry scaling that occurs as the lesions evolve. UV light therapy (UVB) is the only modality that appears to accelerate resolution, but it is seldom indicated.

A "herald patch" precedes the generalized eruption.

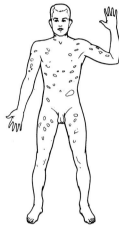

FIGURE 10–15. Distribution of pityriasis rosea. The pattern has been likened to that of a Christmas tree.

For patients with "atypical" pityriasis rosea, a serologic test for syphilis must be performed to rule out secondary syphilis.

Initial treatment:
1. Moisturizers
2. Antihistamines (if needed for itching)

Pityriasis rosea clears spontaneously within 2 months.

Course and Complications. The disease involves spontaneously in a time course ranging from 2 weeks to 2 months, with an average time of approximately 6 weeks. It recurs in only approximately 2% of cases. No complications occur, except for occasional postinflammatory hypopigmentation or hyperpigmentation, which resolves slowly over time, often months.

Pathogenesis. The rash appears to be mediated by a cellular (type IV) immune reaction. A possible viral trigger has been suggested by the increased incidence of disease during the winter months and by the observation that a history of a preceding upper respiratory infection is found more frequently in patients with pityriasis rosea than in control subjects. However, the disease does not occur endemically, and occurrence in household contacts is uncommon. In addition, organisms have never been isolated, and attempts to transmit the disease experimentally have been unsuccessful. In short, the cause remains unknown.

■ SECONDARY SYPHILIS

Definition. The rash of secondary syphilis represents an inflammatory response in the skin and mucous membranes to the hematogenously disseminated *Treponema pallidum* spirochete. Clinically, the rash may appear in various ways, but the most common is scaling papules and plaques (Fig. 10–16).

Incidence. Despite the availability of penicillin, secondary syphilis is still present in our society, and its incidence has been increasing in recent years, both in the general population and in patients infected with HIV.

History. The secondary phase of syphilis starts 6 to 12 weeks after the appearance of the primary chancre. The chancre is usually (but not always) healed by the time the secondary phase develops, but it may be remembered by the patient. Systemic symptoms are usually present and include fever, headache, myalgias, arthralgias, sore throat, and malaise. Pruritus, once thought not to occur in secondary syphilis, is occasionally noted.

Physical Examination. The rash of secondary syphilis is a great imitator. It may appear as macules, nonscaling papules and annular plaques, scaling papules and

The rash of secondary syphilis is a great imitator. Involvement of the palms and soles suggests this diagnosis.

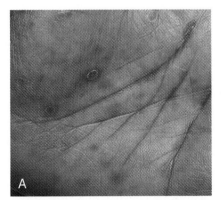
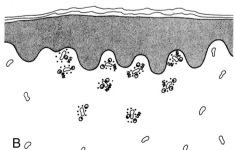

FIGURE 10–16. Secondary Syphilis. **A,** Characteristic palmar papules and plaques. Epidermis—slight scale. Dermis—intense erythema. **B,** Epidermis—slight hyperkeratosis. Dermis—perivascular infiltrate with lymphocytes, plasma cells, and spirochetes (with silver stain).

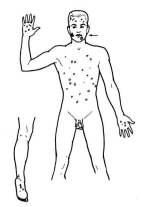

FIGURE 10–17. Distribution of secondary syphilis. Note involvement of the mouth (mucous patches), palms, and soles.

In patients with fever and rash of unknown origin, a serologic test for syphilis should be done.

Therapy: Penicillin

plaques, and, occasionally, pustules or nodules. Vesicles or bullae are not present, however, except in newborns with congenital disease and occasionally in patients with HIV infection. The most common lesions are scaling papules and small plaques in which the color is a clue. Lesions are most frequently not just red but rather reddish brown (ham colored) or yellowish (copper colored). The eruption is often generalized (Fig. 10–17), but palmar and plantar involvement with lesions of these colors is particularly noteworthy. Other possible mucocutaneous features include (1) mucous patches, which are white plaques seen in the mouth; (2) condylomata lata, which are flat-topped, moist, warty-appearing lesions in the genital areas; and (3) spotty alopecia of the scalp, which has been described as "moth-eaten" in appearance. The general physical examination usually reveals the presence of lymphadenopathy.

Differential Diagnosis. As mentioned, the rash of secondary syphilis can mimic many other skin disorders, the most common of which are as follows: *pityriasis rosea*, as has been discussed; *drug eruption*; *viral exanthem*; and (for the annular lesions seen especially in black patients) *sarcoidosis*. A general guideline to remember is that for patients with a generalized rash of unknown origin and systemic complaints, secondary syphilis should be considered and patients should be tested for it.

Laboratory and Biopsy. In secondary syphilis, the serologic test for syphilis (STS) is always positive in immunocompetent hosts. It is usually present in high titer. A positive STS should be followed by a fluorescent treponemal antibody-absorption (FTA-ABS) test, which is a more specific test for syphilis. Positivity of these two blood tests confirms the diagnosis. False-positive tests, usually in low titer, occur in some patients with systemic lupus erythematosus (SLE).

The STS may be negative in a patient with coexisting HIV infection and secondary syphilis. If syphilis is suspected in this setting, a darkfield examination or biopsy of a skin lesion can confirm the diagnosis. These procedures visualize the spirochetes in serous fluid obtained from the lesion or in special stains of biopsy material. The histologic findings otherwise are frequently nonspecific, showing simply an inflammatory infiltrate and, in lesions with scale, hyperkeratosis and mild acanthosis. Plasma cells are often present in the inflammatory infiltrate and may suggest the diagnosis. Patients diagnosed with syphilis should also be tested for HIV infection because the presence of the former indicates a risk factor for acquiring the latter.

Therapy. Penicillin remains the treatment of choice for syphilis. For primary and secondary syphilis in immunocompetent hosts, a single intramuscular injection of 2.4 million units of benzathine penicillin is adequate therapy. HIV-infected patients require more intensive therapy, either with benzathine penicillin injections weekly for 3 weeks or with a course of intravenous aqueous penicillin or intramuscular ceftriaxone. Immunocompetent patients who are allergic to penicillin may be treated with a 15-day course of either tetracycline or erythromycin orally. With therapy, many patients experience a febrile reaction (Jarisch-Herxheimer reaction) beginning within 12 hours and resolving within 1 day.

Course and Complications. Without therapy, the lesions of secondary syphilis spontaneously resolve in 1 to 3 months in the immunocompetent host. With therapy, the lesions resolve promptly, and the titer of the STS is markedly reduced by 12 months. The FTA-ABS test often remains positive indefinitely.

In the secondary phase, the treponemal organism spreads not only to the skin but also to other organs. Hepatitis occurs in approximately 10% of the patients, bone and joint disease in approximately 4%, and nephritis even less often. Central nervous system involvement, as reflected by abnormal cerebrospinal fluid findings, occurs in approximately 10% of immunocompetent patients but is much more frequent in HIV-infected patients, in whom rapid progression to symptomatic neurosyphilis may occur.

Approximately one third of untreated immunocompetent patients develop late (years later) complications of syphilis (tertiary), of which the most important are the cardiovascular and central nervous system manifestations. In patients with HIV infection, progression to tertiary syphilis is more frequent and can occur within months after primary infection.

In patients with HIV infection, syphilis progresses rapidly and requires more intensive therapy.

Pathogenesis. The disease is caused by the spirochete *T. pallidum*. The organism is traumatically inoculated into mucous membranes or skin, most often during sexual intercourse. After a 10- to 90-day incubation period, the *primary* lesion appears as an ulcer (chancre). After another brief latent period, during which the organism continues to multiply, hematogenous dissemination occurs (*secondary* syphilis). Organisms infecting the skin provoke an immunologic response, which is clinically manifested by a variety of inflammatory lesions.

■ MYCOSIS FUNGOIDES

Definition. Mycosis fungoides is not a fungal infection; rather, it is a cutaneous T-cell lymphoma with a misleading label. Cutaneous T-cell lymphoma is a more appropriate name. The skin lesions result from proliferation in the dermis of malignant T-lymphocytes that have a propensity to migrate into the epidermis. The clinical appearance of the lesion depends on the stage of the disease, which may evolve from patch through plaque to noduloulcerative lesions, reflecting the progressive increase of the cellular infiltrate in the skin (Fig. 10–18).

Mycosis fungoides is a cutaneous T-cell lymphoma, not a fungal infection.

Incidence. Mycosis fungoides is uncommon. A survey in Rochester, Minnesota, discovered an annual incidence of 0.5 per 100,000 population. In the United States, mycosis fungoides accounts for less than 1% of all lymphomas and fewer than

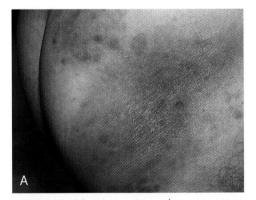
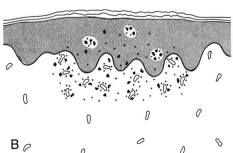

FIGURE 10–18. Mycosis Fungoides. **A,** Epidermis—patch: crinkled, slight scale; plaque: scale. Dermis—patch: erythema; plaque: erythema, often with violaceous hue. **B,** Epidermis—hyperkeratosis; epidermal atrophy (especially in patch stage); exocytosis of malignant lymphocytes, sometimes in focal collections (Pautrier's microabscesses). Dermis—mild to marked infiltrate of mixed inflammation cells, including cerebriform lymphocytes.

200 deaths per year. The disease affects adults, most often those in the older age groups.

History. In the usual case, the eruption slowly evolves over a period of years. It often starts as a nonspecific rash, which may be diagnosed as "atypical" psoriasis or eczema. *Parapsoriasis*, an uncommon idiopathic disorder characterized by salmon-colored, slightly scaling patches, may be a precursor. With evolution, the lesions become more elevated and indurated. In most patients with mycosis fungoides, pruritus is present, ranging from mild to severe.

Mycosis fungoides should be considered in patients with "atypical" eczema or psoriasis.

Physical Examination. The key to the diagnosis rests with the following features. The lesions are irregular in shape, peculiar in color (often reddish brown, violaceous, or orange), and asymmetric in distribution. The degree of elevation of the lesions depends on the stage of the disease. In the patch stage, the lesions are flat, surmounted by a slight scale, and sometimes accompanied by epidermal atrophy, which clinically appears as "cigarette paper" wrinkling of the surface. Other lesions may show *poikiloderma*, a term used to describe a reticulate pattern of hyperpigmentation, hypopigmentation, and erythema with telangiectasia. In poikiloderma, the epidermis also shows atrophy. In the patch stage, the lesions are most frequently found in the girdle area as shown in Figure 10–18**A**. As the disease progresses, increased cellular infiltration of the skin occurs, clinically expressed as elevated, indurated plaques. These plaques are generally more widespread. In advanced disease, nodules appear and frequently ulcerate. Lymphadenopathy is also frequently found in more advanced disease.

Mycosis fungoides should be suspected in rashes with lesions that are:
1. **Irregular in shape**
2. **Peculiar in color**
3. **Asymmetric in distribution**

Sézary syndrome represents a leukemic variant of mycosis fungoides; this syndrome is characterized by total body erythema (erythroderma), lymphadenopathy, and a high number of mycosis (or Sézary) cells in the peripheral circulation.

Differential Diagnosis. Mycosis fungoides may appear as *parapsoriasis, atypical eczema*, or *psoriasis*. In patients with nodular disease, other malignant tumors may be considered. In patients with Sézary syndrome, the differential diagnosis includes other causes of generalized erythema (see Chapter 15).

Laboratory and Biopsy. The most important laboratory test is the skin biopsy. Frequently, multiple biopsies must be performed before a histologic diagnosis can be secured, particularly in patients with early patch stage disease.

Multiple skin biopsies, often over time, are frequently needed to establish the diagnosis.

The most important histologic feature is the presence of *Pautrier's microabscesses* within the epidermis. These represent collections of lymphocytes, many of which are atypical. Atypical lymphocytes are also found in varying numbers in the dermal infiltrate. With high-power examination, the nuclei of these lymphocytes are characteristically highly convoluted or cerebriform. In the early stages of the disease, they may be present only in small numbers; in the nodular stage, one sees a dense infiltrate of malignant cells.

The malignant cells in mycosis fungoides are derived from a monoclonal proliferation of helper T-cells. The *T-cell receptor gene rearrangement test* may be used to determine monoclonality in T-cell infiltrates in skin and other tissues. Differentiated helper T-cells have specific cell surface receptors that possess specificity that is determined by rearrangement of the receptor gene. The T-cell receptor gene rearrangement test detects a population of cells with the same rearrangement, thereby determining monoclonality, a finding that is supportive of malignancy. This test has been used as an aide in diagnosing mycosis fungoides in skin, blood, and lymph nodes. False-positive results occasionally occur.

A complete blood cell count, with careful examination of peripheral smear, should also be performed in looking for circulating mycosis fungoides cells. If lymph nodes are enlarged, a lymph node biopsy should be performed.

Therapy. For disease localized to the skin, external therapy is preferred. Four modalities have been used: (1) for extremely early skin involvement, topical steroids are sometimes successfully employed; the other "external" modalities are (2) UV light, either short-wave (UVB) or long-wave (UVA) in combination with psoralens (PUVA); (3) topical nitrogen mustard, which is applied as a liquid or ointment to the total cutaneous surface; and (4) total body electron beam therapy. Orally administered low-dose methotrexate, isotretinoin and intramuscular interferon-α have been used in patients with recalcitrant skin disease.

In patients with systemic disease, chemotherapy is usually used, sometimes in combination with one of the topical modalities. Some patients with Sézary syndrome also have been successfully treated with extracorporeal photochemotherapy. In this treatment, white blood cells are removed from the patient several hours after psoralen ingestion, are externally exposed to UVA, and are reinfused into the circulation. Treatments are given monthly.

> Initial treatment:
> 1. Topical steroids
> 2. Ultraviolet light
> 3. Topical nitrogen mustard

Course and Complications. In most patients, mycosis fungoides is a chronic, smoldering disease with slow progression over many years. Treatment in the early stages often results in complete clearing of the skin lesions, although relapses are common after therapy is discontinued. Systemic involvement develops in advanced disease, usually affecting the lymph nodes first and the internal organs later. Mean survival in patients with systemic involvement is approximately 2 years.

Pathogenesis. Mycosis fungoides is a neoplastic disease of helper (CD4+) T-cells, with its first manifestation usually appearing in the skin. A debate is ongoing about whether the process starts as malignant or whether it begins as a chronic inflammatory condition in which activated T-cells eventually undergo malignant transformation. Either way, the end result is a monoclonal proliferation of helper T-cells in the skin.

> In mycosis fungoides, there is a monoclonal proliferation of helper T cells in the skin.

THERAPY OF MYCOSIS FUNGOIDES

Topical
- Steroids (e.g., triamcinolone cream 0.1% BID)
- Ultraviolet B light
- Nitrogen mustard

Systemic
- Psoralens with ultraviolet A light (PUVA)
- Methotrexate
- Retinoids (e.g., isotretinoin)
- Interferon alfa-2b
- Extracorporeal photochemotherapy
- Combination chemotherapy

The initiating events in the disease are not well established. The Langerhans cells in the epidermis have been implicated as participating in the initial phases, perhaps themselves stimulated by external factors and, in turn, interacting with T-cells that are subsequently activated. Environmental chemicals have been implicated as a causative factor in some patients, but this has not been well proven. A T-cell lymphotrophic virus (HTLV-I) has been recovered from a subset of patients with aggressive cutaneous T-cell lymphomas. However, for most patients with mycosis fungoides, the underlying origin remains unknown, and the pathogenetic pathway is a matter of debate.

■ DISCOID LUPUS ERYTHEMATOSUS

DLE may be limited to the skin or may be a manifestation of SLE.

Definition. Discoid lupus erythematosus (DLE) is one of several rashes that can occur in lupus. DLE is the rash that scales (Fig. 10–19). Immunoglobulins are found in the skin in this autoimmune disease. Clinically, the lesions appear as disc-shaped plaques surmounted by a white adherent scale that also involves the hair follicles. DLE may be limited to the skin, or it may be one of the manifestations of SLE.

Incidence. The disease primarily affects young and middle-aged adults. It is uncommon, but the exact incidence in the general population is not known. Of all new patients seen in our dermatology clinic, 2 per 1,000 were seen for DLE.

History. The eruption may be slightly pruritic but is more often asymptomatic. Patients may give a history of exacerbation after sunlight exposure. In patients with DLE, a history should be taken for symptoms of possible SLE, including photosensitivity, hair loss, nasal and oral ulcerations, Raynaud's phenomenon, and arthritis.

Physical Examination. The earliest lesion is a purplish-red plaque, which accumulates scale as it matures. The scale is white and usually cohesive, so it can often be removed in one piece. When this is done, the underside of the scale may show small, spiny projections. These have been called "carpet tacks," and they represent the keratinous plugs that had been present in dilated hair follicles. The oldest

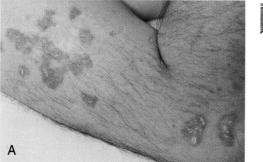
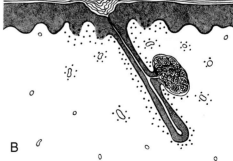

FIGURE 10–19. Discoid Lupus Erythematosus. **A,** Epidermis—scale that when removed shows "carpet tacking" on underside. Dermis—erythema. **B,** Epidermis—hyperkeratosis with follicular plugging; vacuolar degeneration of basal cell layer. Dermis—perivascular and periappendageal inflammatory cell infiltration.

lesions appear as *depressed,* atrophic plaques, often with pigmentary change, usually hypopigmentation in the center with a hyperpigmented rim (Fig. 10–20).

The distribution of the lesion of DLE favors sun-exposed areas (i.e., the face, upper trunk, and arms). An occasional patient has widespread cutaneous involvement. Erosions in the oral cavity, particularly of the palate, are occasionally found in patients with DLE.

Differential Diagnosis. *Psoriasis* may be the most common misdiagnosis. The finding of atrophy helps to differentiate the two. *Lichen planus* lesions are also purplish, but they usually are small (papular), have scant scale, and do not result in depressed sears. The scaling patches and plaques that occur in *subacute cutaneous lupus erythematosus* (SCLE) also do not scar, frequently are annular, and often are accompanied by circulating anticytoplasmic antibodies—anti-Ro (SSA) and anti-La (SSB).

Laboratory and Biopsy. Skin biopsy establishes the diagnosis. With routine processing, the diagnosis is strongly supported by the findings of (1) hyperkeratosis with follicular plugging, (2) vacuolar degeneration of the basal cell layer, and (3) a dermal inflammatory cell infiltrate that is both perivascular and periappendageal. Epidermal atrophy is also seen in older lesions. Diagnosis can be further confirmed with direct immunofluorescent techniques (the lupus band test). In more than 90% of patients with DLE, immunoglobulins (usually IgG or IgM) are deposited as a "band" at the dermal-epidermal junction in lesional skin. Caution must be exercised if the biopsy is taken from facial skin, in which false-positive results may occur.

In addition to the history and physical examination, a laboratory screen for SLE should be done on all patients with DLE. This includes a complete blood cell count, a urinalysis, and an antinuclear antibody (ANA) test. If the latter is positive, an anti-DNA antibody test should be ordered. Patients with DLE who have positive ANA tests or persistent complete blood cell count abnormalities are more likely to develop SLE subsequently.

Therapy. Topical therapy usually is adequate. Steroids, applied topically or injected intralesionally, are used most often. Sun protection is important, and sunscreens that protect against both short-UV (UVB) and long-UV (UVA) light should be strongly recommended to all patients. Patients with extensive or recalcitrant

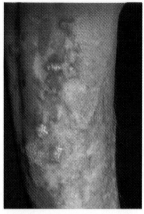

FIGURE 10–20. Discoid lupus erythematosus causes depressed atrophic lesions. It is the only papulosquamous disorder in which this manifestation occurs. (From Helm KF, Marks JG: Atlas of Differential Diagnosis in Dermatology. New York, Churchill Livingstone, 1998.)

Patients with DLE should be screened for SLE with:
1. **Complete blood cell count**
2. **Urinalysis**
3. **Antinuclear antibody test**

Initial therapy:
1. **Topical steroids**
2. **Sunscreens**

THERAPY OF CUTANEOUS LUPUS

Topical
- Steroids (e.g., triamcinolone cream 0.1% BID)
- Sunscreens

Systemic
- Antimalarials (e.g., hydroxychloroquine 200 mg BID)
- Retinoids (e.g., isotretinoin, acitretin)
- Dapsone
- Gold

disease sometimes require systemic therapy; antimalarials, such as chloroquine (250 mg daily) or hydroxychloroquine (200 to 400 mg daily) are used most often. Patients receiving these antimalarial drugs should undergo ophthalmologic examination every 6 months to monitor for the retinal toxicity that rarely is encountered with the dosages used in DLE. For patients with DLE not responding to the foregoing measures, alternative systemic therapies, including retinoids (isotretinoin or acitretin), dapsone, and oral gold (auranofin), may be used.

From 5% to 10% of patients presenting with DLE subsequently develop SLE.

Course and Complications. The course of the disease is chronic but, with therapy, usually controllable. New lesions may continue to appear over a course of years as old ones become inactive. Eventual remission spontaneously occurs in approximately 50% of patients. Scarring and postinflammatory hypopigmentation and hyperpigmentation are common and may result in disfigurement, particularly in blacks. In the scalp, the scarring leads to permanent alopecia; if extensive, this can be a cosmetic problem. In patients presenting with only DLE lesions, the risk of subsequently developing SLE is 5% to 10%.

Pathogenesis. Lupus erythematosus has been called an autoimmune disease because of the autoantibodies found in the disease. In DLE, these are found in the form of IgG and IgM deposited at the dermal-epidermal junction. The cause of this deposition and the role that these immunoglobulins play in the pathogenesis of the skin lesions are not clear. UV light has been implicated as a pathogenic factor. Circumstantial evidence for this includes the localization of lesions mainly in sun-exposed areas, the finding that many patients note that sun exposure exacerbates their skin disease, and experimental induction of skin lesions with UV light. A sequence of pathogenic events has been proposed as follows. UV light damages epidermal cells, releasing their nuclear antigens. These diffuse to the dermal-epidermal junction, where they combine with antibodies from the circulation, initiating an inflammatory reaction resulting ultimately in the clinical lesion.

T-cell dysregulation has also been implicated in the pathogenesis of cutaneous lupus. For example, increased activity of the Th2 subset of helper T-cells has been found in lesional skin. The main function of these cells is to augment humoral immunity. Genetic predisposition to DLE is possible, but familial disease and association with specific HLA phenotypes have been reported more frequently with SLE than with DLE. Current evidence suggests that most patients with DLE have a genetically different disease from that in patients with SLE, a concept that accounts for the observation that most patients with DLE never develop SLE.

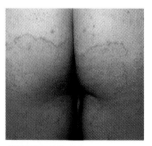

FIGURE 10-21. Unknown.

■ UNKNOWN (Fig. 10-21)

This 50-year-old man was initially seen in dermatology consultation for generalized dry, red, itchy skin of many years' duration. Three skin biopsies were performed and showed an inflammatory infiltrate with some atypical lymphocytes but not in sufficient numbers to diagnose mycosis fungoides (Sézary syndrome). He was treated with a topical steroid cream applied to the entire skin surface. On follow-up 2 weeks later, much of the rash had improved, but a sharply demarcated, scaling eruption persisted on the buttocks and feet.

What is your differential diagnosis?

The differential diagnosis would include any of the papulosquamous disorders listed in Table 10–1, although pityriasis rosea, secondary syphilis, and DLE are not likely. Mycosis fungoides still must be considered for these irregularly shaped, asymmetric plaques, especially in light of the patient's history. Partially treated psoriasis is also possible. For a scaling rash of uncertain origin (especially one in which the lesions have sharp, serpiginous borders), however, fungus infection is the first diagnosis to exclude.

What test would you do next?

A KOH preparation should be the first test. In this case, it was positive, diagnostic for a superficial fungal infection.

Important Point

This case illustrates the general rule that if the diagnosis is uncertain and if the rash scales, scrape it! Adherence to this principle results in many negative KOH examinations, but the effort is rewarded by the positive ones, as in this case. This fast, simple, painless test made the diagnosis and led to the institution of appropriate therapy. Because the eruption was widespread, a systemic antifungal was prescribed, and the rash cleared.

REFERENCES

Psoriasis

Ellis CN, Fradin MS, Messana JM, et al.: Cyclosporine for plaque-type psoriasis. N Engl J Med 324:277–284, 1991.
Greaves MW, Weinstein GD: Treatment of psoriasis. N Engl J Med 332:581–588, 1995.
Ruzicka T: Psoriatic arthritis: new types, new treatments. Arch Dermatol 132:215–219, 1996.
Stern RS: Psoriasis. Lancet 350:349–353, 1997.
Weinstein GD, Kreuger GG, Lowe NS, et al.: Tazarotene gel, a new retinoid, for topical therapy of psoriasis. J Am Acad Dermatol 37:85–92, 1997.

Fungal Infections

DeDoncker P, Gupta AK, Marynissen G, et al.: Itraconazole pulse therapy for onychomycosis and dermatomycoses: an overview. J Am Acad Dermatol 37:969–974, 1997.
Gupta AK, Sauder DN, Shear NH: Antifungal agents: an overview. J Am Acad Dermatol 30:911–933, 1994.
Gupta AK, Shear NH: Terbinafine: an update. J Am Acad Dermatol 37:979–988, 1997.
Rippon JW: Medical Mycology. 3rd Ed. Philadelphia, WB Saunders, 1988.

Pityriasis Rosea

Allen RA, Janniger CK, Schwartz RA: Pityriasis rosea. Cutis 56:198–202, 1995.
Leenutaphong V, Jiamton S: UVB phototherapy for pityriasis rosea: a bilateral comparison study. J Am Acad Dermatol 33:996–999, 1995.

Secondary Syphilis

Fiumara NJ: The diagnosis and treatment of infectious syphilis. Compr Ther 21:639–644, 1995.

Gregory N, Sanchez M, Buchness MR: The spectrum of syphilis in patients with human immunodeficiency virus infection. J Am Acad Dermatol 22:1061–1067, 1990.

Hook EW, Mara CM: Acquired syphilis in adults. N Engl J Med 326:1060–1069, 1992.

Pandhi RK, Singh N, Ramam M: Secondary syphilis: a clinicopathologic study. Int J Dermatol 34:240–243, 1995.

Rudolph AH, Duncan WC, Kettler AH: Treponemal infections: a periodic synopsis. J Am Acad Dermatol 18:1121–1129, 1988.

Mycosis Fungoides

Chuang TY, Su WPD, Muller SA: Incidence of cutaneous T cell lymphoma and other rare skin cancers in a defined population. J Am Acad Dermatol 23:254–256, 1990.

Diamandidou E, Cohen PR, Kurzrock R: Mycosis fungoides and Sezary syndrome. Blood 88:2385–2409, 1996.

Vonderheid EC, Tan ET, Kantor AF, et al.: Long-term efficacy, curative potential, and carcinogenicity of topical mechlorethamine chemotherapy in cutaneous T cell lymphoma. J Am Acad Dermatol 20:416–428, 1989.

Wieselthier JS, Koh HK: Sézary syndrome: diagnosis, prognosis, and critical review of treatment options. J Am Acad Dermatol 22:381–401, 1990.

Zackheim HS, Amin S, Kashani-Sabet M, et al.: Prognosis in cutaneous T-cell lymphoma by skin stage: long-term survival in 489 patients. J Am Acad Dermatol 40:418–425, 1999.

Zackheim HS, Kashani-Sabet M, Amin S: Topical corticosteroids for mycosis fungoides: experience in 79 patients. Arch Dermatol 134:949–954, 1998.

Zelickson BD, Peters MS, Muller SA, et al.: T-cell receptor gene rearrangement analysis: cutaneous T cell lymphoma, peripheral T cell lymphoma, and premalignant and benign cutaneous lymphoproliferative disorders. J Am Acad Dermatol 25:787–796, 1991.

Discoid Lupus Erythematosus

Callen JP: Chronic cutaneous lupus erythematosus: clinical, laboratory, therapeutic, and prognostic examination of 62 patients. Arch Dermatol 118:412–416, 1982.

Callen JP: Management of skin disease in lupus. Bull Rheum Dis 46:4–7, 1997.

George R, Kurlan S, Jacob M, et al.: Diagnostic evaluation of the lupus band test in discoid and systemic lupus erythematosus. Int J Dermatol 34:170–173, 1995.

Sontheimer RD: Lupus erythematosus: clinical-pathogenetic correlations. Prog Dermatol 24:1–12, 1990.

Stein LF, Saed GM, Fivenson DP: T-cell cytokine network in cutaneous lupus erythematosus. J Am Acad Dermatol 37:191–196, 1997.

VESICLES AND BULLAE

HERPES SIMPLEX
HERPES ZOSTER
VARICELLA
BULLOUS IMPETIGO
CONTACT DERMATITIS (ACUTE)
UNCOMMON BLISTERING DISEASES
    Pemphigus Vulgaris
    Bullous Pemphigoid
    Dermatitis Herpetiformis
    Porphyria Cutanea Tarda

Blisters occur:
1. Intraepidermally
2. Subepidermally

Vesicles and bullae, when intact, are easily recognized primary lesions (Table 11–1). Crusts (dried serum and blood) are secondary lesions that should lead one to suspect a preceding vesicle or pustule. The etiology of vesicular and bullous diseases includes viral and bacterial infections, allergic and irritant contact dermatitis, and autoimmune and metabolic diseases. Pathogenesis of the blister formation is helpful in understanding the lesion's location within the skin. The blister may occur within the epidermis (intraepidermal) or beneath it (subepidermal).

The following diseases illustrate the pathogenetic mechanisms involved in blister formation at the different levels of the skin. Detachment of the horny layer by an epidermolytic toxin produced by *Staphylococcus aureus* causes a subcorneal blister. Invasion of epidermal cells by herpesvirus causes degenerative changes and intraepidermal vesicles. Intercellular edema caused by contact dermatitis results in stretching of the intercellular bridges (spongiosis) until they disappear, forming intraepidermal vesicles. Dissolution of the intercellular adhesion molecules secondary to autoantibodies in pemphigus vulgaris causes loss of epidermal cohesion (acantholysis) and blisters within the epidermis.

Damage to the structures within the basement membrane zone causes loss of coherence between basal cells and the dermis. These subepidermal bullae are characteristic of bullous pemphigoid, dermatitis herpetiformis, and porphyria cutanea tarda.

Blisters usually rupture, producing crusting and weeping. If they become filled with purulent material, they are called *pustules*.

TABLE 11–1 ■ COMMON BLISTERING DISEASES

Disease	Frequency*	Etiology	History	Physical Examination	Differential Diagnosis	Laboratory Test
Herpes simplex	1.5	Herpes simplex virus	Itching or pain prodrome	Grouped vesicles Perioral and perineal location most frequent	Impetigo Fungus Contact dermatitis	Tzanck smear Culture
Herpes zoster	0.4	Varicella-zoster virus	Itching or pain prodrome	Grouped vesicles Dermatomal distribution	—	Tzanck smear Culture Immunofluorescence stain
Varicella	<0.1	Varicella-zoster virus	Marked pruritus	Macules, papules, vesicles, pustules Generalized	Rickettsialpox Smallpox	Tzanck smear Culture
Bullous impetigo	0.1	Staphylococcus aureus	Pruritus	Circular yellow crusts, purulent bullae Head, neck, extremities	Contact dermatitis Herpes simplex Fungus	Gram stain Culture
Contact dermatitis	2.8	Allergen Irritant	Irritant: exposure occurs hours to days before rash Allergic: exposure occurs 1–4 days before rash	Papulovesicles Conforms to area of contact with sharp margins Often has a geometric or linear configuration	Atopic dermatitis Cellulitis Fungus	Patch test

*Percentage of new dermatology patients with this diagnosis seen in the Hershey Medical Center Dermatology Clinic, Hershey, PA.

■ HERPES SIMPLEX

Definition. Herpes simplex is an acute, self-limited, intraepidermal vesicular eruption caused by infection with herpes simplex virus (HSV) (Fig. 11–1). HSV is a medium-sized DNA virus that replicates within the nucleus. Based on culture and immunologic characteristics, it is divided into two types—HSV-1 and HSV-2. Usually, HSV-1 causes oral infection, and HSV-2 causes genital infection. Primary infections with these viruses are characteristically followed by recurrent attacks.

Incidence. Investigators estimate that 100 million episodes of oral herpes occur yearly in the United States. Office visits for genital herpes have increased 15-fold over the past 25 years. One-half million new cases of genital herpes occur each year in the United States. Approximately 45 million Americans have circulating antibodies to HSV-2, and 10 million are HSV-1 serology positive. The prevalence of HSV-2 infection has increased 30% in the past two decades; approximately one in five persons more than 11 years old is infected.

History. Primary infection with HSV-1 usually occurs in children, in whom it is subclinical in 90% of cases. The remaining 10% of infected children have acute gingivostomatitis. In contrast, HSV-2 primary infection usually occurs after sexual contact in postpubertal individuals, and it produces acute vulvovaginitis or progenitalis. Primary infections are frequently accompanied by systemic symptoms that include fever, malaise, myalgias, headache, and regional adenopathy. Localized pain and burning may be so severe that drinking and eating or urinating may be compromised.

Infection of the lips (herpes labialis) is usually caused by HSV-1, whereas the genitals and buttocks are more often infected with HSV-2. The risk of a woman's developing genital herpes on exposure to an infected man is estimated to be 80% to 90%. The risk of recurrence after primary genital infections is less with HSV-1 (14%) than with HSV-2 (60%). Recurrent attacks are preceded by localized itching or burning and are characterized by occurrence in the same location. This prodrome usually begins within 24 hours before the appearance of the eruption and occurs in approximately two thirds of patients.

Herpes should be suspected if a vesicular eruption is:
1. **Recurrent in same location**
2. **Preceded by a prodrome**

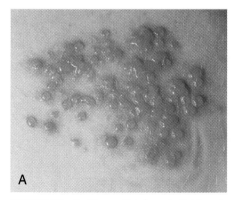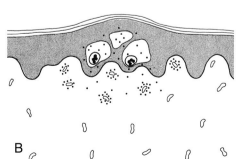

FIGURE 11–1. Herpes Simplex. **A,** Epidermis—grouped vesicles. Dermis—erythema. **B,** Epidermis—bullae, multinucleated giant cells. Dermis—perivasicular inflammation.

Grouped vesicles on an erythematous base are characteristic of HSV infection.

HSV infections are not limited to the lips and genital area; either type can infect any area of skin. Therefore, a history of a vesicular eruption recurring in the *same* location should lead to a suspicion of HSV infection.

Physical Examination. Indurated erythema followed by grouped vesicles on an erythematous base are typical of herpes infections. The vesicles quickly become pustules, which rupture, weep, and crust. Affected skin sometimes becomes necrotic, resulting in punched-out ulceration.

Primary infections—gingivostomatitis or vulvovaginitis—are characterized by extensive vesiculation of the mucous membranes. This results in erosions, necrosis, and a marked purulent discharge. Herpes infections can develop in any area where inoculation has occurred. *Recurrent herpes* infections are characterized by localized grouped vesicles in the same location. *Herpetic whitlow* is infection of the fingers. This is an occupational hazard of medical and dental personnel that can be prevented by wearing gloves. Traumatic herpes simplex has been reported in epidemics among wrestlers (herpes gladiatorum). *Eczema herpeticum* is a generalized cutaneous infection with HSV in individuals with predisposing skin diseases such as atopic dermatitis. It is accompanied by severe toxic symptoms and may be fatal.

Differential Diagnosis. *Impetigo, contact dermatitis,* and, less often, *superficial fungal infections* may be confused with herpes simplex and can be ruled out by history, Gram stain and culture of the blister fluid, patch testing with suspected allergens, and potassium hydroxide (KOH) preparation test of the blister roof.

Tzanck smear confirms a herpetic infection.

Laboratory and Biopsy. The occurrence of grouped vesicles on an erythematous base is characteristic of HSV infection. It can be confirmed with a Tzanck smear, which reveals multinucleated giant cells (Fig. 11–2). The Tzanck smear is a simple yet reliable method of confirming a herpetic infection. Smears from the base of the lesion stained with Giemsa, Wright, or toluidine blue stain demonstrate multinucleated giant cells diagnostic of HSV infection. A detailed description of preparing a Tzanck preparation is presented in Chapter 4. The positivity of the Tzanck preparation varies with the lesion samples: vesicle, 67%; pustule, 55%; and crust-ulcer, 16.7%. A high correlation exists between the Tzanck preparation and viral culture. However, when properly performed, the culture has a greater positivity: vesicle, 100%; pustule, 73%; and crust-ulcer, 33%. A 4-hour HSV antigen test kit (Herpchek) based on enzyme immunoassay is available through clinical laboratories and compares favorably with viral cultures. Although usually not necessary, the biopsy reveals an intraepidermal blister, a necrotic epidermis, multinucleated epidermal giant cells, and an acute inflammatory process.

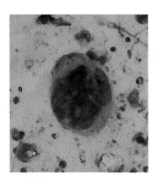

FIGURE 11–2. Multinucleated giant cell in Tzanck smear, characteristic of herpesvirus infection.

Therapy. Acyclovir (Zovirax), valacyclovir (Valtrex), famciclovir (Famvir), and penciclovir (Denavir) are the drugs of choice for HSV infections. Their low toxicity and specificity for HSV have resulted in widespread acceptance. Their unique mechanism of action accounts for their selectivity against HSV. Acyclovir is a synthetic acyclic purine nucleoside analogue. Phosphorylation of acyclovir depends on HSV-specific thymidine kinase. This enzyme converts acyclovir to acyclovir monophosphate, which is further converted into acyclovir triphosphate by cellular enzymes. Acyclovir triphosphate inhibits viral DNA polymerase and replication of viral DNA. It is effective against replicating virus but does not eliminate latent virus. Valacyclovir is a prodrug that is better absorbed than its metabolite acyclovir. Famciclovir, also a prodrug, is metabolized to penciclovir, a synthetic acyclic guanosine derivative. Penciclovir shares similar activation pathways with

> ## THERAPY OF HERPES SIMPLEX
>
> - First Episode—Primary
>   Acyclovir: 400 mg TID × 7 days, 5 mg/kg IV q8h × 5–7 days
>   Valacyclovir: 1,000 mg BID × 7 days
>   Famciclovir: 250 mg TID × 7 days
> - Recurrent
>   Acyclovir: 400 mg TID × 5 days, 5% ointment q2h × 7 days
>   Valacyclovir: 500 mg BID × 5 days
>   Famciclovir: 125 mg BID × 5 days
>   Penciclovir cream 0.1% q2h while awake × 4 days
> - Chronic Suppressive
>   Acyclovir: 400 mg BID
>   Valacyclovir: 500 or 1000 mg QD
>   Famciclovir: 250 mg BID

acyclovir that depend on viral thymidine kinase to form penciclovir triphosphate, which halts DNA synthesis. In active infections, these antiviral drugs decrease the duration of vital shedding, accelerate healing of the lesions, and may reduce local and systemic symptoms.

Treatment does not prevent recurrent infection.

Intravenous acyclovir is indicated in the treatment of severe primary HSV and in initial and recurrent infections in immunocompromised patients. The most important adverse reactions are deposition of drug crystals in the renal tubules of patients with inadequate hydration or impaired renal function. Resistant strains of HSV have emerged in immunocompromised patients and have posed a significant clinical problem. Foscarnet is an alternative drug if acyclovir fails because of acyclovir-resistant thymidine kinase–deficient HSV.

Course and Complications. The incubation period after contact with HSV is approximately 1 week. The clinical course of the primary herpes infection lasts approximately 3 weeks. A prodrome of 1 to 2 days is followed by a vesiculopustular eruption that continues for 1½ weeks. This phase is followed by crusting, ulceration, and healing after an additional 1½ weeks. For most patients, HSV is an asymptomatic chronic infection of sensory ganglia. Overt eruptions recur in a minority of infected persons after varying periods of latency, during which the virus remains dormant within the dorsal nerve root ganglion corresponding to the site of infection. Recurrences have a shorter course of 1 to 2 weeks. Several factors, including fever, ultraviolet light, physical trauma, menstruation, and emotional stress, are attributed to initiating recurrence. Asymptomatic, subclinical shedding of the HSV is common and is instrumental in transmitting HSV to others.

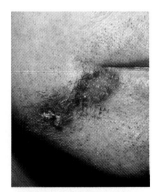

FIGURE 11–3. Chronic cutaneous herpes simplex.

The immunocompromised host is most at risk for developing complications from HSV infections. These complications include the following: chronic ulcerative herpes simplex (Fig. 11–3), which lasts for weeks to months; generalized acute mucocutaneous herpes simplex; and systemic infection involving the liver, lung, adrenal glands, and central nervous system.

Untreated neonatal herpes is frequently fatal.

HSV infection of the neonate, *neonatal herpes,* is a devastating but fortunately uncommon disease. Approximately 1,500 cases occur each year in the United States. The fatality rate without treatment is more than 50%, and at least 50% of the survivors have significant neurologic sequelae. Significant reduction of mortality and morbidity occurs with acyclovir treatment. For women who have evidence of active HSV infection at delivery, cesarean section is recommended. Complicating neonatal HSV infection, however, are the findings that (1) cultures to screen women immediately before delivery do not predict infection for the fetus, (2) more than 70% of mothers of babies with neonatal HSV have no history of genital HSV infection, and (3) symptomatic disease may not occur for as long as 1 month after delivery. Two thirds of affected infants have mucocutaneous manifestations of HSV infection.

In most cases of neonatal herpes, the mothers have no history of genital disease.

A relatively uncommon complication of HSV infection is *erythema multiforme.* Immune complexes composed of antibody and HSV antigen have been found in the serum of patients with erythema multiforme after HSV infection. These immune complexes may be the pathogenesis of the vascular changes seen in erythema multiforme. In addition, HSV DNA has been found in the lesions of erythema multiforme associated with HSV infection.

Erythema multiforme may occur after HSV infection.

Pathogenesis. HSV is a highly contagious virion spread by direct contact with infected individuals who are often asymptomatically shedding the virus. Studies of shedding and survival of HSV from patients with herpes labialis have detected herpesvirus in their saliva (78%) and on their hands (67%), with virus viability on skin, cloth, and plastic for 2 to 4 hours.

The virus penetrates the epidermal cell in which a complex series of steps occurs. The virus undergoes a replicative cycle and induces protein and DNA synthesis with the assembling of intact virions and eventual lysis of the host cell membrane. New copies of viral DNA are packaged into capsids, which are then covered with an amorphous tegument. The viral envelope, which contains viral-specific glycoproteins, is formed by budding through the host nuclear membrane. This process requires an intact host cellular metabolism for substrate synthesis and replication. The destructive effect on epidermal cells results clinically in intraepidermal vesicles.

Latent HSV, undetectable by tissue culture, electron microscopy, and immunofluorescence, presumably resides in the dorsal nerve root sensory or autonomic ganglia in a nonreplicative state. Outbreaks recur with reactivation of the replicative cycle, production of new virus, and spreading back down the nerve. Latency within the ganglion cells is possible apparently because the HSV genomes within these cells are relatively well protected from immunologic attacks.

■ HERPES ZOSTER

Vesicular dermatomal eruption is distinctive for herpes zoster.

Definition. Herpes zoster ("shingles") is an intraepidermal vesicular eruption occurring in a dermatomal distribution (Fig. 11–4). It is caused by the recrudescence of latent varicella-zoster virus in persons who have had varicella.

Incidence. From 10% to 20% of individuals develop herpes zoster during their lifetime. Two thirds of these persons are older than 50 years. The attack rate is age dependent, with a rate of 1 case per 1,000 among healthy people less than 20 years old, 3 cases per 1,000 in patients between 20 and 49 years old, and a peak of 11 per 1,000 at age 80 to 89 years. Patients with cancer and AIDS have a higher incidence than the general population (e.g., 8% to 25% of patients with Hodgkin's disease develop herpes zoster). The frequency of second attacks may be 5%. How-

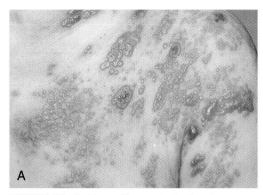
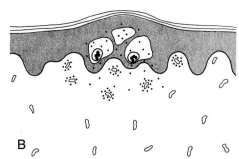

FIGURE 11–4. Herpes Zoster. **A,** Epidermis—grouped vesicles in dermatomal distribution. Dermis—erythema. **B,** Epidermis—bullae, multinucleated giant cells. Dermis—perivascular inflammation.

ever, what is thought to be recurrent zoster may be HSV in a dermatomal distribution.

The prodrome may simulate a migraine, pleurisy, myocardial infarction, or appendicitis.

History. A prodrome of radicular pain and itching precedes the eruption. It can stimulate a migraine, pleurisy, myocardial infarction, or appendicitis.

Physical Examination. The eruption is characterized by groups of vesicles on an erythematous base situated unilaterally along the distribution of a cranial or spinal nerve. Bilateral involvement is rare. Frequently, the eruption involves the immediately adjacent dermatomes.

Differential Diagnosis. The dermatomal distribution of herpes zoster is diagnostic. However, *herpes simplex* may occur in a dermatomal fashion.

Herpes zoster is not a marker for occult malignant disease. It may be the presenting sign of HIV infection.

Laboratory and Biopsy. Usually, no laboratory tests are necessary. The Tzanck preparation, direct immunofluorescence staining of vesicle smears, biopsy, and culture are confirmatory in unusual cases. Although herpes zoster has a higher incidence in patients with established malignant disease, patients presenting with herpes zoster who are otherwise healthy do not have a higher incidence of occult cancer and therefore do not need a screening laboratory examination for malignancy. In patients at risk for HIV infection, herpes zoster may be the presenting sign, and serologic testing for HIV is indicated.

Therapy. When the vesiculopustules of herpes zoster rupture, crusting and weeping are reduced with astringent (Domeboro) compresses. Analgesics commensurate with the amount of pain experienced by the patient are indicated. Acyclovir (Zovirax), at a dosage of 10 mg/kg every 8 hours intravenously or 800 mg five times daily orally for 7 to 10 days, halts the progression of herpes zoster in *immunocompromised* patients and is most effective when started within 3 days of the beginning of the eruption. Effects are less cutaneous and visceral dissemination, cessation of new vesicle formation, and reduced pain. The modest benefit of acyclovir, valacyclovir (Valtrex), and famiclovir (Famvir) for the *otherwise healthy* patient may not justify the expense, except in severe infections and in patients more than 50 years old, to reduce postherpetic neuralgia. The use of corticosteroids in otherwise healthy patients to prevent postherpetic neuralgia has been advocated, but it has not been convincingly proven to be worthwhile. Amitriptyline (Elavil), at a dosage of 50 to 100 mg daily, may be helpful in managing postherpetic neuralgia once it occurs. Capsaicin analgesic cream 0.075% (Zostrix-HP) used topically

Systemic acyclovir is indicated for herpes zoster in immunocompromised patients.

THERAPY OF HERPES ZOSTER

- Antivirals*
  - Acyclovir: 800 mg, 5 times per day × 7 days,
  - 10 mg/kg IV q8h × 5–7 days
  - Valacyclovir: 1 g TID × 7 days
  - Famciclovir: 500 mg TID × 7 days
- Compresses
  - Aluminum acetate
- Pain Medication
  - Analgesics
  - Amitriptyline: 25–100 mg/QHS

*Mild rash or pain, age ≤ 50 years, rash > 72 hours—treatment is optional.

---

three or four times daily on affected skin also can provide pain relief. Caution should be used to avoid inadvertent contact with the eyes or unaffected skin because capsaicin normally produces transient burning.

Course and Complications. The succession of lesions begins with macules, which develop into vesicles. Over the next several days, pustules develop and are followed by crusting and eventual healing in 2 to 3 weeks. Hemorrhagic bullae and gangrenous changes may occur and may result in scarring.

Cutaneous dissemination of herpes zoster from the original dermatome develops in some patients, particularly immunocompromised patients in whom the condition is more likely to be severe and prolonged. It occurs within 5 to 7 days of the initial eruption and may be accompanied by fever, malaise, and prostration. The immunocompromised patient is susceptible to visceral involvement of the liver, lung, and central nervous system.

Postherpetic neuralgia is uncommon in patients less than 40 years old, but 27%, 47%, and 73% of untreated adults older than 55, 60, and 70 years of age, respectively, develop this complication, which frequently is difficult to control and is troubling to the patient. However, 80% of patients with postherpetic neuralgia become asymptomatic in 12 months.

When herpes zoster involves the tip of the nose, suspect eye involvement.

The nasociliary branch of the ophthalmic division of the trigeminal nerve innervates the eye and the tip of the nose. Therefore, herpes ophthalmicus should be suspected when herpes zoster involves the tip of the nose. Scarring of the cornea and conjunctiva may occur. Other occasional complications of herpes zoster are full-thickness skin necrosis and Bell's palsy.

Pathogenesis. After primary varicella infection, the virus becomes latent within the sensory nerve ganglia. With reactivation, replication again occurs with migration of the virus along the nerve to the skin. Viremia frequently occurs, sometimes resulting in disseminated lesions.

■ VARICELLA

Definition. Varicella (chicken pox) is an acute, highly contagious, intraepidermal vesicular eruption caused by varicella-zoster virus. Clinically, it appears as a generalized vesicular eruption (Fig. 11–5).

Incidence. Varicella is predominantly a childhood disease, with 90% of cases occurring before the age of 10 years. Investigators estimate that 3.5 to 4.0 million cases occur annually in the United States. Chicken pox occurs throughout the year, but incidence peaks sharply in March, April, and May.

> **Chicken pox has all types of lesions: macules, papules, vesicles, pustules, and crusts.**

History. After a 2- to 3-week incubation period, a 2- to 3-day prodrome of chills, fever, malaise, headache, sore throat, anorexia, and dry cough precedes the onset of the markedly pruritic vesicular eruption. The patient is infectious for approximately 1 week (1 to 2 days before the rash and an additional 4 to 5 days until the vesicles have become crusted).

Physical Examination. Varicella is a generalized pruritic eruption that is most prominent on the trunk but also involves the head, the extremities including palms and soles, and the mucous membranes of the mouth and conjunctiva. It is characterized by successive crops of rapidly progressive lesions over an 8- to 12-hour period. The lesions begin as macules, which quickly develop into papules, vesicles, and pustules. Crusting and, sometimes, necrosis precede healing. Characteristically, all types of lesions are present at the same time. The vesicles are 2 to 3 mm in diameter, occur on an erythematous base, and have a "dewdrop on a rose petal" appearance. They are often umbilicated and hemorrhagic.

Differential Diagnosis. Before its eradication, *smallpox* was the most important disease to exclude. The presence of lesions in all stages in varicella helped to differentiate it from smallpox, in which all lesions are in the same stage of development. *Disseminated herpes simplex, coxsackievirus,* and *echovirus,* as well as *rickettsialpox,* can produce vesicular eruptions similar to those of varicella. Diagnosing varicella usually is not difficult, but if one is in doubt, cultures can rule out these other infections.

Laboratory and Biopsy. The diagnosis of varicella usually is obvious. A Tzanck preparation reveals multinucleated giant cells typical of herpesvirus infection. Viral cultures, direct fluorescent antibody stain of vesicle smears, and serologic stud-

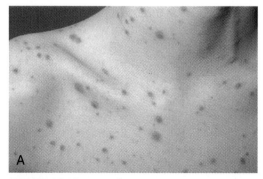 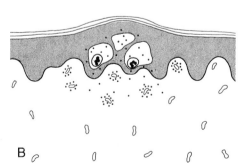

FIGURE 11–5. Varicella. **A,** Epidermis—individual vesicles in generalized distribution. Dermis—erythema. **B,** Epidermis—bullae, multinucleated cells. Dermis—perivascular inflammation.

THERAPY OF VARICELLA

- Prevention
  - Varicella virus vaccine
  - Varicella-zoster immune globulin
  - Acyclovir
- Symptomatic Infection
  - Antihistamines
    - Diphenhydramine: 25–50 mg QID; elixir: 12.5 mg/5 mL–5 mg/kg/day in 4 divided doses
    - Hydroxyzine: 10–25 mg QID; syrup: 10 mg/5 mL, 2 mg/kg/day in 4 divided doses
  - Oatmeal Bath
  - Calamine lotion
- Adults, Severe Infection, Immunosuppression
  - Acyclovir: 20 mg/kg (800 mg max) orally QID × 5 days

---

ies may also be done to confirm the diagnosis, although these usually are not necessary. Culturing the varicella-zoster virus is difficult; therefore, the direct identification of the virus in vesicle smears by immunofluorescence staining is the preferred test.

Therapy. The treatment of chicken pox is largely symptomatic. Antihistamines and topical agents such as calamine lotion are used to reduce itching. Baths (Aveeno) are used for their cleansing and anti-inflammatory actions. Aspirin should be avoided in children because of its association with Reye's syndrome. Acyclovir (Zovirax) reduces complications in adults and immunosuppressed children. The use of acyclovir in immunologically normal children generally is not indicated unless rare visceral involvement is present, such as varicella pneumonia.

Active vaccination with live attenuated virus—the OKA strain—is safe and effective in healthy children and adults. Passive immunization with varicella-zoster immune globulin (VZIG) is used in high-risk patients. VZIG is prepared from plasma containing high titers of varicella-zoster antibody. It is effective in preventing or modifying varicella infection in immunodeficient patients if it is administered shortly after exposure. VZIG is not given to patients with active disease. Patients with leukemia or lymphoma, those with congenital or acquired immunodeficiency, those receiving immunosuppressive medication, and newborns of mothers who have varicella are candidates for treatment.

Varicella-zoster immune globulin (VZIG) is given prophylactically, not for active disease.

Morbidity and mortality are greatly increased in immunocompromised patients.

Course and Complications. Approximately 100 deaths occur each year as the result of varicella. The major complications (pneumonia, encephalitis, and hepatitis) are disproportionately high in adults and in extremely young children. The estimated complication rate in children between the ages of 1 and 14 includes encephalitis in 17 per 100,000 cases, Reye's syndrome in 3.2 per 100,000 cases, and death in 2 per 100,000 cases. Approximately 200 per 100,000 patients with varicella require hospitalization. In adults, death occurs in 50 per 100,000 cases. The immunocompromised patient has a complication rate of 32%, with a 7% death rate.

Varicella during pregnancy poses an approximate 10% risk of intrauterine infection of the fetus, resulting in congenital varicella syndrome or neonatal varicella, with devastating effects on the child.

Pathogenesis. Varicella primary infection begins in the nasopharynx. After local replication, viremia seeds the reticuloendothelial tissue. Secondary viremias cause dissemination to the skin and viscera. Varicella-zoster virus then enters a latent phase in the sensory ganglia.

■ BULLOUS IMPETIGO

Definition and Etiology. Bullous impetigo is an intraepidermal (subcorneal) bacterial infection of the skin caused by certain strains of *S. aureus* (Fig. 11–6). Impetigo is also discussed in Chapter 13.

Incidence. Bullous impetigo occurs most frequently in preschool-age children.

History. Crowding, poor hygiene, chronic dermatitis, and neglected injury of the skin are predisposing factors in the development of impetigo. An initial site of involvement is followed by multiple sites that may be pruritic.

Physical Examination. Large, fragile, clear, or cloudy bullae are characteristic of bullous impetigo. A thin, varnish-like crust occurs after rupture of the bulla. A delicate collarette-like remnant of the blister roof is often present at the rim of the crust. Gyrate lesions may be formed with clear centers and active margins of 0.5 to 2 cm. Autoinoculation results in satellite lesions. The face, neck, and extremities are most often affected. Regional adenopathy may be present, but patients have no systemic symptoms.

Differential Diagnosis. *Contact dermatitis, HSV infection,* and occasionally *superficial fungal infections* may produce vesiculobullous or crusted lesions similar to those of impetigo. The history, patch tests, Tzanck and KOH preparations, and appropriate cultures differentiate these entities. *Pemphigus vulgaris* may also produce crusted lesions and should be suspected in patients with chronic, apparently impetiginized plaques that have not responded to appropriate antibiotics.

Staphylococcal scalded skin syndrome is an uncommon disorder primarily affecting infants and young children. It is characterized by the sudden onset of fever, skin tenderness, and erythema, followed by the formation of large, flaccid bullae

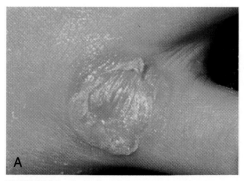 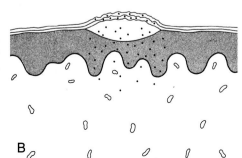

FIGURE 11–6. Bullous Impetigo. **A,** /Epidermis—bulla, crust. **B,** Epidermis—subcorneal bulla, inflammation.

and shedding of large sheets of skin, leaving a denuded, scalded-appearing surface. In contrast to bullous impetigo, in which *S. aureus* may be recovered, the bullae of staphylococcal scalded skin syndrome are sterile. The usual source of infection is in the conjunctiva, nose, or pharynx. In the newborn, an infected umbilical stump may be the source.

Laboratory and Biopsy. Gram stain of the clear or cloudy fluid from a bulla reveals gram-positive cocci. *S. aureus* grows out in more than 95% of the cultures. Biopsy of impetigo, which is usually not done because the diagnosis is obvious, reveals a subcorneal pustule or blister.

Therapy. Most *S. aureus* cultured from impetigo lesions is penicillin resistant. Therefore, a cephalosporin such as cephalexin (Keflex), erythromycin (Ilosone), or a penicillinase-resistant semisynthetic penicillin such as dicloxacillin (Dynapen) should be chosen. Mupirocin (Bactroban) ointment 2% applied three times daily is as effective as oral antibiotics in treating impetigo that is limited to a small area.

General hygiene should also be implemented to prevent spread. Cleansing with antibacterial soaps and gentle removal of crust hasten healing. Daily changing of items that contact the area of impetigo such as towels, washcloths, and shavers is recommended.

Course and Complications. Even without treatment, impetigo spontaneously heals in 3 to 6 weeks. Antibiotics hasten healing (within 1 week of starting therapy) and reduce contagiousness.

Pathogenesis. An epidermolytic toxin causes the subcorneal cleavage characteristic of bullous impetigo and staphylococcal scalded skin syndrome. This toxin is from pathogenic phage group II *S. aureus*. In bullous impetigo, the toxin is produced at the site of the lesion. In staphylococcal scalded skin syndrome, it is produced remotely and then is hematogeneously carried to the skin.

> **Epidermolytic toxin causes bullae.**

■ CONTACT DERMATITIS (ACUTE)

Because acute contact dermatitis is characterized by a vesicular eruption, it is briefly mentioned here. In Chapter 9, it is discussed in more detail, along with other eczematous eruptions.

Contact dermatitis is an inflammatory reaction of the skin caused by an irritant or allergenic chemical. It may be an acute or chronic process. Intraepidermal

---

THERAPY OF BULLOUS IMPETIGO

- Antibiotics
    Cephalexin: 25–50 mg/kg/day in oral suspension, 500 mg BID
    Erythromycin: 30–50 mg/kg/day in oral suspension, 500 mg BID
    Dicloxacillin: 500 mg BID
    Mupirocin ointment: applied TID
- General Hygiene
    Antibacterial soaps: Lever 2000, Dial, Hibiclens
    Changing of towel, washcloth, shaver, etc., daily

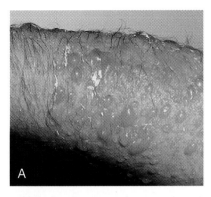
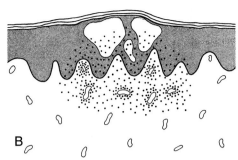

FIGURE 11–7. Contact Dermatitis (acute). **A,** Epidermis—bullae. Dermis—erythema. **B,** Epidermis—bulla, spongiosis. Dermis—perivascular infiltrate.

vesicles are the hallmark of acute contact dermatitis (Fig. 11–7). Additional characteristics are weeping, crusting, edema, and erythema. The areas involved frequently have sharp margins with geometric and linear configurations. Poison ivy and other plants characteristically cause linear streaks of papulovesicles. Treatment is with steroids (topical or systemic), antihistamines, and wet dressings or soaks.

■ UNCOMMON BLISTERING DISEASES

Pemphigus vulgaris, bullous pemphigoid, dermatitis herpetiformis, and porphyria cutanea tarda are rare blistering disorders that are important because of their significant mortality or morbidity (Table 11–2). They should be considered when the more common causes of blistering disease have been ruled out and appropriate laboratory data have been collected. Three of the four diseases—pemphigus vulgaris, bullous pemphigoid, and dermatitis herpetiformis—are examples of immunologically mediated disorders. Porphyria cutanea tarda is a metabolic disorder characterized by defective heme synthesis and excessive porphyrin production.

Pemphigus Vulgaris

The bullae break easily, leaving erosions and crusts.

Pemphigus vulgaris is an autoimmune disease characterized by blistering of the skin and mucous membranes. It predominantly occurs in middle and old age, with an estimated incidence of 1 per 100,000. The bullae are flaccid, superficial, and range from 1 to 10 cm. They rupture easily, leaving large denuded, bleeding, weeping, and crusted erosions (Fig. 11–8). Pressure applied laterally to the bulla results in extension (Nikolsky's sign). The oral mucosa (erosions of the mouth) is almost always involved and frequently is the presenting site.

The bulla of pemphigus vulgaris occurs intraepidermally just above the basal layer. It is formed by the loss of cohesion between epidermal cells (acantholysis). Direct (with patient skin) and indirect (with patient serum) immunofluorescence studies are positive, showing deposits of immunoglobulins (Ig) (predominantly IgG) or complement C3 between epidermal cells (intercellular space) (Fig. 11–9). Experimental evidence suggests that the interaction between the circulating IgG autoantibodies and epidermal cell surface antigens (adhesion molecule-desmo-

TABLE 11–2 ■ UNCOMMON BLISTERING DISEASES

Disease	Pathogenesis	Physical Examination	Blister Location	Laboratory Test	Therapy
Pemphigus vulgaris	Autoimmune	Flaccid bullae, erosions, and crusts Generalized	Intraepidermal	DIF (+) IgG and C3 inter-cellular in epidermis IIF (+)	Prednisone Azathioprine Methotrexate Gold
Bullous pemphigoid	Autoimmune	Tense bullae on inflamed or noninflamed skin Flexor surfaces	Subepidermal	DIF (+) IgG and C3 base-ment membrane zone IIF (+)	Prednisone Azathioprine Methotrexate
Dermatitis herpeti-formis	Immune complex?	Excoriated, crusted papules, ves-icles, and urticarial plaques Elbows, knees, back, buttocks	Subepidermal	DIF (+) IgA dermal papil-lae IIF (+)	Dapsone Sulfapyridine Gluten-free diet
Porphyria cutanea tarda	Metabolic	Tense bullae, crusted erosions, milia Dorsum of the hands	Subepidermal	Elevated urine uropor-phyrin DIF (+) IIF (−)	Phlebotomy Antimalarials

DIF, direct immunofluorescence; C3, complement; Ig, immunoglobulin; IIF, indirect immunofluorescence; +, positive; −, negative.

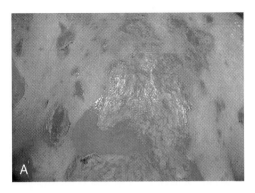

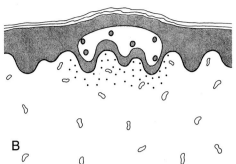

FIGURE 11–8. Pemphigus Vulgaris. **A,** Epidermis—flaccid bullae. **B,** Epidermis—suprabasal bulla, acantholytic epidermal cells.

glein 3) contained in intercellular adhering junctions (desmosomes) leads to blister formation. In addition, the production of proteolytic enzymes that hydrolyze the cell surface proteins causes loss of adhesion between keratinocytes.

Before the introduction of systemic steroids, pemphigus vulgaris had an extremely high mortality. Systemic steroids and immunosuppressive agents such as methotrexate, cyclophosphamide, azathioprine, and gold are used. The overall mortality rate is 8% to 10%, now occurring more frequently as a result of steroid-induced complications than of the disease.

Initial therapy: Steroids

Untreated pemphigus vulgaris has a high mortality.

Bullous Pemphigoid

Bullous pemphigoid is an autoimmune disorder characterized by subepidermal bullae. It occurs in elderly patients (sixth, seventh, and eighth decades). The preferred sites of involvement are the groin, axillae, and flexural areas. Approximately one third of patients have oral involvement. The blisters are large and tense and occur on normal or erythematous skin (Fig. 11–10). The bullae do not extend laterally (negative Nikolsky's sign) like those of pemphigus vulgaris. Healing usually occurs without scarring.

Direct and indirect immunofluorescence studies reveal a linear band of IgG and complement C3 deposited along the basement membrane zone, where blister formation occurs (Fig. 11–11). The IgG autoantibodies are directed against a normal-appearing antigen (the bullous pemphigoid antigen) in the basement mem-

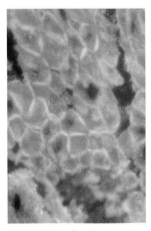

FIGURE 11–9. Direct and indirect immunofluorescence shows intercellular staining for immunoglobulin G or complement characteristic of pemphigus vulgaris.

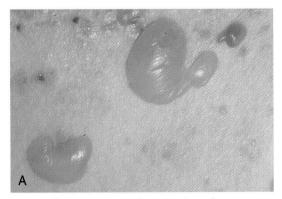

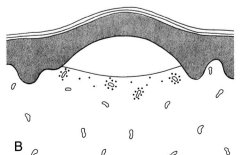

FIGURE 11–10. Bullous pemphigoid. **A,** Dermis—tense bullae. **B,** Dermis—subepidermal bulla.

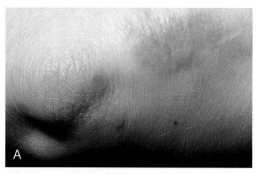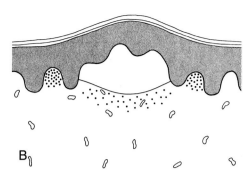

FIGURE 11-12. Dermatitis Herpetiformis. **A,** Dermis—tense bullae. **B,** Dermis—subepidermal bulla, neutrophils in dermal papillae.

brane zone. This antigen is found intracellularly in association with the hemidesmosome and extracellularly in the lamina lucida, which is the uppermost portion of the basement membrane zone between the epidermis and dermis.

The prognosis is excellent, and the disease usually subsides after months or years. The tendency for the blistered skin to heal results in a low mortality rate. However, the morbidity caused by widespread blistering requires treatment with systemic steroids and immunosuppressive agents.

Initial therapy: Steroids

Dermatitis Herpetiformis

Dermatitis herpetiformis is a chronic, intensely pruritic, vesicular disease characterized by grouped (herpetiform) papules, vesicles, and urticarial plaques, which are distributed symmetrically on the elbows, knees, buttocks, low back, and shoulders (Fig. 11–12). The vesicles often are not intact, secondary to scratching as a result of intense pruritus. The disease usually begins in early adult life, and the general health of the patient is otherwise excellent.

Because of scratching, excoriations, rather than vesicles, may be all that is seen

Initial therapy: Dapsone

The typical histologic change of dermatitis herpetiformis is a subepidermal blister with neutrophilic abscesses in the dermal papillae. Direct immunofluorescence testing demonstrates granular deposits of IgA at the tips of the dermal papillae (Fig. 11–13). Indirect immunofluorescence testing for IgA antiendomysial antibodies is also sensitive and specific.

Dermatitis herpetiformis characteristically clears rapidly after treatment with dapsone or sulfapyridine, but the disease promptly recurs when therapy is stopped. Approximately 75% of patients have associated (but usually asymptomatic) gluten-sensitive enteropathy. In these patients, a strict gluten-free diet causes remission or allows a significant reduction of the medication dose.

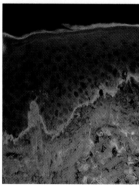

FIGURE 11-11. Direct and indirect immunofluorescent staining shows linear deposit of immunoglobulin G or complement at the dermal-epidermal junction characteristic of bullous pemphigoid.

Porphyria Cutanea Tarda

The porphyrias are a group of disorders characterized by abnormalities in the heme biosynthetic pathway resulting in abnormal porphyrin metabolism and excessive accumulation of various porphyrins. Porphyria cutanea tarda is the most common form of porphyria. It is characterized by subepidermal blisters on the hands and excessive uroporphyrin excretion in the urine. Bullae, vesicles, erosions,

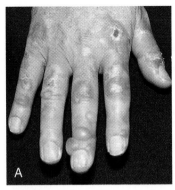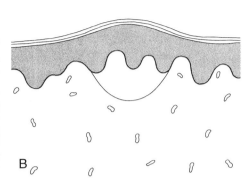

FIGURE 11–14. Porphyria Cutanea Tarda. **A,** Dermis—tense bullae. **B,** Dermis—subepidermal bulla.

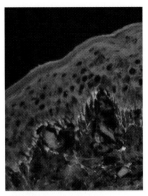

FIGURE 11–13. Direct and indirect immunofluorescent staining shows granular deposits of immunoglobulin A in the tips of dermal papillae characteristic of dermatitis herpetiformis.

crusts, milia, and mild scarring occur on sun-exposed skin, especially the dorsum of the hands (Fig. 11–14). Facial hair, predominantly on the temples and cheeks, and mottled facial pigmentation resembling melasma also occur.

The bullae of porphyria cutanea tarda occur subepidermally. Direct immunofluorescence reveals Ig and complement around the dermal blood vessels and at the dermal-epidermal junction. The metabolic changes in porphyria cutanea tarda are diagnostic, so immunofluorescent testing is not warranted. Characteristically, urine uroporphyrins and coproporphyrins are markedly elevated, with a ratio of urine uroporphyrin to urine coproporphyrin of at least 3:1. Liver function tests and serum iron levels are usually elevated. The urine is dark brown and fluoresces orange red under Wood's light. *Variegate porphyria* has neurologic and abdominal symptoms as well as the same cutaneous findings as porphyria cutanea tarda. The ratio of urine uroporphyrin to coproporphyrin is 1 : 1 in variegate porphyria.

Porphyria cutanea tarda is familial or sporadic. It is often precipitated by alcohol, hepatitis C, or birth control pills. The biosynthetic pathway for heme requires the conversion of uroporphyrinogen to coproporphyrinogen by the enzyme uroporphyrinogen decarboxylase. When this enzyme is absent, uroporphyrins accumulate and produce porphyria cutanea tarda. Treatment of choice is phlebotomy or antimalarials when these drugs are used in extremely low dosage.

Variegate porphyria and porphyria cutanea tarda have identical skin findings.

Initial treatment:
1. **Removal of precipitant—alcohol, birth control pills, etc.**
2. **Phlebotomy**
3. **Antimalarials**

■ UNKNOWN (Fig. 11–15)

This 32-year-old woman had a history of a recurrent vesicular eruption on the upper portion of her leg. It started 5 years ago and recurs five or six times yearly. A tingling sensation precedes the onset of the rash.

What is your diagnosis?

These grouped vesiculopustules on an erythematous base are typical of HSV infection. In addition, the history of a recurrent vesicular eruption in the same place is classic for this viral infection. No other diagnosis should be seriously considered.

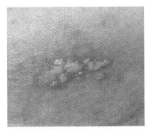

FIGURE 11–15. Unknown.

What laboratory tests would you do?

A Tzanck preparation is all that is necessary to confirm the clinical diagnosis. If one is still in doubt, a viral culture can be obtained.

What are your recommendations to the patient?

Acyclovir, valacyclovir, or famciclovir may be used in patients with frequent recurrences. These medications reduce the duration of viral shedding and time to healing of lesions when they are administered early in the course of a recurrent episode.

Important Points

1. The Tzanck preparation is an easy laboratory test that confirms the diagnosis of HSV infection.
2. Acyclovir, valacyclovir, and famciclovir are the current treatments of choice for HSV infection, but they are not curative.

REFERENCES

Herpes Simplex

Abramowicz M (ed): Drugs for non-HIV viral infections. Med Lett *41*:113–120, 1999.

Benedetti JK, Zeh J, Corey L: Clinical reactivation of genital herpes simplex virus infection decreases in frequency over time. Ann Intern Med *131*:14–20, 1999.

Brice SL: Cutaneous infection with herpes simplex virus: a review. Curr Concepts Skin Disord *12*:5–15, 1991.

Busso M, Berman B: Antivirals in dermatology. J Am Acad Dermatol *32*:1031–1040, 1995.

Corey L, Adams HG, Brown ZA, et al.: Genital herpes simplex virus infections: clinical manifestations, course and complications. Ann Intern Med *98*:958–972, 1983.

Engel JP: Long-term suppression of genital herpes. JAMA *280*:928–929, 1998.

Fleming DT, McQuillan GM, Johnson RE, et al.: Herpes simplex virus type 2 in the United States, 1976 to 1994. N Engl J Med *337*:1105–1111, 1997.

Langenberg AGM, Corey L, Ashley RL, et al.: A prospective study of new infections with herpes simplex virus type 1 and type 2. N Engl J Med *341*:1432–1438, 1999.

Pereira FA: Herpes simplex: evolving concepts. J Am Acad Dermatol *35*:503–520, 1996.

Safrin S, Crumpacker C, Chatis P, et al.: A controlled trial comparing foscarnet with vidarabine for acyclovir-resistant mucocutaneous herpes simplex in the acquired immunodeficiency syndrome. N Engl J Med *325*:551–555, 1991.

Straus SE, Rooney JF, Sever JL, et al.: Herpes simplex virus infection: biology, treatment, and prevention. Ann Intern Med *103*:404–419, 1985.

Wald A, Zeh J, Selke S, et al.: Virologic characteristics of subclinical and symptomatic genital herpes infections. N Engl J Med *333*:770–775, 1995.

Westheim AI, Tenser RB, Marks JG: Acyclovir resistance in a patient with chronic mucocutaneous herpes simplex infection. J Am Acad Dermatol *17*:875–880, 1987.

Whitley R, Arvin A, Prober C, et al.: Predictors of morbidity and mortality in neonates with herpes simplex virus infections. N Engl J Med *324*:450–454, 1991.

Herpes Zoster

Abramowicz M (ed): Drugs for non-HIV viral infections. Med Lett *41*:113–120, 1999.

Balfour HH, Bean B, Laskin OL, et al.: Acyclovir halts progression of herpes zoster in immunocompromised patients. N Engl J Med *308*:1448–1453, 1983.

Fueyo MA, Lookingbill DP: Herpes zoster and occult malignancy. J Am Acad Dermatol *11*: 480–482, 1984.

Huff JC, Bean B, Balfour HH, et al.: Therapy of herpes zoster with oral acyclovir. Am J Med 85:84–89, 1988.

Kost RG, Straus SE: Postherpetic neuralgia: pathogenesis, treatment, and prevention. N Engl J Med 335:32–42, 1996.

Ragozzino MW, Melton LJ, Kurland LT, et al.: Risk of cancer after herpes zoster: a population-based study. N Engl J Med 307:393–397, 1982.

Straus SE, Ostrove JM, Inchause G, et al.: Varicella-zoster virus infections. Ann Intern Med 108:221–237, 1988.

Varicella

Abramowicz M (ed): Drugs for non-HIV viral infections. Med Lett 41:113–120, 1999.

Advisory Committee on Immunization Practices: Prevention of varicella. MMWR Morb Mort Wkly Rep 45:1–36, 1996.

Dunkle LM, Arvin AM, Whitley RJ, et al.: A controlled trial of acyclovir for chickenpox in normal children. N Engl J Med 325:1539–1544, 1991.

Fleisher G, Henry W, McSorley M, et al.: Life-threatening complications of varicella. Am J Dis Child 135:896–899, 1981.

Krause PR, Klinman DM: Efficacy, immunogenicity, safety, and use of live attenuated chickenpox vaccine. J Pediatr 127:518–525, 1995.

Weibel RE, Neff BJ, Kuter BJ, et al.: Live attenuated varicella virus vaccine efficacy trial in healthy children. N Engl J Med 310:1409–1415, 1984.

Weller TH: Varicella and herpes zoster: changing concepts of the natural history, control, and importance of a not-so-benign virus. N Engl J Med 309:1362–1368, 1434–1440, 1983.

Impetigo

Demidovich CW, Wittier RR, Ruff ME, Bass JW, Browning WC: Impetigo: current etiology and comparison of penicillin, erythromycin, and cephalexin therapies. Am J Dis Child 144:1313–1315, 1990.

Eells LD, Mertz PM, Piovanetti Y, et al.: Topical antibiotic treatment of impetigo with mupirocin. Arch Dermatol 122:1273–1276, 1986.

Lyell A: The staphylococcal scalded skin syndrome in historical perspective: emergence of dermopathic strains of Staphylococcus aureus and discovery of the epidermolytic toxin. J Am Acad Dermatol 9:285–294,1983.

Uncommon Blistering Diseases

Ahmed AR, Graham J, Jordan RE, et al.: Pemphigus: current concepts. Ann Intern Med 92:396–405, 1980.

Anhalt G J, Patel H, Diaz LA: Mechanisms of immunologic injury: pemphigus and bullous pemphigoid. Arch Dermatol 119:711–714, 1983.

Fine JD: Management of acquired bullous skin diseases. N Engl J Med 333:1475–1484, 1995.

Helm KF, Peters MS: Dermatology: immunodermatology update. The immunologically mediated vesiculobullous diseases. Mayo Clin Proc 66:187–202, 1991.

Katz SI: Dermatitis herpetiformis. Int J Dermatol 7:529–535, 1978.

Korman NJ: Bullous pemphigoid: the latest in diagnosis, prognosis, and therapy. Arch Dermatol 134:1137–1141, 1998.

Roujeau JC, Lok C, Bastuji-Garin S, et al.: High risk of death in elderly patients with extensive bullous pemphigoid. Arch Dermatol 134:465–469, 1998.

Thiers BH: The porphyrias. J Am Acad Dermatol 5:621–625, 1981.

12 INFLAMMATORY PAPULES

SCABIES
INSECT BITE REACTIONS
LICHEN PLANUS
MILIARIA

The diseases discussed in this chapter are characterized by discrete, small, erythematous papules that do *not* become confluent. Most of these disorders are pruritic, some markedly so. As a result, the papules are often crusted secondary to excoriation. Papules are common primary lesions found in numerous skin diseases, including acne, eczematous diseases, and the scaling disorders. However, in these diseases, other features are present that allow for their characterization. For example, comedones and pustules accompany papules in acne, eczematous papules are confluent, and plaques as well as papules are present in the scaling disorders. The diseases in this chapter feature individual papules as the predominant finding (Table 12–1). The papules are not scaling, except in lichen planus, in which the scale often is not obvious. Therefore, lichen planus is included in this chapter rather than in Chapter 10.

■ SCABIES

Definition. Scabies is an infestation of the epidermis with the "itch" mite, *Sarcoptes scabiei* var. *hominis*. Clinically, a few burrows are usually found and are diagnostic. Inflammatory papules resulting from host hypersensitivity, however, constitute the more frequent and obvious findings (Fig. 12–1).

Incidence. Scabies is a common disease, but the incidence fluctuates over the years. In the 20th century, incidence peaks have followed 30-year cycles, occurring during World War I, World War II, and the middle to late 1970s, although this latest scourge has persisted through the 1990s. Scabies can occur endemically among school-age children and institutionalized patients, particularly those in nursing homes.

Itching is often severe enough to interrupt sleep.

Family members and friends often also itch.

History. Pruritus is the major complaint. It is often severe enough to interrupt sleep. Frequently, a history of itching can be elicited in family members and other close personal contacts. The incubation time from inoculation to the onset of pruritus is usually approximately 1 month, so in early cases, other contacts may not yet be symptomatic. Because scabies also occurs in pets (canine scabies), a pet history should be elicited, particularly in patients with recurrent disease.

TABLE 12–1 ■ PAPULES

	Frequency*	Etiology	History	Physical Examination	Differential Diagnosis	Laboratory Test
Scabies	1.5	Mite	Other close contacts often affected	*Burrows* (when found) diagnostic Generalized distribution sparing head Genitalia often affected	Eczematous dermatitis	Scraping
Insect bite reactions	0.7	Stinging and biting arthropods	Insect often not seen by patient	Papules with central puncta, and often *grouped* *Asymmetric* distribution	Urticaria Impetigo Mucha-Habermann disease	—
Lichen planus	0.6	Unknown	—	Purple, polygonal flat-topped papules with Wickham's striae Can be generalized: wrists, ankles, and *mucous membranes* favored	Lupus erythematosus Lichen planus–like drug eruption Graft versus host disease	Biopsy
Miliaria	0.1	Sweat duct occlusion	Fever or occlusion of affected skin	Numerous small papules Trunk, especially back, usually affected	Contact dermatitis Folliculitis Candidiasis	Biopsy (not usually necessary)

*Percentage of new dermatology patients with this diagnosis seen in the Hershey Medical Center Dermatology Clinic, Hershey, PA.

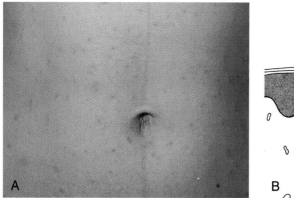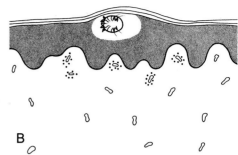

FIGURE 12–1. Scabies. **A,** Widespread, discrete papules. Epidermis—normal or excoriated. Dermis— erythema. **B,** Epidermis—mite burrowed in the superficial epidermis. Dermis—inflammation.

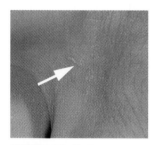

FIGURE 12–2. Diagnostic burrow.

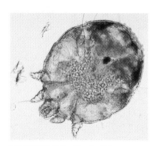

FIGURE 12–3. Scabies mite (400×).

The entire body is treated.

Physical Examination. Small inflammatory papules predominate. They are often excoriated. The distribution is generalized, but favored locations include the finger webs, wrists, elbows, axillae, girdle area, and feet. In addition, the male genitalia are usually involved. Itching papules and small nodules on the penis should be considered the result of scabies unless proved otherwise. In temperate climates, the head is almost always spared in adults but may be involved in children. In infants, vesicles may also be present, particularly on the palms and soles.

The diagnostic finding is a burrow, which appears as a 2- to 5-mm, delicate, white, serpiginous, superficial, thread-like line (Fig. 12–2). The most common location for burrows is on the hands. With close inspection, a tiny black speck can often be seen at the end of the burrow. This black dot represents the adult mite, which is best visualized under the microscope. In some patients with scabies, particularly if the condition has been longstanding, scattered nodules may also be found.

Differential Diagnosis. Because of the intense pruritus, in some patients only excoriations are seen. In these patients, a misdiagnosis of neurotic excoriations could be made. Widespread disease may be misdiagnosed as *eczematous dermatitis*.

Laboratory and Biopsy. The presence of mites or eggs is diagnostic (Fig. 12–3). This is accomplished by a skin scraping with a No. 15 blade, as described in Chapter 4. The highest yield is from a burrow, but mites and eggs also can be recovered from papules and nodules.

A biopsy is usually not necessary but may provide the diagnosis when it previously had not been suspected. Microscopically, one sees edema in the epidermis, which may be sufficient to result in a microvesicle. An inflammatory reaction occurs in the superficial dermis with lymphocytes and eosinophils. A fortuitous but diagnostic finding is the presence of a mite in the stratum corneum.

Therapy. In Roman times, therapy was accomplished with hot sulfur spring baths. Today, therapy remains topical but must be applied to the *entire body surface*. A *single application* of either 1% lindane lotion or 5% permethrin (Elimite) cream is applied at bedtime from the head to the toes and is washed off in the morning. Some physicians recommend a single reapplication after 1 week, but the medication should not be used more often than that. Treatment also is recommended for household contacts; those who are asymptomatic require only one application.

THERAPY OF SCABIES

- Topical: overnight application
  Lindane lotion 1%
  Permethrin cream 5%
- Systemic
  Ivermectin: 0.2 mg/kg in single dose

Rare cases of neurotoxicity have been reported from the absorption of lindane in infants and in patients who overuse this medication. Accordingly, instructions to patients must be clear, and permethrin cream is preferred for infants.

Most recently, systemic ivermectin has been successfully used for treating scabies. A single oral dose of 0.2 mg/kg is sufficient for cure in most patients, although residual itching may persist for up to 1 month after this systemic treatment.

Course and Complications. When untreated, itching progresses and may become unbearable. After treatment, many patients continue to itch for 1 to 2 weeks. This possibility must be explained so the patient avoids overuse of the medication. Residual itching can be treated symptomatically with topical steroids and oral antihistamines. Nodules, if present, may last for 1 month or longer.

Itching may persist for 1 to 2 weeks after treatment.

Complications are uncommon. Secondary bacterial infection may occur in excoriated skin. In immunocompromised and institutionalized patients (particularly patients with AIDS), scabies may appear as a widespread scaling eruption that often *does not* itch. This uncommon variant is called Norwegian scabies and is easily misdiagnosed as eczema or psoriasis. On close inspection, however, burrows and mites are usually numerous, and their presence confirms the diagnosis.

Norwegian scabies occurs in immunosuppressed patients, particularly those with AIDS.

Pathogenesis. The discovery in 1687 of the "itch mite" made this parasite one of the first causes of human disease to be identified. The *S. scabiei* mite lives in and on human skin, where it completes its life cycle in approximately 2 weeks. The impregnated female burrows into the stratum corneum, where she lays two or three eggs daily for as long as 30 days. Each egg produces a larva, which leaves the burrow and molts to produce a nymph. Several additional moltings result in a mature mite, which then mates. After mating, the male dies, and the female completes the life cycle by burrowing back into the stratum corneum. Secretions from the burrowing female mite cause intraepidermal edema fluid, on which she feeds.

The itching and inflammation are thought to be a result of a hypersensitivity reaction by the host to the foreign material (i.e., mites, eggs, and feces) in the skin. This may account for the persistence of the itching for 1 to 2 weeks after successful treatment; it may take that long for the stratum corneum to turn over and to shed the foreign material and for the hypersensitivity reaction to subside.

During World War II, studies were performed on the natural history and the contagious nature of scabies. From these studies, the following were found:

1. It is difficult to transmit scabies through fomites such as bedding and clothing (human-to-human transmission is most common).

2. The incubation time from inoculation to itching usually is approximately 1 month.

3. Untreated, the course is one of progressive itching.

4. Previously infested individuals are more difficult to reinfest, possibly because the hypersensitivity reaction is partially protective.

■ INSECT BITE REACTIONS

Definition. Insect bites and stings produce local inflammatory reactions (Fig. 12–4) in response to injected foreign chemicals and protein. Acute skin reactions appear as hives, and more chronic reactions appear as inflammatory papules. Insects that sting (usually out of anger) include bees, wasps, and fire ants. Insects that bite (usually out of hunger) include mosquitoes, fleas, flies, bedbugs, and lice. Spiders, ticks, and chiggers are other arthropods that sometimes attack human skin.

Incidence. Insect bites are common. Most are recognized as such and are not brought to a physician's attention. Physicians may be consulted when the reaction is severe or produces chronically recurring pruritic papules.

"Indoor" insects:
1. Fleas
2. Spiders
3. Bedbugs
4. Lice

History. When someone is stung by an insect, the insult is usually remembered because the sting induces immediate pain. This is not always the case for biting insects; some delay may occur between the actual bite and the itching that follows. If the physical examination suggests insect bites (even if the patient is unaware of having been bitten), the history should be carefully pursued for possible exposures. For indoor exposure, fleas are common offenders. We inquire not only about pets currently living in the dwelling but also about whether pets had recently occupied the premises. If a house had been previously occupied by flea-infested pets, the abandoned hungry fleas may form a welcoming party for the newly arrived human guests. We also ask about pets in homes the patient visits. Spiders are sometimes responsible for indoor bites; their presence requires a careful search of the home. Bedbugs are a less common problem. Infestations with head lice often occur epidemically in school children, so a history of affected playmates should be sought and the school nurse should be consulted.

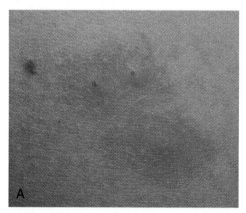
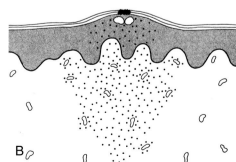

FIGURE 12–4. Insect bite reaction. **A,** Grouped papules. Epidermis—small central puncta or crusts. Dermis—wheal or erythema. **B,** Epidermis—crust; spongiosis; inflammation cell infiltrate. Dermis—dense infiltrate of mixed inflammatory cells, often including eosinophils.

Contrary to some misconceptions, it is not necessary for other persons dwelling in the same household to be affected. For insect bite reactions, two factors are required: a biting insect and a host who is allergic to the bite. Not all people are sensitive.

Physical Examination. The reaction to a sting is usually an immediate hive, often with a central punctum. Of the stinging insects, only the honey bee leaves behind its stinger, which on close inspection appears as a sharp barb projecting from the skin. If found, this stinger should be removed gently to prevent release of additional venom from the attached venom sack. Fire ants produce multiple itching hives, which quickly progress to painful papulovesicles and pustules. The bite of a recluse spider is unique in that it produces a severe local necrotic reaction with ulceration (Fig. 12–5). Although the bite may be "quiet," the reaction that ensues over the following days is not. Chiggers favor the legs and areas of tight-fitting clothing where they produce inflammatory papules, vesicles, and occasionally even bullae (Fig. 12–6). Ticks burrow their heads in the skin, and pubic lice (pediculosis pubis) attach to hair; both can be macroscopically visualized. Head lice (pediculosis capitis) may be difficult to find but should be suspected in the presence of itching of the scalp, particularly the occiput. The eggs (nits) are most often found and appear as small, 2- to 3-mm, oval, translucent concretions affixed to hair shafts.

Physicians are most often consulted for insect bites that produce itching papules. These typically are grouped and asymmetric. Flea bites frequently occur in streaks of three: "breakfast, lunch, and dinner." Sometimes, a central punctum can be identified in the papule; this is diagnostic. If the offending insects remain in the environment, new lesions will continue to appear. Occasionally, only excoriations are found.

Differential Diagnosis. For patients with urticarial reactions, other causes of urticaria (see Chapter 17) may be considered. When the hive has a central punctum, however, its cause is an insect bite. *Other foreign bodies* can induce pruritic papules in the skin. Fiberglass is an example. This diagnosis can be suggested by the history and can be confirmed by the presence of refractile material in the epidermis on biopsy or skin scraping. *Dermatitis herpetiformis* (see Chapter 11) is in the differential diagnosis, particularly when only excoriations are found. Excoriation may also lead to secondary infection and a diagnosis of impetigo (see Chapter 13). An uncommon idiopathic disorder, *Mucha-Habermann disease*, presents with scattered necrotic papules and vesicles that can resemble insect bites but usually are more generalized and symmetric. A skin biopsy helps to distinguish Mucha-Habermann disease from an insect bite reaction.

Laboratory and Biopsy. The diagnosis usually is made clinically. A biopsy, if performed, shows a wedge-shaped superficial and deep cellular infiltrate so dense that it may be mistaken for malignant lymphoma. An insect bite is suggested by virtue of a mixed inflammatory cell infiltrate, which includes numerous eosinophils.

Therapy. The primary therapy is to remove the offending insect from the environment of the patient or vice versa. Insects that are attached to the skin can be gently removed with tweezers (e.g., ticks) or killed chemically (e.g., lice) with agents such as lindane shampoo and permethrin creme (Nix) rinse. For fleas, not only must the pet be treated, but also the house must be professionally fumigated.

Papules occur only in people who are allergic.

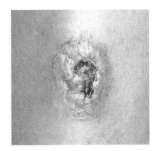

FIGURE 12–5. Necrotic skin reaction to a recluse spider bite.

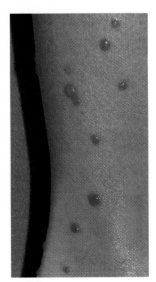

FIGURE 12–6. Papules and vesicles from chigger bites.

Successful treatment of flea bites includes fumigation of the home.

THERAPY OF INSECT BITE REACTIONS

- Separation of host from insect
- Lindane or permethrin (lice)
- House fumigation and treatment of pet (fleas)
- Symptomatic therapy for itching
    Topical steroids
    Antihistamines

Treatment of the inflammatory reaction of the skin is symptomatic. Topical steroids and systemic antihistamines may be helpful in relieving the itching.

Course and Complications. In highly sensitive individuals, stings can produce serious anaphylactic reactions that occasionally result in death. Patients with anaphylactic reactions require prompt therapy with epinephrine, antihistamines, and, often, systemic steroids. Subsequent "desensitization" immunotherapy is frequently indicated for future prophylaxis. Immunotherapy is not necessary, however, in most children with urticarial reactions, even if these reactions are severe and generalized, as long as symptoms are confined to the skin. It is advisable, however, for such patients to carry injectable epinephrine (Ana-Kit, EpiPen) when picnicking, hiking, or camping.

Most insect bite reactions resolve spontaneously and uneventfully. Secondary infection may occur, particularly when the patient has been scratching excessively. Scratching and infection also can lead to scars. A persistent local reaction to the bite of an infected deer tick is a characteristic finding in Lyme disease and is called *erythema migrans* (see Chapter 17).

Pathogenesis. Most insect bite reactions are the result of host allergy to injected secretions, including venoms (from stinging insects) and enzymes. Histamine, acetylcholine, and other vasoactive chemicals have also been isolated from the venom of stinging insects, and these, too, may play a role in the immediate reaction. However, the primary mechanism for insect bite reactions is allergic. The degree of host allergy determines the intensity of the reaction, which ranges from none to severe. As exemplified by *erythema migrans*, cutaneous reactions to insect bites also may be caused by microorganisms transmitted by the bite.

■ LICHEN PLANUS

Definition. Lichen planus is an idiopathic inflammatory disorder of the skin. Clinically, the papules are flat (planus) and are surmounted by subtle, fine white dots and lines that, with imagination, resemble the appearance of lichen (Fig. 12–7).

Incidence. The disorder is uncommon but not rare. It is the presenting problem in 6 per 1,000 of our new dermatology patients. The prevalence of lichen planus in the United States is estimated at 4.4 per 1,000. Women are more often affected than are men.

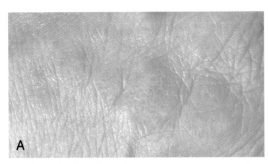 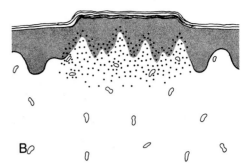

FIGURE 12–7. Lichen planus. **A,** Flat-topped purple papules with Wickham's striae. Epidermis—slight, adherent scale. Dermis—violaceous erythema. **B,** Epidermis—hyperkeratosis; degeneration of the basal cell layer; "saw-tooth" pattern of rete pegs. Dermis—dense, band-like lymphocytic infiltrate in the upper dermis.

History. The major complaint is itching, which is often severe. Mucous membrane involvement sometimes results in painful erosions. Lichen planus–like eruptions can be induced by drugs, so a careful drug history should be elicited.

Physical Examination. The primary lesion is a purple, polygonal, pruritic, flat-topped papule. Its surface has a fine reticulate pattern of white dots and lines (Wickham's striae) that can be visualized on *close* inspection. Wickham's striae are more readily visible through a hand-held lens after the application of a drop of oil on the surface of the papule. The papules are sometimes arranged in streaks, presumably resulting from the trauma of scratching (Koebner phenomenon, Fig. 12–8). The wrists and ankles are favored locations for lichen planus, but any area may be affected, including the palms, soles, and genitalia. Patients may have only a few papules or innumerable ones in a generalized distribution. Uncommonly, individual lesions may attain plaque size. Residual hyperpigmented macules typically result from the inflammatory process. The nails and hair follicles are occasionally involved with dystrophic changes and even scarring.

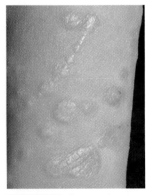

FIGURE 12–8. Papules in streaks—Koebner phenomenon.

Mucous membrane involvement is common and, in some patients, is the sole manifestation of the disease. Most often, this condition appears as white streaks in a reticulate pattern (see Chapter 23). Blisters and erosions also sometimes occur. The buccal mucosa is affected most often, but the tongue, lips, and gums also may be involved.

Differential Diagnosis. The white lines on the surface of violet lichen planus papules are usually subtle, so the disease usually does not appear as a scaling disorder. Occasionally, however, more scale can be present, in which case the papulosquamous disorders (see Chapter 10) must be considered, including *psoriasis, fungal infection, pityriasis rosea,* and *discoid lupus erythematosus.* Of these, *discoid lupus* is the most commonly confused, and in some patients the two diseases may overlap. Lichen planus presenting with only a few scattered papules can be confused with *insect bites. Drug eruptions* can mimic lichen planus. Drugs that most often cause lichenoid eruptions are thiazides, phenothiazines, gold, quinidine, and the antimalarials quinacrine and chloroquine. When the palms and soles are involved, a serologic test for syphilis should be performed to rule out *secondary syphilis.* Some patients with *graft-versus-host disease* also develop a skin eruption that closely resembles lichen planus both clinically and histopathologically. The differential diagnosis for mucous membrane involvement with lichen planus includes *"leukoplakia," candidiasis,* and *secondary syphilis* (see Chapter 23).

Drugs that can cause lichen planus–like eruptions:
1. **Thiazides**
2. **Phenothiazines**
3. **Gold**
4. **Quinidine**
5. **Quinacrine**
6. **Chloroquine**

Laboratory and Biopsy. If the clinical diagnosis is in doubt, a biopsy may be performed. In lichen planus, the histologic features are characteristic. The typical constellation of findings includes hyperkeratosis, thickened granular layer, degeneration of the basal cell layer, colloid bodies (necrotic basal cells), and dense, "band-like" inflammatory infiltrate in the papillary dermis that obscures and disrupts the dermal-epidermal junction.

Therapy. The treatment is nonspecific and often is not totally successful. The inflammatory reaction is suppressed with steroids. Localized disease is treated with strong topical steroids such as fluocinonide 0.05% cream. For severe widespread disease, a course of systemic steroids is sometimes required, but caution is advised when administering these agents on a long-term basis because of the well-known side effects. Antihistamines are used with varying success for the pruritus. Topical and systemic retinoids (e.g., tretinoin gel and oral acitretin) have been successful in some patients with mucous membrane lesions. Cyclosporine has been used as a treatment of last resort in selected patients with severe disease.

Course and Complications. The course may be chronic, ranging from months to years. Almost two thirds of patients experience spontaneous resolution within 1 year. Patients with mucous membrane involvement usually have a more prolonged course, often lasting years. Recurrences are uncommon, occurring in less than 20% of patients.

Serious complications are uncommon. Postinflammatory hyperpigmentation may be cosmetically unpleasing but usually fades with time. Complications of mucous membrane lichen planus include candidiasis and squamous cell carcinoma (see Chapter 23).

Pathogenesis. The cause of lichen planus remains unknown. Evidence that immune factors play a role includes (1) the finding of immunoglobulins at the dermal-epidermal junction in 95% of lichen planus lesions, (2) the observation that certain drug reactions can mimic lichen planus, and (3) the occurrence of lichen planus–like eruptions in patients who have undergone bone marrow transplantation and who are experiencing a graft-versus-host reaction.

Cellular immune mechanisms appear to be primarily involved in lichen planus. Activated helper T-cells are present in early lesions and appear to target the basal cells that may have been antigenically altered. Cytokines and macrophages also play a role. In older lesions, suppressor T-cells have been shown to predominate. Several epidemiologic studies have shown a higher prevalence of hepatitis C virus infection in patients with lichen planus than in normal control subjects. The pathogenetic link between these two disorders, however, is not known.

THERAPY OF LICHEN PLANUS

- Topical steroids (e.g., fluocinonide cream 0.1% BID)
- Antihistamines (e.g., hydroxyzine: 10–25 mg TID)
- Systemic steroids
- Retinoids (acitretin)
- Cyclosporine

■ MILIARIA

Definition. Miliaria, or heat rash, represents an inflammatory reaction around a sweat duct. The reaction is caused by occlusion of the duct with extravasation of its contents into the surrounding tissue. Clinically, miliaria most often appears as multiple small papules (Fig. 12–9).

Incidence. Miliaria is an uncommon presenting complaint in our outpatients. In the infant, heat rash is recognized by the parents and seldom causes them to seek a dermatologic consultation. However, we frequently see it in hospitalized patients, in whom it is responsible for approximately 1% of our inpatient consultations. It is more common in warm, humid environments, particularly in skin that has been occluded.

History. In the ambulatory patient, miliaria results from exposure to a hot, humid environment. In the bedridden patient, fever, sweating, and occlusion of the skin are predisposing factors. Pruritus often is the presenting complaint.

Physical Examination. *Miliaria rubra* is the most common form of miliaria and appears as multiple discrete, small, red papules. It occurs most often on the trunk, particularly the back. Although sweat ducts are not visible, miliaria is suspected when a patient has multiple small, discrete, uniform-size papules not associated with hair follicles. Less common variants are *miliaria crystallina*, with superficial noninflamed vesicles containing crystal-clear fluid ("dewdrops"), and *miliaria pustulosa*, with erythematous pustules.

Differential Diagnosis. Miliaria rubra may be confused with *contact dermatitis*, but in contact dermatitis the papules tend to be confluent rather than discrete, and itching is often more pronounced. Miliaria pustulosa may be confused with *folliculitis*. In miliaria, the pustules are usually smaller and more numerous and do not have a centrally placed hair. Sometimes, however, the two conditions coexist because they may share the same predisposing factor of occlusion. Candidiasis also occurs in moist occluded skin, but the eruption is usually "beefy red," confluent, scaling, and surrounded by satellite papules and pustules. The word *milia* sounds similar to miliaria, but the condition it denotes is different. Milia are small, non-

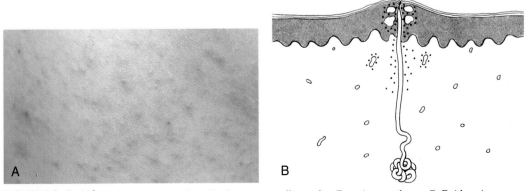

FIGURE 12–9. Miliaria. **A,** Miliaria rubra. Epidermis—small papules. Dermis—erythema. **B,** Epidermis—occluded sweat duct with underlying intraepidermal edema and inflammation. Dermis—superficial inflammatory cell infiltrate.

Miliaria is heat rash— milia are small, keratin-filled cysts.

inflamed, superficial epidermal keratin cysts often found on the face in young infants and adults.

Laboratory and Biopsy. The diagnosis is usually made clinically. For pustules, a Gram stain and culture rule out bacterial folliculitis. A potassium hydroxide preparation enables one to identify *Candida.* If a biopsy is performed, serial sections must be done to reveal the intraepidermal portion of the sweat duct, which is surrounded by spongiosis and a chronic inflammatory cell infiltrate in the epidermis and superficial dermis.

Therapy. Therapy is directed at removing the predisposing conditions. Most important are cooling measures and air exposure for occluded skin. For ambulatory patients, this is easily accomplished. For bedridden patients, this means ensuring that the beds are dry and that the patients are frequently turned. Hydrocortisone lotion 1% can be applied to help relieve the itching, but this must be done sparingly to avoid any further contribution to the occlusive process.

Course and Complications. With decreasing heat and increasing air exposure, the condition resolves spontaneously within days. Complications are uncommon. Conditions that predispose to miliaria, however, also can contribute to coexisting infection with bacterial and candidal organisms.

Pathogenesis. Occlusion of the sweat duct is the primary event in the pathogenesis of miliaria. In miliaria rubra, this occurs within the epidermis at the level of the granular cell layer. Increased hydration appears to play the major role, resulting in swelling of the stratum corneum and compromise of the ductal lumina. After occlusion, sweat extravasates into the epidermis, where it produces an irritant reaction. Experimentally, stripping of the stratum corneum with adhesive tape restores sweat flow, providing evidence that the occlusive process occurs in the stratum corneum. Bacteria and increased sweat tonicity have also been implicated pathogenetically in miliaria, but their pathogenetic roles have not been proved conclusively.

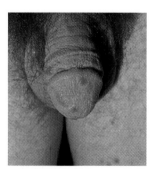

FIGURE 12–10. Unknown.

■ UNKNOWN (Fig. 12–10)

This 30-year-old man presented with a 2-month history of itching that has become progressively more severe. The itching spares the head but is otherwise generalized, including involvement of the genitalia, as shown in Figure 12–10.

What do you see?

Physical examination reveals discrete papules, many of which are excoriated.

What is the most likely diagnosis?

The most likely diagnosis is scabies. Scabies should be suspected for any generalized pruritic process. For pruritic papules on the penis, the diagnosis is scabies until proved otherwise.

How would you confirm it?

The diagnosis is secured if a mite can be found. For this, careful examination of the entire cutaneous surface should be carried out in the search for burrows. The patient's hands, particularly the finger webs, should be scrutinized. Even if a burrow is not found, scraping of several of the papules may reveal a mite or mite products. In this patient, scraping of the penile papules was positive.

Important Points

1. Suspect scabies for any generalized itching condition.
2. The index of suspicion should be greatly heightened if pruritic papules are found on the penis.
3. Although burrows are diagnostic and are the best place to scrape, the mite can also be recovered from scrapings of the papules.

R E F E R E N C E S

Scabies

Chouela EN, Abeldano AM, Pellerano G, et al.: Equivalent therapeutic efficacy and safety of ivermectin and lindane in the treatment of scabies. Arch Dermatol 135:651–655, 1999.
Meinking TL, Taplin D, Hermida JL, et al.: The treatment of scabies with ivermectin. N Engl J Med 333:26–30, 1995.
Mellanby K: The development of symptoms, parasitic infection and immunity in human scabies. Parasitology 35:197–206, 1944.
Yonkosky D, Ladia L, Gackenheimer L, Schultz MW: Scabies in nursing homes: an eradication program with permethrin 5% cream. J Am Acad Dermatol 23:1133–1136, 1990.

Insect Bite Reactions

Brown M, Hebert AA: Insect repellents: an overview. J Am Acad Dermatol 36:243–249, 1997.
Burkhart CG, Burkhart CN, Burkhart KM: An assessment of topical and oral prescriptions and over-the-counter treatments for head lice. J Am Acad Dermatol 38:979–982, 1998.
DeShazo RD, Butcher BT, Banks WA: Reactions to the stings of the imported fire ant. N Engl J Med 323:462–466, 1990.
Honig PJ: Bites and parasites. Pediatr Clin North Am 30:563–581, 1983.
Krinsky WL: Dermatoses associated with the bites of mites and ticks (Arthropoda: *Acari*). Int J Dermatol 22:75–91, 1983.
Valentine MD, Schuberth KC, Kagey-Sobotka A, et al.: The value of immunotherapy with venom in children with allergy to insect stings. N Engl J Med 323:1601–1603, 1990.

Lichen Planus

Altman J, Perry HO: The variations and course of lichen planus. Arch Dermatol 84:179–191, 1961.
Boyd AS, Neldner KH: Lichen planus. J Am Acad Dermatol 25:593–619, 1991.

Ho VC, Gupta AK, Ellis CN, Nickoloff BJ, Voorhees JJ: Treatment of severe lichen planus with cyclosporine. J Am Acad Dermatol 22:64–68, 1990.

Laurberg G, Geiger JM, Hjorth N, et al.: Treatment of lichen planus with acitretin: a double-blind, placebo-controlled study in 65 patients. J Am Acad Dermatol 24:434–437, 1991.

Sanchez-Perez J, DeCastro M, Buezo GF: Lichen planus and hepatitis C virus: prevalence on clinical presentation of patients with lichen planus and hepatitis C virus infection. Br J Dermatol 134:715–719, 1997.

Saurat JH, Gluckman E, Bussel A, et al.: The lichen planus–like eruption after bone marrow transplantation. Br J Dermatol 93:675–681, 1975.

Miliaria

Shuster S: Ductal disruption: a new explanation of miliaria. Acta Derm Venereol 77:1–3, 1997.

Wenzel FG, Horn TD: Nonneoplastic disorders of eccrine glands. J Am Acad Dermatol 38: 1–17, 1998.

PUSTULES 13

ACNE
ACNE ROSACEA
FOLLICULITIS
IMPETIGO
CANDIDIASIS
RARE CAUSES OF PUSTULES

Pustules are collections of neutrophils that are situated superficially usually in a hair follicle (e.g., acne and folliculitis) or just below the stratum corneum (e.g., impetigo and candidiasis). Although pustules represent the unifying clinical feature of these disorders, they may not always be the predominant finding; sometimes, they are not even present. For example, in some patients with acne, only comedones or papules are found. In impetigo, often only crusts are found because the pustules have been broken and dried. Pus often indicates infection. For pustules (and crusts) in the skin, infection is an appropriate diagnostic consideration, but as can be seen from Table 13–1, not all pustular dermatoses are caused by pathogenic microorganisms. However, if infection is suspected, simple laboratory tests can be performed for confirmation.

The most common pustular diseases are listed in Table 13–1. Other rare causes of pustules are briefly mentioned at the end of the chapter.

■ ACNE

Definition. Acne vulgaris (common acne) is a disorder affecting pilosebaceous units in the skin (Fig. 13–1). The cause is multifactorial. Clinical lesions range from noninflamed *comedones* to *inflammatory papules*, *pustules*, *nodules*, and *cysts*.

Incidence. Acne is the most common disease seen by a dermatologist. It begins at a surprisingly young age; comedones can be found on examination in 50% of boys age 9 to 11 years. The incidence and severity of the disease increase in the teenage years. In a survey of 1,085 high school students, 85% responded that they had acne. Contrary to popular belief, acne is not confined to teenagers. It may continue into the third and fourth decades of life; in some patients, it does not begin until then.

History. The patient usually makes the diagnosis and often has attempted therapy with over-the-counter medication. A history of hirsutism or irregular menses in a woman with acne should lead to the consideration of possible androgen excess.

TABLE 13–1 ■ COMMON PUSTULAR DISEASES

			Physical Examination			
	Frequency*	Etiology	Appearance of Lesions	Distribution	Differential Diagnosis	Laboratory Test
Acne	13	Multifactorial	Pustules, papules, nodules, and comedones	Face and upper trunk	Folliculitis Rosacea	None
Rosacea	1.3	Unknown	Papules and pustules on a background of erythema and telangiectasia	Central portion of face	Acne Lupus erythematosus Seborrheic dermatitis	None
Folliculitis	1.1	Infection (S. aureus)	Scattered pustules, many with centrally placed hairs	Buttocks and thighs, beard area, scalp	Acne Fungal infection	Gram stain Culture
Impetigo	0.6	Infection (S. aureus)	Crusts (often honey-colored) predominant	Anywhere, most common on face	Ecthyma Herpes simplex	Gram stain Culture
Candidiasis	0.3	Infection (C. albicans)	Satellite pustules around a "beefy red" erythematous area	Moist areas, particularly the groin	Tinea cruris Intertrigo Miliaria Folliculitis Contact dermatitis	Potassium hydroxide preparation

* Percentage of new dermatology patients with this diagnosis seen in the Hershey Medical Center Dermatology Clinic, Hershey, PA.

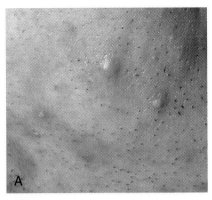

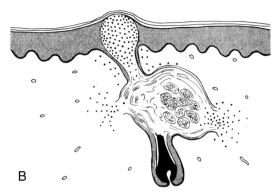

FIGURE 13–1. Acne. **A,** Epidermis—pustule. Dermis—erythema. **B,** Epidermis—intraepidermal, intrafollicular collection of neutrophils. Dermis—occluded pilosebaceous unit with accumulation of keratin, sebum, and inflammatory cells. Extravasation of material through the ruptured wall leads to further dermal inflammation.

Self-administered androgenic steroids aggravate acne in athletes and others who illicitly use these hormonal agents. Topical or systemic corticosteroids can also cause an acneiform eruption.

Physical Examination. The noninflamed lesions in acne are called comedones and are of two types: (1) the *open comedo* or "blackhead," which appears as a dilated pore filled with black keratinous material (not dirt), and (2) the *closed comedo* or "whitehead," which is a small, flesh-colored, dome-shaped papule that often is difficult to see (Fig. 13–2). Inflammatory acne lesions are more easily seen by both patient and physician. They appear as papules, pustules, nodules, or "cysts," depending on the magnitude of the inflammatory response. Acne is found in areas with numerous sebaceous glands, usually the face and upper trunk. The lower trunk is much less often involved, and the distal extremities are always spared.

Differential Diagnosis. The diagnosis of acne is rarely difficult, particularly in teenagers. Occasionally, acne comedones may be confused with *flat warts*, which are small, flesh-colored, flat-topped papules usually located on the face. On close inspection, the flat wart is seen to have a sharp right-angle edge and a finely textured surface, whereas a closed comedone has a dome-shaped, smooth surface.

Steroid acne is caused by use of corticosteroids and is distinguished from acne vulgaris by its sudden onset (usually within 2 weeks of starting high-dose systemic or potent topical corticosteroid therapy) and appearance (uniform, 2- to 3-mm, red, firm papules and pustules). Steroid acne caused by topically applied agents most often occurs on the face. With systemic corticosteroids, the eruption is most prominent on the upper trunk.

Pustular acne vulgaris can be confused with bacterial folliculitis or rosacea. In *bacterial folliculitis*, hairs are visible in some of the pustules, and a bacterial culture is positive, usually for *Staphylococcus aureus* or, less often, a gram-negative organism. *Rosacea* is distinguished from acne vulgaris by the presence of a background blush of erythema and telangiectasia and the absence of comedones. Rosacea also usually occurs later in life.

Papular acne is occasionally confused with *adenoma sebaceum*, a misnomer for lesions that are angiofibromas. Adenoma sebaceum is a skin manifestation of tuberous sclerosis. Clinically, the lesions appear as firm, pink papules that are clus-

Noninflammatory lesions:
1. **Open comedones**
2. **Closed comedones**
Inflammatory lesions:
1. **Papules**
2. **Pustules**
3. **Nodules and "cysts"**

FIGURE 13–2. Closed comedones or "whiteheads."

tered primarily in the center of the face, are persistent, and are, of course, resistant to acne therapy.

Laboratory and Biopsy. The diagnosis is almost always made clinically. Occasionally, a bacterial culture is indicated to rule out infection. A biopsy is not indicated.

Therapy. Four categories of medication have been proved efficacious in the treatment of acne: topical agents, systemic antibiotics, systemic retinoids, and hormonal agents. For the majority of patients, systemic retinoids and hormonal therapy are not required.

Topical Agents. Topical agents are most effective for superficial lesions. The topical comedolytic agents are benzoyl peroxide, available in 2.5%, 5%, and 10% concentrations, and topical retinoids—tretinoin (Retin-A Micro cream) and adapalene (Differin gel). The topical retinoids are particularly helpful for comedones, whereas benzoyl peroxide also exerts an antibacterial effect. Topical antibiotics (erythromycin, clindamycin) also are available but are used less frequently.

We usually start treatment with a topical retinoid at bedtime and a 5% benzoyl peroxide emollient gel (e.g., Desquam-E 5%, Benzac-W 5%) in the morning. The patient should apply these medications to the *entire affected area* (e.g., the entire face) rather than just to individual lesions. In addition, patients must be advised that retinoids and benzoyl peroxide preparations can cause skin irritation, which usually is worst during the first 1 to 2 weeks of use and afterward diminishes. In part because of the irritation, the patient may notice that the condition appears worse rather than better after the first several weeks of use.

Systemic Antibiotics. Systemic antibiotics are indicated in patients with inflammatory lesions. Tetracycline (500 mg twice daily) is the antibiotic of first choice because of its low cost, efficacy, and relative safety, even when it is administered

---

THERAPY OF ACNE

Topical
- Benzoyl peroxide 5% gel daily
- Retinoids
    Retin-A Micro cream daily
    Adapalene gel daily
- Antibiotics
    Erythromycin 2% solution or gel daily
    Clindamycin 1% lotion or gel daily

Systemic
- Antibiotics
    Tetracycline: 500 mg BID
    Erythromycin: 500 mg BID
- Isotretinoin:
    1 mg/kg daily for 20 weeks
- Hormonal therapy
    (e.g., Ortho Tri-Cyclen oral contraceptive pills)

for a prolonged period. Because foods, particularly dairy products, interfere with the absorption of tetracycline, this drug must be taken on an empty stomach. Other antibiotics used in treating acne include erythromycin (500 mg twice daily), doxycycline (100 mg twice daily), and minocycline (100 mg twice daily).

Systemic Retinoids. The oral retinoid isotretinoin (Accutane) became commercially available in September 1982 for use in the treatment of patients with severe acne (Fig. 13–3). This potent vitamin A analogue decreases follicular keratinization, sebum production, and intrafollicular bacterial counts. Side effects are common. Almost all patients experience chapped lips and dry skin, and extracutaneous complications also occur—for example, elevations in liver enzymes and plasma lipids. Most important, systemic retinoids are *teratogenic*. It is mandatory that female patients not be pregnant when taking isotretinoin. Special consent forms, strict birth control measures, and monthly pregnancy tests are required for women taking isotretinoin. Because of these restrictions, the drug is recommended only for the treatment of selected patients with severe, therapy-resistant scarring or debilitating disease. The drug should be prescribed only by physicians who are familiar with its use.

Isotretinoin is teratogenic.

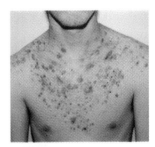

FIGURE 13–3. Severe nodular "cystic" acne with scarring.

Hormonal Therapy. Birth control pills with low androgenicity improve acne in many patients. Several products are available including Ortho Tri-Cyclen for which the U.S. Food and Drug Administration has approved acne as an indicated use.

Antiandrogens have also been used for treating therapy-resistant acne in women. Cyproterone acetate is available in Europe, whereas spironolactone has been used in the United States. Again, these agents should be prescribed only by physicians who are fully aware of their potential side effects.

Patient Education. The most important aspect of a successful acne treatment program is patient compliance. Instructions should be given both verbally at the time of the patient's initial visit and on a written take-home sheet that reinforces what was said. Patients will be best able to comply if medications are used only twice daily so the medication schedule can be centered on an already established daily habit such as teeth brushing. At the time of the initial visit, answers can also be given to several common questions (often unasked) that acne patients or their parents frequently have regarding the following:

1. *Diet.* Some evidence indicates that a "Western" diet may have an adverse effect on acne, but specific foods have not been specifically implicated. For most patients, a sensible diet is all that is suggested.

2. *Cleanliness.* Acne is not a function of poor hygiene. In general, acne cleansing agents are also not recommended because they cause irritation that unnecessarily compounds the irritation from the recommended topical comedolytics.

3. *Cosmetics.* If cosmetics are used, they should be water based and used sparingly.

4. *Picking.* In many patients with acne, much of the skin damage is self-inflicted. Although the temptation to squeeze a fresh pustule is often overwhelming, it should be vigorously discouraged because it can produce more tissue damage, sometimes resulting in scars.

Course and Complications. With therapy, the prognosis for acne is good, if not excellent. The patient should understand that most therapies provide control of the disease rather than cure and that improvement does not occur overnight. If improvement has not been noted after 2 months, more intensive therapy can be prescribed, including increased concentrations of the topical agents, increased dosage of the oral antibiotic, or change in the antibiotic therapy. Continued improvement in the disease is expected with continued therapy. Many patients can discontinue systemic antibiotics after a number of months, but most patients require prolonged (often lasting years) maintenance therapy with topical agents, and some also require continued antibiotics. However, bacterial resistance to antibiotics is becoming more frequent, thereby limiting the usefulness of long-term antibiotic therapy for acne. Isotretinoin induces prolonged remissions, if not "cures," in many patients.

Acne spontaneously remits with time, the amount of which varies widely. For individual patients, we have no way to predict in advance when they will "outgrow" their acne. The goal of therapy is to keep the condition under control as long as it is active.

The major complication of acne is its psychosocial ramifications, which can be devastating for some patients. Patients with severe cystic acne may even be socially ostracized. In an ironic quirk of timing, acne occurs at a time of life when personal appearance is a prime concern and self-consciousness is at its peak. Some young people appear to be psychologically more severely affected by their acne than others, but none view it as a blessing. Regardless of the severity of the acne, for patients seeking help (even those with apparently mild disease), the disease is important and deserves serious attention. Patients are not impressed with soothing advice that trivializes their disease and reassures them that they will eventually "outgrow it."

In addition to the cosmetic liability of active lesions, scars further compound and perpetuate a poor self-image in some patients long after the acne has remitted. Scars are difficult to treat. Dermabrasion, laser "resurfacing," chemical peels, and surgery have all been employed, with varying results. Because scars are more easily prevented than treated, the emphasis in acne is on early and aggressive medical therapy.

Factors involved in acne pathogenesis:
1. **Androgens**
2. **Follicular obstruction**
3. *Propionibacterium acnes*

Pathogenesis. Multiple factors are involved in the pathogenesis of acne. The three most significant are the following:

1. *Androgenic hormones.* Under androgen stimulation, sebaceous glands enlarge and increase their sebum production. Before puberty, the responsible androgens are secreted by the adrenal gland. During puberty, the addition of gonadal androgens provides further sebaceous gland stimulation.

2. *Follicular obstruction.* For acne to occur, outlet obstruction of the follicular canal is required. This obstruction occurs because of accumulation of adherent keratinized cells within the canal, to form an impaction. The cause of follicular obstruction is not known, but it may also be influenced by androgens.

3. *Bacteria.* Proximal to the follicular outlet obstruction, sebum and keratinous debris accumulate. This provides an attractive environment for the growth of anaerobic bacteria, specifically *Propionibacterium acnes*. These bacteria produce lipase enzymes that hydrolyze the sebaceous lipids, resulting in the release of free fatty acids, which are presumed to cause inflammation. *P. acnes* bacteria play other roles in the pathogenesis of acne; for example, these bacteria are chemotactic for neutrophils. Regardless of the mechanism, the therapeutic benefit of antibiotics supports the notion that bacteria play a pathogenetic role in acne.

■ ACNE ROSACEA

Definition. Rosacea or "middle-age acne" is a chronic inflammatory disorder affecting the blood vessels and pilosebaceous units of the face (Fig. 13–4). The etiology is unknown. Clinically, papules and pustules are superimposed on a background of erythema and telangiectasia.

Incidence. Rosacea is a relatively common disorder that primarily affects middle-aged adults. Approximately 1% of our new patients are seen for this disease.

History. The disorder often has a gradual onset. Usually, the patient first notices erythema; with time, telangiectasia appears. The development of papules and pustules is usually sufficient for the patient to bring the problem to a physician's attention.

Papules and pustules are superimposed on a background of erythema and telangiectasia.

Physical Examination. Typically, papules and pustules are superimposed on a background of erythema and telangiectasia. Sometimes, only the erythema and telangiectasia are present. Characteristically, comedones are not found. The disease affects the central third of the face and spares the lateral aspects of the forehead and cheeks.

Differential Diagnosis. Rosacea is distinguished from *acne vulgaris* by the absence of comedones, the background of erythema and telangiectasia, the onset in middle life, and the distribution in the central third of the face. Rashes that may be confused with the vascular element in rosacea occur in lupus erythematosus, photodermatitis, and seborrheic dermatitis, but none of these exhibit pustules. In patients with rosacea with a prominent flushing component, the *carcinoid syndrome* sometimes enters the differential diagnosis.

Laboratory and Biopsy. The diagnosis is almost always made clinically. A biopsy is rarely needed, but if performed it shows vascular dilatation, often with degenerative changes in the collagen and elastic fibers in the upper dermis. The papules and pustules in rosacea are histologically similar to those found in acne vulgaris, but in rosacea the inflammatory infiltrate is more likely to have a granulomatous component. This represents a foreign body reaction in the dermis to the extravasated contents of affected pilosebaceous units. The granulomatous response can

Histologically, a granulomatous reaction often is present and may be confused with sarcoidosis or tuberculosis.

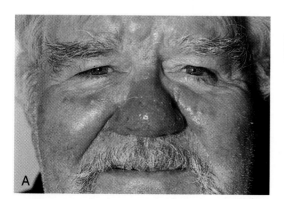
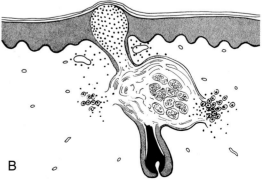

FIGURE 13–4. Rosacea. **A,** Epidermis—pustules and papules. Dermis—erythema and telangiectasia. **B,** Epidermis—intrafollicular inflammation; granulomatous reaction to the contents of a ruptured pilosebaceous unit.

be impressive and occasionally has been confused with granulomatous disorders such as sarcoidosis and tuberculosis.

Therapy. Systemic antibiotics are frequently used for the papular and pustular components. Sometimes, the erythema is also improved. Low-dose tetracycline (500 mg daily) is the usual treatment, and most patients respond within 1 month, after which the drug often can be tapered. Topical metronidazole 0.75% (MetroGel, MetroCream) applied twice daily also is effective in treating the papules, pustules, and erythema of rosacea. The mechanism of action is unknown. Systemic isotretinoin (Accutane) is reserved for the rare patient with severe disease that has resisted all other therapy.

Strong topical steroids are contraindicated.

Topical steroids should not be used because they are well known to aggravate the disease. Sun exposure can also be an aggravating factor, and sun protective measures should be recommended.

Course and Complications. The disease is usually chronic, but most patients respond well to therapy. In many, however, therapy must be continued for months to years. The erythematous component may be improved by therapy, but the telangiectasia persists.

Rhinophyma sometimes develops in patients with rosacea. As the name suggests, this disease involves hyperplasia of the sebaceous glands, connective tissue, and vascular bed of the nose. The hyperplasia can be striking, resulting in a bulbous nose. The nose of W. C. Fields was a prototype, but contrary to popular belief, rosacea is not a sign of excessive alcohol intake. Ocular complications occur in some patients with rosacea. Eye findings range from blepharitis to conjunctivitis and even keratitis. The latter can be severe and has been known to result in visual impairment. Oral tetracycline is helpful for the ocular complications.

Pathogenesis. The pathogenetic mechanisms in this disease are not well understood. For the vascular component, investigators have suggested that sun exposure damages the collagen support of the vascular network, thereby resulting in vasodilatation. Other aggravating factors that have been incriminated, but not well proved, include the ingestion of foods that cause vasodilatation (e.g., hot liquids, caffeinated beverages, alcohol, and spicy foods) and psychologic stress. Immune mechanisms have also been implicated, with immunoglobulin deposition occurring at the dermal-epidermal interface. The pathogenetic significance of this finding remains unclear. The cause of the pustular component is not known, although the pathogenesis may be similar to that of acne vulgaris.

THERAPY OF ROSACEA

Topical
- Metronidazole gel or cream BID

Systemic
- Tetracycline: 500 mg daily
- Isotretinoin

■ FOLLICULITIS

Definition. Folliculitis is an inflammatory reaction in the hair follicle caused by bacteria, usually *S. aureus*. Clinically, the lesion appears as a pustule, often with a central hair (Fig. 13–5).

Incidence. Folliculitis is relatively common, representing approximately 1% of our new patients. The disorder primarily affects young adults.

History. Folliculitis is usually asymptomatic; occasionally, patients complain of mild discomfort associated with the lesions. The process may be chronic or recurrent.

Physical Examination. A pustule is the predominant lesion, although papules may be found. The lesions are individual and do not become confluent. They are usually distributed on the buttocks and thighs but also may occur in the beard area and sometimes on the scalp. The key to the diagnosis is appreciated only on close inspection, whereby hairs can be seen in the exact center of many of the lesions.

FIGURE 13–6. Pseudofolliculitis barbae.

Differential Diagnosis. The distribution, absence of comedones, and presence of a hair growing from the pustules help to differentiate folliculitis from *acne*. Gram-negative organisms can cause *gram-negative folliculitis*, mainly in two settings: patients with acne who are receiving antibiotic therapy in whom gram-negative pathogens are selected out, and individuals exposed to hot-tubs and swimming pools contaminated with *Pseudomonas aeruginosa*. Both types are uncommon. *Pseudofolliculitis barbae* is a disorder of the neck and jaw of men whose beard hairs are sharply curved. This configuration causes the hairs to reenter the skin, where they induce an inflammatory reaction resulting in papules and pustules (Fig. 13–6). The ingrowing hairs can often be visualized. *Keratosis pilaris* is a common follicular disorder that presents as tiny, rough, scaling follicular papules (*no* pustules) on the backs of the upper arms, buttocks, and thighs (Fig. 13–7). Rarely, *fungal infections* can result in follicular pustules. These are usually associated with scaling plaques and therefore are not usually confused with the individual pustules of bacterial folliculitis. *Eosinophilic folliculitis* is manifested by pruritic papules on the trunk. It is most frequently found in HIV-infected patients.

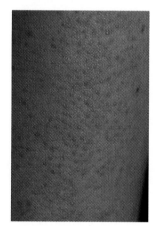

FIGURE 13–7. Keratosis pilaris.

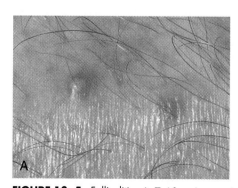
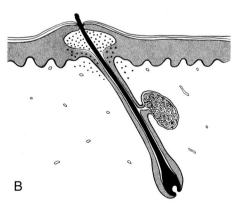

FIGURE 13–5. Folliculitis. **A,** Epidermis—pustule with centrally placed hair. Dermis—erythema. **B,** Epidermis—subcorneal pustule at the opening of a hair follicle. Dermis—inflammation in the upper dermis.

Laboratory and Biopsy. In staphylococcal folliculitis, Gram stain of the pus reveals gram-positive cocci, and bacterial culture confirms the diagnosis. A biopsy is not necessary but if done would reveal a collection of neutrophils in the superficial portion of the hair follicle.

Therapy. Most cases of staphylococcal folliculitis are mild and can be managed with an antiseptic cleanser such as povidone-iodine (Betadine) or chlorhexidine (Hibiclens) used daily or every other day for at least several weeks. For more extensive involvement, a 10-day course of a systemic antibiotic such as dicloxacillin (250 mg four times daily) is suggested in addition to the cleansers.

Course and Complications. Response to therapy usually is good, but recurrences are common. Such patients may be carriers of *S. aureus*, and more prolonged use of the antiseptic cleansers is recommended. In addition, we often ask these patients to apply an antibiotic ointment (e.g., bacitracin) twice daily in their nares because this is a common site for *S. aureus*. Complications are uncommon and local. Occasionally, the follicular infection can extend more deeply, resulting in a furuncle that requires incision and drainage.

Pathogenesis. In folliculitis, the bacteria gain entry into the skin through the follicular orifice and establish low-grade infection within the epidermis surrounding the follicular canal. Patients who carry *S. aureus* on their skin are more susceptible to this disorder. Occlusion and maceration sometimes also are predisposing factors.

Patients with recurrent folliculitis may be chronic "carriers" of S. aureus.

■ IMPETIGO

Definition. Impetigo represents a superficial skin infection caused by gram-positive bacteria, usually *S. aureus*. The early lesions are pustules, which quickly break to form crusts (Fig. 13–8). Crusts are the most commonly encountered clinical lesions. Some strains of *S. aureus* can also cause blisters (bullous impetigo), as discussed in Chapter 11.

Most impetigo is caused by S. aureus.

Incidence. Impetigo occurs most often in children. Although less than 1% of our new patients present with impetigo, this rate would be higher in a general medical practice, particularly a pediatric practice.

History. The eruption often starts as a single lesion, but patients and parents often do not seek medical help until multiple new lesions develop. Other family members are sometimes affected. Staphylococcal bacterial infection also occurs secondarily (impetiginization) in association with certain skin diseases, especially atopic dermatitis.

THERAPY OF FOLLICULITIS

- Antiseptic cleansers: Betadine, Hibiclens
- Antibiotics
     Dicloxacillin: 250 mg QID

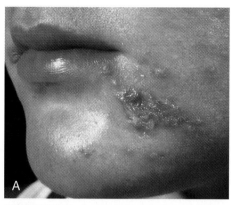
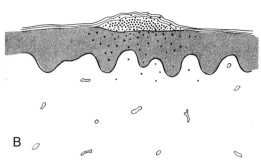

FIGURE 13-8. Impetigo. **A,** Epidermis—pustules and crusts. Dermis—minimal erythema. (Courtesy of O. Fred Miller, M.D.) **B,** Epidermis—subcorneal pustules. Dermis—mild inflammatory reaction in upper dermis.

Physical Examination. The most commonly encountered clinical finding is a honey-colored crust. Intact pustules usually are not found. When the crust is removed, a superficial glistening base is revealed. Impetigo does not extend deeply, so ulcerations are not present. Lesions can be found anywhere but most often are located on the face. Brown or honey-colored crusts also are the hallmark of secondary bacterial infection.

Differential Diagnosis. Different from the staphylococcal impetigo described previously, *ecthyma* is caused by group A streptococci, but much confusion exists regarding these two types of bacterial skin infections. In both, the presenting lesion usually is a crust, but the more important clinical difference is the depth of the infection. With staphylococcal impetigo, the process is superficial (just below the stratum corneum), so when the crust is removed, only a shallow, glistening erosion is seen (Fig. 13–9). In streptococcal pyoderma, the infection is deep, extending through the epidermis, so when the crust is removed, a deeper defect (i.e., an ulcer) is noted (Fig. 13–10). In addition, with staphylococcal impetigo, one usually sees little or no surrounding erythema, whereas with streptococcal infection, erythema is moderate to marked. Finally, staphylococcal impetigo is most common on the face, whereas ecthyma is usually found on the lower extremities, occurring after a scratch or an insect bite.

When the vesicles in *herpes simplex* age, they become cloudy and eventually form crusts. At this stage, herpes is often misdiagnosed as impetigo. Features favoring herpes include the recognition (by patient or physician) of clear vesicles present at the start and a history of recurrence in the same location. Inflammatory *fungal infections* can cause pustules and are in the differential diagnosis for "sterile" pustular processes. Potassium hydroxide (KOH) examination and fungal cultures are indicated in patients with negative Gram stains and bacterial cultures or poor response to antibiotic therapy.

Laboratory. A Gram stain reveals gram-positive cocci. Bacterial culture typically grows *S. aureus*. In obtaining material for Gram stain and culture, the clinician should first remove the crust so the specimen can be obtained from the weeping, glistening erosion.

Therapy. Both topical and systemic antibiotics have been advocated for treating impetigo. Topical preparations such as bacitracin have long been used, especially

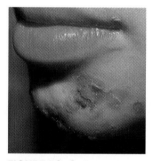

FIGURE 13-9. Impetigo on the chin. "Honey-colored" crusts are characteristic. Culture taken from the glistening base beneath the crust grew *Staphylococcus aureus*.

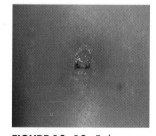

FIGURE 13-10. Ecthyma on the lower leg. Streptococcal skin infection extends more deeply, often forming an ulcer (ecthyma).

THERAPY OF IMPETIGO

- Antibiotics
    Cephalexin: 25–50 mg/kg/day in oral suspension, 250 mg QID
    Erythromycin: 30–50 mg/kg/day in oral suspension, 250 mg QID
    Dicloxacillin: 250 mg QID
    Mupirocin ointment—applied TID
- General hygiene
    Antibacterial soaps: Lever 2000, Dial, Hibiclens
    Changing of towel, washcloth, shaver, etc. daily

Penicillinase-resistant antibiotics are needed.

for small lesions. Mupirocin (Bactroban) ointment is a topical preparation that in several studies compared favorably with systemic antibiotics. Nevertheless, for more extensive lesions, systemic antibiotic therapy is preferred. Most *S. aureus* strains, including those encountered in outpatients, produce penicillinase, so penicillin is not appropriate treatment. The preferred antibiotics are oral cephalexin or penicillinase-resistant penicillins such as dicloxacillin used over a 7- to 10-day course. Older children and adults are treated with 250 mg four times daily. Younger children and infants are treated with cephalexin suspension, 25–50 mg/kg/daily in divided doses. The increasing resistance of *S. aureus* to erythromycin may limit the usefulness of this agent in impetigo. Methicillin-resistant strains of *S. aureus* have also been encountered. Although this situation remains uncommon, it may become more problematic with time.

Course and Complications. With appropriate antibiotic therapy, prompt healing is to be expected, with marked improvement within several days in most patients. Bacteriologic cure is achieved in 7 to 10 days in nearly all cases. If a rapid response to therapy does not occur, the physician should consider the possibility that the infection is caused by an antibiotic-resistant strain. In such instances, the result of the initial culture, if obtained, serves as a guide in selecting an alternative antibiotic.

Complications are rare. Acute glomerulonephritis may occur as a sequela to skin infection from streptococcal but not from staphylococcal infections. This emphasizes the importance of discriminating between these two types of skin infections.

Honey-colored crusts indicate that the skin is secondarily infected.

Pathogenesis. *S. aureus* is ubiquitous in our environment. The bacteria can colonize skin without causing actual infection. This is particularly true in patients with chronic dermatoses such as atopic dermatitis or psoriasis. More than 10% of patients with atopic dermatitis have *S. aureus* colonizing their eczematous skin. Impetiginization, characterized by honey-colored crusts, occurs more often in these patients than in those with psoriasis. Experimentally, it is relatively easy to create skin infection by inoculation with *S. aureus* compared with infection with group A streptococci, which is much more difficult to reproduce experimentally. Clinically, moisture and trauma may cause breaks in the stratum corneum, through which the bacteria can gain entry and can establish clinical infection. With staphylococcal infection, however, this "trauma" is often subclinical, and most patients cannot recall obvious trauma to their skin. Once bacteria have gained entry, they establish infection in the uppermost layer of the viable epidermis just below the stratum corneum. Inflammatory cells, primarily neutrophils, respond and are responsible for the pus that is clinically evident and eventuates into the characteristic crusts.

Infection with group A streptococci is more difficult to establish. These organisms do not colonize normal skin but must be inoculated through a damaged surface such as a scratch or insect bite. Once established, the organism produces proteolytic enzymes, which are in part responsible for the surrounding inflammation.

■ CANDIDIASIS

Definition. Candidiasis represents an inflammatory reaction in the skin resulting from infection of the epidermis with *Candida albicans*. Clinically, the infection appears as a "beefy red" erythematous area with surrounding satellite papules and pustules (Fig. 13–11). The pustules, when present, help in the diagnosis. In this section, candidiasis of the skin is discussed. Mucous membrane infection is discussed in Chapter 23.

Incidence. Candidiasis can affect people of all ages. Although only 0.3% of our new patient visits are for candidiasis, in some situations this disease is much more common. It is particularly common in diaper-clad infants and in hospitalized patients. Two percent of our in-hospital consultations are for candidiasis.

History. Patients usually complain of itching and burning of the skin. A moist environment is the most important local predisposing factor for the development of this disease. For infections in the perineal area, diapers and excessive skin folds help to provide this moist environment. Wet surgical dressings can do the same in other locations. On the hands, *C. albicans* infection between the fingers occurs in patients who frequently have their hands in water, such as bartenders and dishwashers. In women with recurrent candidal vulvovaginitis, a history should be taken for predisposing factors, such as pregnancy, diabetes mellitus, birth control pills, and antibiotics.

Moisture predisposes to candidiasis.

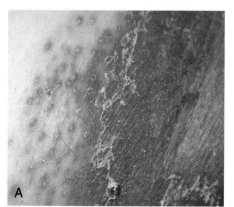
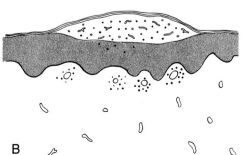

FIGURE 13–11. Candidiasis. **A,** "Beefy red" erythema with satellite papules and pustules. Epidermis—pustules and scales. Dermis—erythema. (Courtesy of O. Fred Miller, M.D.) **B,** Epidermis—subcorneal pustules: note associated hyphae and spores. Dermis—perivascular inflammation.

Physical Examination. The most consistent finding in cutaneous candidiasis is bright red erythema of the affected skin, characteristically surrounded by satellite pustules and papules. Pustules are not always present, but often their residua are noted. These appear as small, 2- to 3-mm, erythematous macules rimmed with a collarette of scale that represents the remnant of the pustule roof. As noted, the distribution of candidiasis favors moist areas. Perineal infection is most common in diapered infants and in women, in whom it is often accompanied by candidal vaginitis. In bedridden patients, especially those taking antibiotics, perianal involvement occurs and often extends up the back with multiple papules and pustules. Other favored locations are the intertriginous areas under the breasts, in the axillae, between the fingers, and under wet dressings.

> **Cutaneous candidiasis is "beefy red" with satellite papules and pustules.**

Differential Diagnosis. The differential diagnosis depends in part on the location of the infection. In the groin area, candidiasis may be confused with *tinea cruris* or *intertrigo*, an irritant dermatitis caused by maceration and rubbing in intertriginous folds, usually the inguinal folds in obese patients. Compared with candidiasis, tinea cruris is much more sharply demarcated, and intertrigo is less likely to be so brightly erythematous. Neither exhibits the satellite papules and pustules of candidiasis.

On the back of a bedridden patient, candidal infection may be confused with *miliaria* (heat rash) or *folliculitis*. In candidiasis, however, the papular and pustular lesions are usually accompanied by confluent erythematous involvement in the perianal and, often, perineal areas from which the infection spread. A KOH preparation is negative in miliaria and folliculitis. Candidiasis developing under wet dressings can be confused with contact dermatitis. The finding of pustules favors candidiasis. The KOH preparation confirms the diagnosis.

Laboratory and Biopsy. The important laboratory test is the KOH examination of scrapings from pustules or peripheral scale. If a pustule is present, a scraping of its roof and contents has a high positive yield. The finding of hyphae and pseudohyphae is diagnostic for infection. Spores alone are not, because *C. albicans* and other yeast organisms can colonize skin without causing infection. For this reason, a skin culture for *C. albicans* is less helpful than a positive KOH scraping; a positive culture from skin does not distinguish between colonization and infection, whereas the KOH preparation does, because the KOH examination detects the infectious filamentous form of the organism. It can be difficult, if not impossible, to distinguish between the hyphae and pseudohyphae of candidiasis and the hyphae of dermatophytic infections. Usually, however, the clinical picture is sufficient to distinguish between the two. A biopsy is not needed.

> **Hyphae and pseudohyphae are found on the KOH examination.**

Therapy. Topical nystatin-containing preparations have long been used, but candidiasis is better treated with one of the topical imidazole creams. Over-the-counter creams include clotrimazole (Lotrimin) and miconazole (Micatin). Creams containing econazole (Spectazole), ketoconazole (Nizoral), or sulconazole (Exelderm) require a prescription. The imidazole cream should be applied twice daily. The clinician should instruct the patient to apply the medication *sparingly*, because excessive application of creams to already moist areas can contribute to maceration and may cause further irritation.

> **The topical medication should be applied sparingly.**

Widespread candidiasis is treated with systemic therapy. Ketoconazole (Nizoral; 200 mg daily) and fluconazole (Diflucan; 100 mg daily) are effective oral agents, but they are seldom needed for local cutaneous infection. These oral agents

---

THERAPY OF CANDIDIASIS

- Topical creams BID
    - Clotrimazole
    - Miconazole
    - Ketoconazole
- Systemic
    - Ketoconazole: 200 mg daily
    - Fluconazole: 100 mg daily

---

are more often indicated for severe, persistent, or recurrent mucous membrane candidiasis.

Attention should also be given to predisposing factors, especially moisture. Drying measures depend on the situation. For example, an infant with candidal diaper dermatitis should have more frequent diaper changes, and a bedridden patient should be turned more frequently to increase air exposure to the back and buttocks.

Widespread candidiasis is treated systemically.

Course and Complications. In most instances, response to topical therapy is prompt, and if the predisposing factors have been corrected, recurrence is unlikely. In patients with recurrent disease, both local (e.g., occlusion, moisture) and systemic (e.g., diabetes, AIDS) predisposing factors should be considered. Most patients with local candidiasis are not immunologically deficient, and the disease resolves with treatment of the infection and correction of the predisposing factors. *Systemic candidiasis* occurs exclusively in severely immunocompromised patients, particularly those with hematologic malignant diseases. In such patients, mucous membrane or cutaneous candidal infection may serve as the portal of entry for the systemic infection. *Chronic mucocutaneous candidiasis* is another rare disorder, and it represents chronic infection of the skin and mucous membranes in patients who are deficient in cellular immunity against *C. albicans*.

Pathogenesis. No special pathogenic strains of *C. albicans* exist. The organism commonly colonizes skin and bowel, particularly the colon. Pathogenicity in tissue is associated with conversion of the organism from its yeast to its filamentous form. The most important local factor that encourages this conversion is moisture. Accordingly, skin folds are most commonly involved, as are areas occluded with wet dressings, including diapers. After penetration of the stratum corneum barrier, the organism elicits a complement-mediated acute inflammatory response that produces the dermatitis as well as prevents deeper tissue invasion.

Other predisposing host factors may contribute to candidal infection, including pregnancy, in which local changes in the acidity and glycogen content of the vaginal epithelium make that environment more supportive of candidal growth. Birth control pills can have the same effect. Increased sugar content in the urine of women with poorly controlled diabetes provides another local factor conducive to candidal growth. By eliminating bacterial competitors in the bowel, systemic antibiotics can permit *C. albicans* to flourish there instead, and this situation can contribute to cutaneous infection in the perianal area.

TABLE 13-2 ■ RARE CAUSES OF PUSTULES

Infection
    Bacterial sepsis
        Gonococcal infection
        Staphylococcal infection

Fungal
    Dermatophyte (kerion)
    Blastomycosis

Sterile
    Pustular psoriasis
    Drugs: iodides, bromides, haloperidol

Pustules in bacterial sepsis are purpuric.

FIGURE 13-12. Pustular psoriasis. Multiple superficial sterile pustules.

■ RARE CAUSES OF PUSTULES (Table 13–2)

Pustules in bacterial sepsis usually are few in number and are *purpuric*. Therefore, in a patient with fever and purpuric pustules, the diagnosis of bacterial sepsis must be excluded. In gonococcemia, purpuric pustules are frequent findings and are distally distributed. Their presence, in a setting of fever, arthralgias or arthritis, and tenosynovitis, strongly suggests the diagnosis of *gonococcemia*. Purpuric pustules are less common in staphylococcal septicemia.

Dermatophytes can infect hair follicles and may result in pustules. This condition sometimes is confused with bacterial folliculitis. A *kerion* is a dermatophytic infection, frequently of the scalp, that appears as an indurated boggy inflammatory plaque studded with pustules. Kerions are frequently confused with bacterial pyodermas. *Blastomycosis* is a systemic fungal infection and a rare cause of pustules in the skin.

An uncommon variant of psoriasis is *pustular psoriasis* (Fig. 13–12). This disease can be limited to the palms and soles, superimposed on typical psoriatic plaques, or generalized, with multiple pustules on large areas of erythematous skin. The generalized form is a rare but striking disease and frequently is accompanied by fever. Finally, pustular eruptions can be induced by *drugs*, particularly halogens, including iodides, bromides, and halogenated compounds, of which haloperidol (Haldol) is an example.

■ UNKNOWN (Fig. 13–13)

This 38-year-old woman was receiving wet dressings to her leg ulcer. After 1 week, a rash developed around the ulcer.

Describe what you see.

Surrounding the ulcer is an erythematous eruption with satellite pustules and papules.

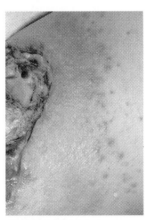

FIGURE 13-13. Unknown.

What is your differential diagnosis?

The differential diagnosis includes contact dermatitis from the medications used in the dressings. However, with the satellite pustules and papules, candidiasis also needs to be considered.

What is the first diagnostic test you would do?

The first diagnostic test should be a KOH examination of a scraping from the border of the lesion. In this patient's case, it was positive for hyphae. It is difficult to distinguish microscopically between candidal and dermatophytic hyphae, but the clinical picture favors candidiasis.

How would you treat it?

Local therapy with a topical imidazole cream, applied sparingly twice daily, and discontinuation of the wet dressings resulted in prompt clearing of the eruption.

R E F E R E N C E S

Acne

Cunliffe WJ: Acne. Chicago, Year Book, 1989.

Goulden V, Clark SM, Cunliffe WS: Post-adolescent acne: a review of clinical features. Br J Dermatol *136*:66–70, 1997.

Hurwitz RM: Steroid acne. J Am Acad Dermatol *21*:1179–1181, 1989.

Jansen T, Burgdorf WHC, Plewig W: Pathogenesis and treatment of acne in childhood. Pediatr Dermatol *14*:17–21, 1997.

Koo JYM, Smith LL: Psychologic aspects of acne. Pediatr Dermatol *8*:185–188, 1991.

Leyden JJ: New understandings of the pathogenesis of acne. J Am Acad Dermatol *32*:S15–S25, 1995.

Leyden JJ: Topical treatment of acne vulgaris: retinoids and cutaneous irritation. J Am Acad Dermatol *38*:S1–S4, 1998.

Lucky AW, Biro FM, Huster GA, Morrison JA, Elder N: Acne vulgaris in early adolescent boys: correlations with pubertal maturation and age. Arch Dermatol *127*:210–216, 1991.

Thiboutot DM, Lookingbill DP: Hormonal therapy of acne. Dermatol Ther *6*:39–43, 1998.

Acne Rosacea

Bleicher PA, Charles JH, Sober AJ: Topical metronidazole therapy for rosacea. Arch Dermatol *123*:609–614, 1987.

Helm KF, Menz J, Gibson LE, Dicken CH: A clinical and histopathologic study of granulomatous rosacea. J Am Acad Dermatol *25*:1038–1043, 1991.

Plewig G, Kligman AM: Acne and Rosacea. 2nd ed. Berlin, Springer-Verlag, 1993.

Quarterman MJ, Johnson DW, Abele DC, et al.: Ocular rosacea: signs, symptoms and tear studies before and after treatment with doxycycline. Arch Dermatol *133*:49–54, 1997.

Wilkin JK: Rosacea: pathophysiology and treatment. Arch Dermatol *130*:359–362, 1994.

Folliculitis

Back O, Faergemann J, Hornqvist R: Pityrosporum folliculitis: a common disease of the young and middle-aged. J Am Acad Dermatol *12*:56–61, 1985.

Chandrasekar PH, Rolston KVI, Kannangara DW, LeFrock JL, Binnick SA: Hot tub associated dermatitis due to *Pseudomonas aeruginosa*: case report and review of the literature. Arch Dermatol *120*:1337–1340, 1984.

Plewig G, Jansen T: Acneiform dermatoses. Dermatology *196*:102–107, 1998.

Impetigo

Bass JW, Chan DS, Creamer KM, et al.: Comparison of oral cephalexin, topical mupirocin, and topical bacitracin for treatment of impetigo. Pediatr Infect Dis J 16:708–710, 1997.

Brook I, Frazier EH, Yeager JK: Microbiology of nonbullous impetigo. Pediatr Dermatol 14: 192–195, 1997.

Sadick NS: Current aspects of bacterial infections of the skin. Dermatol Clin 15:341–349, 1997.

Candidiasis

Heddenwick S, Kauffman CA: Opportunistic fungal infections: superficial and systemic candidiasis. Geriatrics 52:50–54, 59, 1997.

Hoppe JE: Treatment of oropharyngeal candidiasis and candidal diaper dermatitis in neonates and infants: review and reappraisal. Pediatr Infect Dis J 17:267, 1998.

WHITE SPOTS

14

TINEA VERSICOLOR
VITILIGO
PITYRIASIS ALBA
POSTINFLAMMATORY HYPOPIGMENTATION
TUBEROUS SCLEROSIS

W hite spots in the skin result from decreased melanin pigmentation. This can be caused by a decrease in the number of melanocytes or a decrease in their melanin production. Inflammatory events are frequently responsible, even though the inflammation may not be clinically appreciated. Table 14–1 lists the four most common causes of white spots as well as one uncommon cause. Determination of the degree (partial versus complete) of pigment loss and identification of the presence or absence of scale are helpful distinguishing clinical features.

The degree of pigment loss can be roughly assessed with a Wood's light examination, which helps to accentuate pigment contrast. In a darkened room with a Wood's light, lesions that are completely depigmented appear almost chalk white. This finding is characteristic in vitiligo. The Wood's light examination is also helpful in identifying white spots in lightly pigmented individuals; in patients with extremely fair complexions, white spots may not be evident under bright illumination.

The admonition "If it scales, scrape it!" also pertains to white spots. The two common hypopigmentary conditions that scale (i.e., tinea versicolor and pityriasis alba) can be distinguished with a potassium hydroxide (KOH) preparation.

White spots should be examined for:
1. **Partial versus complete pigment loss**
2. **The presence or absence of scale**

White spots are seen more easily under Wood's light examination.

■ TINEA VERSICOLOR

Definition. Tinea versicolor is a superficial fungal infection of the stratum corneum that results in pigment alteration in the epidermis. The fungal hyphae are transformed *Pityrosporum* yeast organisms. Clinically, the lesions appear as finely scaling patches, which, as the name versicolor implies, can be pink, tan, or white (Fig. 14–1). Of these, white is the most common.

Incidence. Tinea versicolor is a common disease, affecting nearly 1% of the general population. In our clinic, 1.4% of new patients are seen for tinea versicolor. The incidence is higher in tropical climates. Any age group may be affected, but the disease is most common in young adults. Immunosuppression, including that

Lesions in tinea versicolor can be of varying colors, the most common being white.

TABLE 14–1 ▨ WHITE SPOTS

| | | | **Physical Examination** | | | | |
	Frequency*	Etiology	Degree of Pigment Loss†	Presence of Scale	Distribution	Differential Diagnosis	Laboratory Test
Tinea versicolor	1.4	Fungus	Partial	+	Trunk	Vitiligo	Potassium hydroxide preparation
Vitiligo	0.6	Unknown	Complete	–	Anywhere		—
Pityriasis alba	0.4	Unknown	Partial	+	Face, upper arms	Tinea versicolor	—
Postinflammatory hypopigmentation		Nonspecific sequelae of skin inflammation	Partial	–	Anywhere (sites of prior inflammation)	Vitiligo	—
Tuberous sclerosis	Rare	Genetic	Partial	–	Trunk	Vitiligo	CNS imaging

*Percentage of new dermatology patients with this diagnosis seen in the Hershey Medical Center Dermatology Clinic, Hershey, PA.
† As assessed by Wood's light examination.

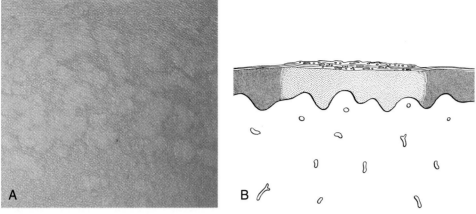

FIGURE 14-1. Tinea versicolor. **A,** Epidermis—fine, often barely perceptible scale; hypopigmented. Dermis—normal. **B,** Epidermis—slight hyperkeratosis; decreased pigmentation. Dermis—normal.

from systemic corticosteroids (either endogenous or exogenous), can be predisposing factors, but most patients are healthy.

History. Tinea versicolor occasionally is associated with mild pruritus, but more often it is asymptomatic. Most patients seek medical attention because of its cosmetic appearance. Because the affected areas do not tan, the patient often first becomes aware of the condition after sun exposure. The surrounding normal skin tans, providing a contrast to the "white spots." During the winter months and in persons with darker complexions, the lesions appear more deeply pigmented than the normal skin (Fig. 14-2).

Physical Examination. The usual lesion is a round, hypopigmented, slightly scaling patch. It often starts as multiple small follicular macules, which subsequently become confluent. The scale usually is subtle and sometimes is appreciated only with gentle scraping of the skin, which reveals a fine, crumbly scale. If a Wood's light examination is performed, the lesions will appear hypopigmented but not chalk white. With Wood's light examination, sometimes the scale fluoresces pale yellow or orange, but this finding is not universal and should not be relied on for diagnosis.

The usual distribution for tinea versicolor is the neck, trunk, and upper arms—that is, the distribution of a short-sleeved turtleneck sweater. Distal extremity and facial involvement is uncommon except in tropical climates.

Differential Diagnosis. In adults, the white spots of tinea versicolor are most often misdiagnosed as *vitiligo*. Tinea versicolor appearing as pink or tan scaling patches on the chest may be misdiagnosed as *seborrheic dermatitis*.

Laboratory Examination. The organism cannot be grown on routine fungal cultures; therefore, the diagnosis rests with the KOH examination. Examination of the scale with a KOH preparation reveals short hyphae, which are often mixed with spores, giving an appearance of "spaghetti (chopped-up spaghetti) and meatballs" or "hot dogs and baked beans" (Fig. 14-3).

Therapy. Topical selenium sulfide has been commonly used. It is effective, easy to apply to a widespread area, and relatively inexpensive. This medication can be used in several ways, but our preference is to apply the 2.5% selenium sulfide

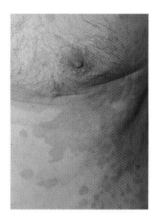

FIGURE 14-2. Pink-tan patches in tinea versicolor.

In tinea versicolor, the scaling may be subtle.

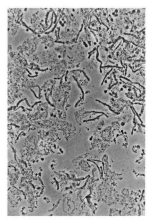

FIGURE 14-3. The potassium hydroxide examination is diagnostic, showing short hyphae and spores.

THERAPY OF TINEA VERSICOLOR

- Selenium sulfide 2.5% or zinc pyrithione shampoo (see text for directions)
- Ketoconazole: 400 mg orally in a single dose

---

shampoo (Selsun, Exsel) in the shower in a "turtleneck sweater" distribution, leave it on for 10 minutes, and then rinse it off. This is done for 3 nights in a row, then weekly for a month, and then once every 3 months to prevent recurrence. Zinc pyrithione shampoo (e.g., Head & Shoulders) has also been successfully used. The topical imidazole antifungal creams are effective against the organism, but this approach is expensive when the eruption is widespread, which it often is. Terbinafine (Lamisil) spray is also effective but expensive.

Oral ketoconazole (Nizoral) is the simplest and most effective therapy. In most adult patients, the fungus is eradicated with a single 400-mg dose. Efficacy is enhanced if the patient works up a sweat 2 hours after ingesting the ketoconazole, thereby delivering the drug, which is concentrated in sweat, to the stratum corneum. For patients with recurrent disease, this regimen can be repeated every 3 months for 1 year.

Course and Complications. The fungus is killed rapidly with therapy, but it takes months for the pigmentation to return to its normal color. It is important to explain this so the patient will not view the treatment as a failure. After topical therapy, the recurrence rate is more than 50%, but this rate can be reduced to less than 15% with the every-3-month retreatment program. Recurrences occur less often with oral ketoconazole therapy.

> **After the initial therapy, it takes months for the white spots to regain pigment.**

Pathogenesis. Tinea versicolor is caused by infection with the yeast *Pityrosporum orbiculare*. This organism is frequently present in its yeast form as a colonizer of normal skin. In tinea versicolor, the spores proliferate in the outer layers of the stratum corneum, often beginning in the areas of follicular openings. When the spore forms are transformed to hyphae, infection occurs. The hyphal forms were called *Malassezia furfur* when it was originally thought that the yeast and hyphae represented different organisms. It is now clear that it is the same organism in different forms. The hyphal structures may invade more deeply into the stratum corneum, but they do not penetrate the viable epidermis. They cause thickening and disruption of the stratum corneum, which is clinically expressed as the fine scale. The hypopigmentation may result from two mechanisms:

1. Fungal enzymes act on surface lipids and produce dicarboxylic acids that diffuse into the epidermis. These acids inhibit tyrosinase, the enzyme in melanocytes that is responsible for melanin production.
2. The infected thickened stratum corneum may serve as a sunscreen, thus preventing ultraviolet light from reaching and stimulating the underlying melanocytes.

Not all patients exposed to this ubiquitous organism develop infection. In fact, conjugal cases are uncommon. Some individuals may be more susceptible by virtue of a genetic predisposition, the nature of which is not known.

■ VITILIGO

Definition. Vitiligo is an acquired condition in which melanocytes have disappeared from the affected skin. The cause is unknown. Lesions clinically appear as totally white, nonscaling, sharply demarcated macules (Fig. 14–4).

Incidence. The reported incidence of vitiligo varies with the population studied. Higher incidence rates in dark-skinned individuals may reflect the observation that vitiligo is more noticeable in more darkly pigmented skin. In the United States, vitiligo is estimated to occur in almost 1% of the general population. Vitiligo represents the presenting complaint in 0.6% of our new patients. The disease can begin at any age, but the peak incidence is in the 10- to 30-year age group.

History. Vitiligo is usually asymptomatic. It begins as one or more small spots that gradually enlarge. The affected areas sunburn easily. Most patients seek medical help because of cosmetic disfigurement.

Physical Examination. The primary lesion is a white macule that is usually totally depigmented. This feature can be appreciated best by Wood's light examination, which accentuates the pigment contrast and also may make evident previously undetected areas in lightly pigmented skin. The skin otherwise is normal; specifically, no scale is present. Macules of vitiligo are round or oval. They may become confluent as they enlarge, resulting in a large macule that has an irregular border but remains sharply demarcated from the surrounding normal skin.

> In vitiligo, depigmentation is complete; this is best seen by Wood's light examination.

Vitiligo can affect any area of the skin and mucous membranes, but the most common areas are the extensor bony surfaces (backs of the hands, elbows, and knees) and the periorificial areas (around the mouth, eyes, rectum, and genitalia). Involvement of hairy areas often results in depigmentation of the hair.

Differential Diagnosis. Vitiligo is more often overdiagnosed than underdiagnosed. Any of the conditions listed in Table 14–1 may be misdiagnosed as vitiligo. Less often, vitiligo is misdiagnosed as one of these conditions. However, vitiligo is the only one of the common white spot diseases that results in total depigmentation. In addition, it can be clinically differentiated from *tinea versicolor* and *pityriasis alba* by the absence of scale.

Laboratory and Biopsy. The laboratory is not helpful for diagnosing vitiligo. Serum thyroid tests and a complete blood count with differential may be ordered to screen for occasionally associated thyroid disease and rarely associated pernicious anemia and Addison's disease. Biopsy usually is not necessary. If performed,

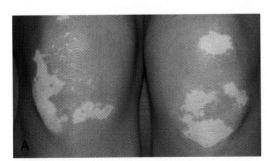
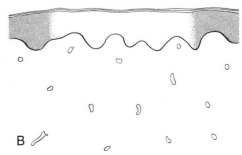

FIGURE 14–4. Vitiligo. **A,** Epidermis—pure white macule. Dermis—normal. **B,** Epidermis—complete absence of pigment and melanocytes. Dermis—normal.

it will show an absence of melanocytes, sometimes with accompanying inflammation. The presence or absence of melanocytes may be difficult to appreciate with routine hematoxylin and eosin stain. Special stains and techniques are required for definitive identification.

Therapy. The goal of therapy is to deal with the cosmetic disfigurement caused by the disease. Therapy for repigmentation is prolonged, and the results often are suboptimal. One treatment involves the administration of a psoralen medication (trimethylpsoralen or 8 methoxypsoralen) followed by exposure to long-wave ultraviolet A light (PUVA). The psoralens can be administered topically or systemically, more frequently the latter, especially for widespread disease. One hundred or more treatments are often required to achieve the end result, which in some patients is complete repigmentation; in others, only partial pigmentation occurs, and in the remainder, treatment fails. For limited disease, topical high-potency steroids (e.g., clobetasol [Temovate]) have been successful in some patients when these agents are applied for one to three 6-week courses.

Initial therapy:
PUVA or topical steroids

Surgical therapies have also occasionally been employed. Normally pigmented skin is harvested (by suction blisters or punch biopsies) and is transplanted into vitiliginous areas. Experimental transplantation of cultured melanocytes has also been reported.

Cosmetic covering agents
may be helpful.

An alternative is to cover the lesions with a cosmetic that is blended to match the color of the patient's normal skin. The products most frequently used for this are CoverMark and Dermablend.

In selected patients with extensive disease, the best cosmetic result may be obtained by depigmenting the remaining normal skin. Topical application of 20% monobenzyl ether of hydroquinone (Benoquin) is used for this, but the patient must be aware that the resulting depigmentation is irreversible.

Course and Complications. The course of vitiligo is unpredictable. In most patients, it is chronic and often slowly progressive. Occasionally, it involves the total body surface, resulting in complete depigmentation. Spontaneous repigmentation occurs in a minority of patients but usually is incomplete. Repigmentation begins around the hair follicles, so it appears as freckles that become confluent as they enlarge.

Ocular involvement with discrete areas of depigmentation of the retina occurs in as many as 30% of patients, and uveitis was reported in 3% of patients in one

---

THERAPY OF VITILIGO

- Covering cosmetics
    CoverMark, Dermablend
- Topical steroids
    Clobetasol cream daily for 6 weeks
- PUVA, systemic
- PUVA, topical
- Epidermal grafting
- Autologous minigrafting
- Transplantation of cultured melanocytes

series. Associated systemic disorders occur in some patients with vitiligo. Thyroid abnormalities, including Graves' disease and thyroiditis, are the most common, with a frequency ranging from 1% to 30%, depending on the series. Addison's disease, pernicious anemia, and alopecia areata are other "autoimmune" disorders uncommonly found in association with vitiligo.

Many patients with vitiligo, particularly deeply pigmented patients, suffer social stigmatization. In some cultures, vitiligo has been confused with the white spots of leprosy and has resulted in social ostracism.

Pathogenesis. Melanocytes are absent in vitiligo. The mechanism for their disappearance is not known. However, three theories, not necessarily mutually exclusive, have been proposed:

1. *Autoimmune.* Investigators have proposed that melanocytes are destroyed by an immune mechanism. Antibodies against melanocyte antigens have been detected in patients with vitiligo. These may be the primary cause of the disease, or they may occur secondary to an initial injury to the melanocytes that results in production of antigens with subsequent antibody formation. Cellular immune mechanisms have also been implicated in melanocyte destruction.

2. *Neural.* This theory proposes that a neurochemical mediator is responsible for the destruction of the melanocytes. Some animal models have clear-cut neural control mechanisms for pigment formation.

3. *Self-destruction.* The intermediate compounds in melanin synthesis are cytotoxic when they are present in sufficient concentrations. The self-destruction theory holds that in vitiligo, these compounds accumulate in melanocytes and eventually destroy them.

Proposed pathologic mechanisms:
1. **Autoimmune**
2. **Neural**
3. **Self-destruction**

■ PITYRIASIS ALBA

Definition. Pityriasis alba is an idiopathic hypopigmentary condition that clinically appears as white (alba) patches surmounted by fine, "bran-like" (*pityron* is Greek for bran) scales (Fig. 14–5).

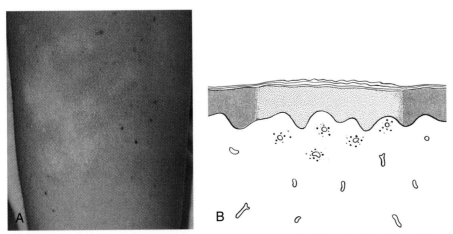

FIGURE 14–5. Pityriasis alba. **A,** Epidermis—hypopigmented; slight scale. Dermis—mild erythema occasionally. **B,** Epidermis—hyperkeratosis; decreased pigmentation. Dermis—mild inflammation around superficial blood vessels.

Pityriasis alba is common in black children.

Incidence. The disease is extremely common but usually not disturbing enough for most patients to seek medical attention. It mainly affects children between the ages of 3 and 16 years and is most common (or most noticeable) in blacks.

History. Pityriasis alba is usually asymptomatic, although an occasional patient may complain of mild itching. Patients or parents are most concerned about the appearance of the lesions.

Physical Examination. The early lesion is a mildly erythematous, slightly scaling patch with an indistinct margin. Most often, only the subsequent lesion is seen, which is a 1- to 4-cm white patch with a fine, powdery scale. In children, the face is the most common area of involvement and may have one to several lesions. Pityriasis alba can occur in other locations. In young women, the most common area is the upper arms (see Fig. 14–5). Rarely, widespread involvement occurs.

Differential Diagnosis. The disease is most often misdiagnosed as *tinea versicolor*. In temperate climates, adults with tinea versicolor seldom have facial involvement, but in children (in whom the disease is much less common), the face is affected in approximately one third of cases. Accordingly, a KOH preparation should be performed on all scaling white spots to rule out tinea versicolor. The white spots in *vitiligo* are distinguished by sharp demarcation, complete depigmentation, and lack of scale.

Laboratory and Biopsy. No specific laboratory test is available to establish the diagnosis. The KOH preparation is negative. The histologic picture is nonspecific, showing slight hyperkeratosis, decreased pigmentation in the basal cell layer, and a mild inflammatory reaction in the upper dermis.

Therapy. Treatment often is not necessary. Emollients can be used for the dry scaling, and 1% hydrocortisone cream is used for the inflammatory reaction.

Course and Complications. The patient must understand that repigmentation will be slow. In most patients, the disease resolves spontaneously, but this takes months and, sometimes, years. For affected children, the disease rarely persists into adulthood. The disorder has no complications.

Pityriasis alba may be a low-grade eczema.

Pathogenesis. The origin of this common disorder is unknown. Most investigators believe that the decreased pigment is a postinflammatory phenomenon and that the initial event is a low-grade eczematous reaction. One study has shown that spongiosis is present in pityriasis alba and that this condition is accompanied by a decrease in the number of melanocytes and melanosomes in the affected skin. Thus, pityriasis alba may be simply another (although clinically characteristic) form of postinflammatory hypopigmentation caused by mild eczematous dermatitis.

THERAPY OF PITYRIASIS ALBA

- Emollients (e.g., Eucerin cream)
- 1% Hydrocortisone cream daily

■ POSTINFLAMMATORY HYPOPIGMENTATION

Definition. Postinflammatory hypopigmentation is the result of melanocyte destruction or suppressed melanin production secondary to inflammation of the skin (Fig. 14–6). It appears as a hypopigmented macule. The inflammation may be due to physical trauma, a chemical agent, or a primary skin disease.

Causes of postinflammatory hypopigmentation:
1. **Physical agents**
2. **Chemicals**
3. **Skin diseases**

Incidence. Inflammation-induced white spots are common incidental findings. Occasionally, they are the patient's primary complaint.

History. The inflammatory event responsible for the white spots is almost always remembered by the patient. Physical agents that often induce white spots include x-irradiation and frostbite. Industrial exposure to chemicals such as phenolic and sulfhydryl compounds can also produce hypopigmentation. Some inflammatory skin diseases can leave residual hypopigmentation. Common examples are discoid lupus erythematosus, eczematous dermatitis (particularly atopic dermatitis), and psoriasis.

Physical Examination. White macules, without scale, conform to areas of prior inflammation.

Differential Diagnosis. Postinflammatory hypopigmentation may be confused with *vitiligo*, particularly if hypopigmentation is profound. However, the pigment loss is rarely complete as it is in vitiligo. Moreover, in vitiligo, the depigmentation is only rarely preceded by recognizable inflammation.

Laboratory and Biopsy. No specific laboratory test is available. The biopsy is not specific, showing decreased pigmentation in the epidermis and occasional mild residual inflammation in the dermis.

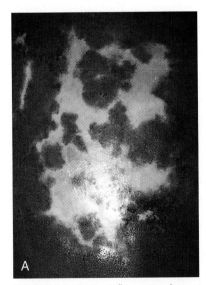
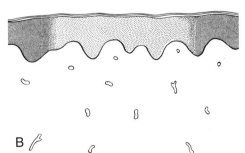

FIGURE 14–6. Postinflammatory hypopigmentation. **A,** Postinflammatory hypopigmentation associated with discoid lupus erythematosus of the scalp. Epidermis—hypopigmented macule. Dermis—normal. **B,** Epidermis—hypopigmented. Dermis—may show some residual inflammation.

**Therapy:
None or cosmetic cover-
ing**

**Repigmentation, if it oc-
curs, takes months and,
sometimes, years.**

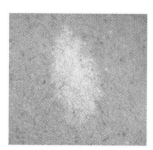

FIGURE 14–7. Tuberous sclerosis. A white "ash leaf" spot.

**The skin of all infants
with seizures should be
examined for white spots
with Wood's light exami-
nation.**

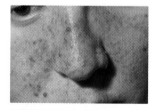

FIGURE 14–8. Tuberous sclerosis. Adenoma sebaceum (angiofibromas) of the face.

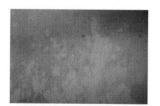

FIGURE 14–9. Unknown.

Therapy. Treatment usually is not required. No effective agents for repigmentating skin are available. Cosmetically troublesome areas can be disguised with an opaque cosmetic such as CoverMark. To avoid future hypopigmentation, patients are advised to avoid contact with any responsible physical or chemical agents and to treat inflammatory skin disease promptly.

Course and Complications. Usually, pigmentation returns gradually. Patients need to understand that this process takes months and sometimes longer. However, if the damage has been severe, the hypopigmentation may be permanent.

■ TUBEROUS SCLEROSIS

Definition. Tuberous sclerosis is a rare, inherited, neurocutaneous disorder with several skin manifestations, including white macules (Fig. 14–7). The classic triad of this disease consists of seizures, mental retardation, and adenoma sebaceum. *Adenoma sebaceum* is a misnamed disorder consisting of angiofibromas that begin in childhood and appear clinically as red papules on the face (Fig. 14–8).

White spots also often occur in this disease and diagnostically are important because they are usually present at birth. They appear as hypopigmented macules, ranging in size from 1 to 3 cm. They are often shaped like a "thumbprint" or an "ash leaf "—that is, oval at one end and pointed at the other. They are most often found on the trunk and less often on the face and extremities. Patients may have as few as 3 or as many as 100 lesions. The spots are most easily seen with Wood's light examination, and sometimes (particularly in infants with extremely fair skin) this is the only method of detection. Therefore, all infants with a seizure disorder should be screened for white spots with a Wood's light examination. Tuberous sclerosis is strongly suspected if more than 3 white spots are detected.

The nervous system is often affected. Calcification of intracranial nodules ("tubers") is common and can be detected early in patients and in apparently unaffected carriers with computed axial tomography or magnetic resonance imaging. Central nervous system involvement is the most debilitating. Mental retardation may be severe, and seizure disorders may be severe and difficult to control. Brain tumors occur in some patients. More than 10% of affected individuals die of internal organ involvement, including brain tumors, renal cysts and tumors, heart rhabdomyomas, and lung lymphangiomas. More mildly affected patients have slow progression of their disease over years.

■ UNKNOWN (Fig. 14–9)

This 25-year-old woman was seen in a dermatology clinic in October with a 4-month history of white spots on her upper trunk. With sun exposure over the summer, the spots had become more noticeable. They had not been red or symptomatic.

What is the most likely diagnosis?

This patient has a typical history for tinea versicolor. Scratching of the affected areas elicited a fine, crumbly scale, further heightening the suspicion of tinea versicolor.

What test would you do?

The KOH preparation is diagnostic, revealing numerous short hyphae and spores.

How would you treat her?

Ketoconazole was prescribed in a single 400-mg dose. The patient was instructed to work up a sweat after 2 hours. The skin gradually repigmented over the following 3 months.

Important Points

1. If it scales, scrape it.
2. It takes months for repigmentation to occur.

REFERENCES

Tinea Versicolor

Borelli D, Jacobs PH, Nall L: Tinea versicolor: epidemiologic, clinical, and therapeutic aspects. J Am Acad Dermatol 25:300–305, 1991.

Savin A: Diagnosis and treatment of tinea versicolor. J Fam Pract 43:127–132, 1996.

Schmidt A: *Malassezia furfur:* a fungus belonging to the physiological skin flora and its relevance in skin disorders. Cutis 59:21–24, 1997.

Sunenshine PJ, Schwartz RA, Janniger CK: Tinea versicolor: an update. Cutis 61:65–68, 71–72, 1998.

Terragni L, Lasagni A, Oriani A, Gelmetti C: Pityriasis versicolor in the pediatric age. Pediatr Dermatol 8:9–12, 1991.

Vitiligo

Bystryn JC: Immune mechanisms in vitiligo. Clin Dermatol 15:853–861, 1997.

Castanet J, Ortone JP: Pathophysiology of vitiligo. Clin Dermatol 15:845–851, 1997.

Falabella R: Surgical therapies for vitiligo. Clin Dermatol 15:927–939, 1997.

Kovacs SO: Vitiligo. J Am Acad Dermatol 38:647–666, 1998.

Schwartz RA, Janniger CK: Vitiligo. Cutis 60:239–244, 1997.

Pityriasis Alba

Galan EB, Janniger CK: Pityriasis alba. Cutis 61:11–13, 1998.

Wells BT, Whyte MB, Kierland RR: Pityriasis alba: a 10-year survey and review of the literature. Arch Dermatol 82:183–189, 1960.

Zaynoun ST, Aftimos BG, Tenekjian KK, et al.: Extensive pityriasis alba: a histological histochemical and ultrastructural study. Br J Dermatol 108:83–90, 1983.

Tuberous Sclerosis

Fitzpatrick TB, Szabo G, Yoshiaki H, et al.: White leaf-shaped macules: earliest visible sign of tuberous sclerosis. Arch Dermatol 98:1–6, 1968.

Schnur RE: Tuberous sclerosis: the persistent challenge of clinical diagnosis. Arch Dermatol 131:1460–1462, 1995.

Webb DW, Osborne JP: Tuberous sclerosis. Arch Dis Child 72:471–474, 1995.

Zvulunov A, Esterly NB: Neurocutaneous syndromes associated with pigmentary skin lesions. J Am Acad Dermatol 32:915–935, 1995.

4

DERMAL

RASHES

■

C H A P T E R

GENERALIZED ERYTHEMA

15

■

DRUG ERUPTIONS
VIRAL EXANTHEMS
TOXIC ERYTHEMA
LUPUS ERYTHEMATOSUS

The rashes discussed in this chapter are composed of erythematous macules and papules that are widespread and sometimes confluent. Various terms have been used to describe this type of eruption, including maculopapular, exanthematous, and morbilliform (measles-like). The major causes of generalized erythematous eruptions are listed in Table 15–1 in the order of relative frequency.

■ DRUG ERUPTIONS

Definition. The expression, "For any rash, think drug!" reflects the finding that drug eruptions can appear in a variety of ways. However, the two most common eruptions are hives (discussed in Chapter 17) and morbilliform rashes. Of these two, morbilliform rashes are more common. A morbilliform drug rash appears as a generalized eruption of erythematous macules and papules, often confluent in large areas (Fig. 15–1).

Incidence. Only 0.6% of our new outpatients are seen for a drug eruption. The frequency, however, is much higher among hospitalized patients, each of whom receives an average of 9 drugs! Drug rashes lead the list for our hospital consultations and account for 7% of all dermatology consultations. Data gathered from 37,665 consecutive medical inpatients in the two Boston Collaborative Drug Studies showed that skin reactions occurred in 865 (2.3%). The reaction rates of the most common offenders in the more recent study (Bigby et al., 1986) are given in Table 15–2.

Approximately 2% of all medical inpatients experience drug-induced skin reactions.

History. The onset of a drug-induced morbilliform eruption usually is not immediate but rather begins within several days of the initiation of the drug. Onset sometimes is delayed as long as 1 week but seldom longer. Because no laboratory tests are available by which to identify the responsible drug, reliance is placed on the history. For patients receiving multiple drugs, this obviously presents a problem. In selecting a single drug from a list of many, the two variables to be considered are the temporal relationship between the initiation of the drug and the onset of the rash and the odds that a given drug is likely to cause a drug eruption. In selecting a putative drug, it is helpful to construct a graph that depicts the patient's

Suspect drugs that are:
1. **New (started within 1 week of the rash)**
2. **Frequent offenders**

TABLE 15–1 ■ GENERALIZED ERYTHEMA

	Frequency*	Etiology	History	Physical Examination	Differential Diagnosis	Laboratory Test
Drug eruption	0.6†	Drug	Recent new drug Pruritus Usually no fever	Rash bright red and confluent	Exfoliative erythroderma (chronic)	—
Viral exanthem	0.2	Rubeola Rubella Enteroviruses, etc.	Associated "viral" symptoms	Erythema mild to moderate Mucous membranes occasionally involved	Drug reaction	Acute and convalescent viral titers
"Toxic" erythema	<0.1	Group A streptococci S. aureus Unknown	Patient feels extremely ill ("toxic") No pruritus	Rash accentuated in flexural folds and often feels like sandpaper Mucous membranes often involved	Drug reaction	Bacterial cultures
Systemic lupus erythematosus (SLE)	Autoimmune	Other symptoms of SLE	"Butterfly" distribution on face Sun-exposed areas favored Rarely total body	Drug reaction	Antinuclear antibody Anti-DNA antibodies Complete blood count Urinalysis	

*Percentage of new dermatology patients with this diagnosis seen in the Hershey Medical Center Dermatology Clinic.

†Frequency in outpatients. For an inpatient, a drug eruption is the most common dermatologic problem acquired in the hospital.

drug history (Fig. 15–2). In this example, drugs A, B, and C are unlikely to be implicated because the patient had been receiving these agents for months. Drug D was stopped 4 days before the rash began, thus making it a less likely cause. Drug G was started 6 hours *after* the rash appeared, and drug H was started the

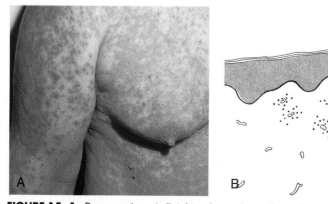

FIGURE 15–1. Drug eruption. **A,** Bright red macules and papules confluent in large areas. Epidermis—normal. Dermis—marked erythema. **B,** Epidermis—normal. Dermis—superficial and deep perivascular inflammatory cell infiltrate that includes eosinophils.

TABLE 15–2 ■ ALLERGIC SKIN REACTIONS TO DRUGS

Drugs	Reaction Rate (Reactions/100 Recipients)
Amoxicillin	5.1
Trimethoprim-sulfamethoxazole	3.4
Ampicillin	3.3
Ipodate	2.8
Blood	2.2
Semisynthetic penicillins	2.1
Cephalosporins	2.1
Erythromycin	2.0
Dihydralazine hydrochloride	1.9
Penicillin G	1.9
Quinidine	1.3
Cimetidine	1.3

following day. Drugs E and F were started 2 days before the rash and therefore have the best temporal relationship. Drug E is a cephalosporin, a well-known cause of rash, and drug F is codeine, a rare cause of morbilliform eruptions. Therefore, drug E is the probable cause and is the first to be discontinued.

In patients with drug rashes, itching is usually present but is not helpful as a diagnostic marker. Fever is rarely found.

Physical Examination. The eruption is generalized and is composed of brightly erythematous macules and papules that tend to be confluent in large areas. Characteristically, the erythema is intense or "drug red." Drug rashes usually start proximally and proceed distally, with the legs being the last to be involved as well as the last to clear.

Differential Diagnosis. The differential diagnosis includes viral exanthem, toxic erythema, and chronic exfoliative erythroderma.

A *viral exanthem* and a drug eruption can be clinically indistinguishable. Often, a drug eruption is much more erythematous, more confluent, and more

Drug rashes usually are:
1. **Bright red**
2. **Confluent in large areas**

Differential diagnosis for acute morbilliform eruptions:
1. **Drug**
2. **Viral**
3. **"Toxic"**

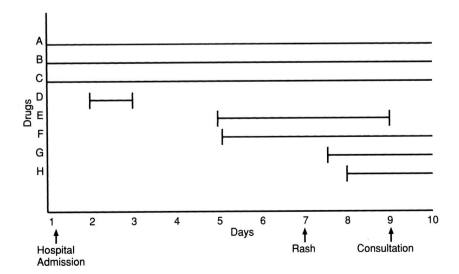

FIGURE 15–2. Graphic depiction of drug history. See text for discussion.

pruritic. The presence of viral signs and symptoms favors a diagnosis of a viral exanthem.

Toxic erythemas include scarlet fever, staphylococcal scarlatiniform eruptions, and Kawasaki syndrome (mucocutaneous lymph node syndrome). Features that help to distinguish these rashes from drug eruptions include a sandpaper-like texture of the "toxic" rash, mucous membrane involvement (scarlet fever and Kawasaki syndrome), the presence of fever, and a focus of infection or the presence of lymphadenopathy.

When a generalized erythema becomes chronic, it is called an *exfoliative erythroderma*—exfoliative because of the prominent desquamation (Fig. 15–3). Long-term administration of an offending drug is one cause. The other three causes are generalization of a benign dermatosis (most often, psoriasis or atopic dermatitis), malignancy (most often, the Sézary variant of cutaneous T-cell lymphoma; see Chapter 10), and an idiopathic disorder.

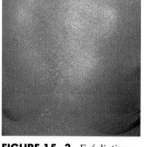

FIGURE 15–3. Exfoliative erythroderma.

Laboratory and Biopsy. No laboratory tests can enable one to diagnose a drug eruption or to incriminate a specific drug. Peripheral blood eosinophilia is sometimes present and may heighten the suspicion of a drug reaction. Skin biopsy is most often performed in patients with chronic exfoliative erythrodermas. A drug eruption shows a superficial and deep perivascular inflammatory cell infiltrate. The presence of eosinophils in the infiltrate is an important clue suggesting a drug-related cause. Skin tests for penicillin may be useful for the diagnosis of immediate hypersensitivity reactions (hives and anaphylaxis) but not for morbilliform eruptions.

Therapy. When the offending drug is identified, it should be discontinued. If the patient is taking multiple drugs and it is not possible to be certain of the offending drug, the number of administered drugs should be reduced to an absolute minimum, and any remaining possible offenders should be changed to alternative agents when possible.

Therapy otherwise is symptomatic, with antihistamines (e.g., hydroxyzine, 10 to 25 mg four times daily) most often used for the pruritus. Moisturizing lotions are helpful during the late desquamative phase of the reaction. Topical steroids are of little value, and systemic steroids are rarely required.

THERAPY OF DRUG ERUPTIONS

- Discontinuance of the offending drug
- Antihistamines
  - Hydroxyzine (Atarax): 10–25 mg QID
  - Diphenhydramine (Benadryl): 25–50 mg QID
- Moisturizers
  - Eucerin cream BID

Drug eruptions take 1 to 2 weeks to clear.

Course and Complications. Drug eruptions clear slowly with *time* after discontinuation of the responsible agent. The time required for total clearing is usually 1 to 2 weeks. For several days after the offending drug has been stopped, the eruption may actually worsen.

Complications are uncommon and primarily cutaneous. When large areas of skin are inflamed, increased body heat and water loss occur. In a patient already seriously ill, this could be a problem, but for most patients it is not.

The risks of continuing an offending agent in the presence of a drug eruption are cutaneous and renal. The cutaneous risk involves progressive worsening of the rash, possibly eventuating in toxic epidermal necrolysis, which is characterized by the loss of large sheets of epidermis. Fortunately, this complication rarely occurs. In fact, sometimes a drug eruption clears despite continued treatment with the offending agent, although this approach is not desirable if an alternative drug is available. The renal risk is allergic interstitial nephritis, an uncommon development usually associated with penicillins and cephalosporins and, rarely, with other drugs. If the responsible drug has been identified, the patient should be advised to avoid the drug in the future, and the medical record should be clearly labeled.

Potential consequences of continuing the offending drug:
1. Worsening rash
2. Interstitial nephritis

Pathogenesis. Although specific immunologic and nonimmunologic mechanisms have been documented for some types of drug-induced cutaneous reactions (e.g., hives and vasculitis), the mechanism for the morbilliform eruption remains unclear. Increasing experimental evidence points to a major role for cellular immune (type IV) processes. The clinical course with delayed onset and prolonged duration of the rash also favors this mechanism.

■ VIRAL EXANTHEMS

Definition. Viral exanthems are caused by hematogenous dissemination of virus to the skin, in which a vascular response is elicited (Fig. 15–4). The clinical appearance of a virus-induced generalized erythema is not specific for a given virus; other signs and symptoms, however, may indicate a particular etiologic agent. The viruses that are most often associated with exanthems are rubeola (measles), rubella (German measles), herpesvirus type 6 (roseola), parvovirus B19 (erythema infectiosum), and the enteroviruses (ECHO and coxsackievirus).

Major viruses producing exanthems:
1. Measles (rubeola)
2. German measles (rubella)
3. Herpesvirus type 6 (roseola)
4. Parvovirus B19 (erythema infectiosum)
5. Enteroviruses (ECHO and coxsackievirus)

Incidence. Exanthem-producing viral infections rank high among the classic "common childhood diseases." Widespread immunization for rubella and rubeola have significantly reduced the incidence of these diseases. However, in the United States occasional outbreaks of measles still occur in schools and on college campuses, as well as in other populations with a low rate of immunization.

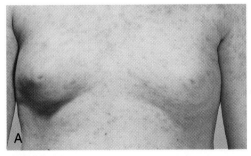 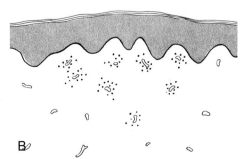

FIGURE 15–4. Viral exanthem. **A,** Erythematous macules and papules. Epidermis—normal. Dermis—mild to moderate erythema. **B,** Epidermis—normal. Dermis—perivascular inflammation.

Viral exanthems occur in adults but much less often than in children. In children less than 2 years of age, roseola is the most common viral exanthem. Erythema infectiosum ("fifth" disease) occurs in young school-age children, often in epidemics.

History. Most viral exanthems are preceded by a prodrome of fever and constitutional symptoms. In *measles*, the prodrome is characterized by the three Cs: cough, coryza, and conjunctivitis. A history of previous exposure to infected individuals may be elicited. Incubation times vary from days to weeks, depending on the virus. Drug history may also be important, especially in patients with infectious mononucleosis. *Mononucleosis* alone is associated with rash only about 3% of the time, but with the administration of ampicillin the frequency of rash approaches 100%.

In patients with infectious mononucleosis, ampicillin increases the likelihood of rash from 3% to nearly 100%.

Physical Examination. The generalized eruption is composed of erythematous macules and papules. In *measles* and German measles, the rash typically begins on the head and proceeds to involve the trunk and extremities. In measles, individual lesions tend to become confluent on the face and trunk but remain discrete on the extremities. The macules and papules in *rubella* are discrete, even on the trunk. In *roseola* (exanthem subitum), rose-red macules and papules develop primarily on the trunk and proximal extremities. *Erythema infectiosum* characteristically begins with red cheeks that have a "slapped" appearance followed by a reticulated (net-like) erythema on the trunk and proximal extremities. The rashes associated with *enterovirus infections* most often are rubella-like but occasionally are purpuric. Vesicular eruptions also occur with some types of enterovirus infections—for example, hand, foot, and mouth disease from coxsackievirus A-16 infection.

Mucous membranes are sometimes involved. In rubella, red spots occur on the soft palate. In measles, Koplik's spots are characteristic and often precede the rash. *Koplik's spots* are found on the buccal mucosa and appear as tiny gray-white papules on an erythematous base. In roseola, erythematous macules develop on the soft palate 48 hours before the exanthem.

In roseola, fever subsides just before the rash appears.

Fever is almost always present. In patients with roseola, the fever characteristically subsides abruptly just before the rash appears. Lymphadenopathy is also common. In rubella, enlarged lymph nodes are found in the head and neck; in measles, lymphadenopathy is often generalized. Aseptic meningitis occasionally occurs in enterovirus infections.

Differential Diagnosis. Drug rashes are usually pruritic and are redder and more confluent than viral exanthems. *Toxic erythemas* favor flexural folds, may feel like sandpaper, and often have more extensive mucous membrane involvement. The rash in *Rocky Mountain spotted fever* begins as erythematous macules and papules but typically starts distally (hands and feet) and becomes *purpuric* as it progresses (see Chapter 18).

Laboratory and Biopsy. Routine laboratory tests are of no help. Usually, no tests are ordered; however, serologic tests can confirm the diagnosis by detecting a rise in antibody titer in convalescent compared with acute serum samples. Viral cultures are available but are not often obtained.

Skin biopsy is not indicated; histologic examination usually shows a nonspecific lymphocytic perivascular infiltrate. In measles, the infection also involves the epidermal cells, resulting in intranuclear inclusions, multinucleated giant cells, and individual cell necrosis.

Therapy. Treatment of acute disease is symptomatic. Rubeola and rubella can be prevented through vaccination with live attenuated virus.

Course and Complications. Spontaneous, complete resolution usually occurs over several days to a week. Systemic complications are uncommon. Encephalitis is the most serious, occurring in patients with measles at a rate of approximately 1 in 1,000, and it results in death in 10% to 20% of affected patients. Before the availability of effective vaccines, measles encephalitis accounted for approximately 500 deaths per year in the United States. The rate is much higher in some developing countries, where it remains a leading cause of death in children. Secondary bacterial infections (e.g., bronchopneumonia) can also complicate measles infection. Worldwide, measles continues to cause about 1 million deaths per year among children less than 5 years of age.

Encephalitis is the most serious complication of measles.

Rubella and erythema infectiosum are frequently complicated by arthritis in adults. Infection with parvovirus B19 has also been associated with acute aplastic crises in patients with a history of prior chronic hemolytic anemia, such as sickle cell disease. The most important complication of rubella is the *congenital rubella syndrome*, which occurs in babies born of mothers who were infected during the first trimester of pregnancy. With rubella vaccination in widespread use, this condition is rare.

Pathogenesis. For all the viral exanthems, the virus gains entry through the upper respiratory (e.g., rubella and rubeola) or gastrointestinal (enteroviruses) route, incubates "silently" for a period of days to weeks, and then enters a viremic phase that causes the febrile prodrome and results in dissemination of virus to other tissues, including the skin. The pathogenesis of the inflammatory reaction in the skin is not known with certainty, but possibilities include the following:

1. Direct invasion of the blood vessel walls by the virus.
2. Deposition of immune complexes in which the virus serves as the antigen. This concept is supported by the observation in measles that the appearance of the rash coincides with the detection of circulating antibodies. These antibodies are also responsible for preventing future infection.
3. Cell-mediated immune responses. Cellular immunity probably plays the most important role for recovery from primary infection and may also be the dominant factor in the inflammatory response. In support of this concept, patients with agammaglobulinemia, although deficient in antibodies, show a normal inflammatory skin reaction to measles infection.

■ TOXIC ERYTHEMA

Definition. Toxic erythema is a cutaneous response to a circulating toxin. In scarlet fever, erythrogenic toxin is elaborated by group A streptococci (*Streptococcus pyogenes*), usually infecting the pharynx. For staphylococcal scarlatiniform eruption, staphylococcal scalded skin syndrome, and toxic shock syndrome, the responsible toxins are elaborated by a focus of *Staphylococcus aureus* infection or colonization. Cases of toxic shock–like syndrome have also been reported in association with severe infections with group A streptococci. In mucocutaneous lymph node syndrome (Kawasaki syndrome, Fig. 15–5), a toxin is presumed but has not been identified. For all toxic erythemas, the skin becomes generally red, often feels like

Toxic erythemas:
1. **Scarlet fever**
2. **Staphylococcal scarlatiniform eruption, scalded skin syndrome, toxic shock syndrome**
3. **Kawasaki syndrome**

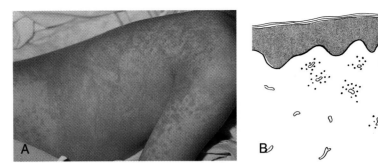

FIGURE 15–5. Kawasaki syndrome. **A,** Generalized erythema with sandpaper texture. Epidermis—normal. Dermis—erythema. **B,** Epidermis—normal, except in scalded skin syndrome. Dermis—perivascular inflammation.

sandpaper, and undergoes postinflammatory desquamation. Mucous membrane involvement is also common.

Incidence. Toxic erythemas are still uncommon, although they have been increasing in frequency in recent years. Children are affected most often, except for toxic shock syndrome, which usually occurs in adults. After the advent of antibiotics, scarlet fever had become a less common and generally less serious disease, although this trend has been reversing in recent years.

> **Except for toxic shock syndrome, toxic erythemas occur most often in children.**

History. Fever is common to all toxic erythemas. Patients with scarlet fever have a history of a sore throat preceding the rash by 1 to 2 days. In the staphylococcal scarlatiniform eruption and staphylococcal scalded skin syndrome, patients may have a history of a local staphylococcal infection causing conjunctivitis, cutaneous abscess, or external otitis. Patients with toxic shock syndrome and mucocutaneous lymph node syndrome look and feel the most seriously ill. Staphylococcal toxic shock syndrome was first described in menstruating women who used occlusive tampons that allowed staphylococcal organisms to proliferate in the occluded vaginal tract. This disorder is now more frequently found in postoperative patients. The focus of infection for staphylococcal toxic shock syndrome is usually the skin, most commonly an area of painful cellulitis on an extremity. The onset of toxic shock syndrome is abrupt. As the name suggests, hypotension is common, as are vomiting, diarrhea, severe myalgias, and encephalopathy with mental confusion. Patients with Kawasaki syndrome frequently experience abdominal pain, diarrhea, arthralgias, and other systemic symptoms.

> **Toxic erythemas are usually:**
> 1. **Sandpapery**
> 2. **Accentuated in flexural folds**
> 3. **Followed by desquamation**

Physical Examination. Toxic erythemas are characterized by a generalized, usually brightly erythematous eruption that frequently feels sandpapery and is accentuated in flexural folds. Postinflammatory desquamation, particularly of the hands and feet, is common but not pathognomonic.

Mucous membrane involvement is usually striking, occurring in all toxic eruptions except staphylococcal scarlatiniform eruption and scalded skin syndrome. Patients with scarlet fever have acute streptococcal pharyngitis and a "strawberry tongue," which starts with a white exudate studded with prominent red papillae ("white strawberry"). After several days, the tongue becomes "beefy red" ("red strawberry"). In toxic shock syndrome, mucous membrane hyperemia frequently affects the conjunctivae, oral pharynx, or vagina. In Kawasaki syndrome, patients usually have marked erythema of the lips ("cherry red" lips), tongue ("strawberry" tongue), and conjunctivae. In this disease, asymmetric lymphadenopathy occurs in approximately 75% of patients—hence the name mucocutaneous lymph node syndrome.

Differential Diagnosis. The differential diagnosis includes *drug eruption, viral exanthem*, and *toxic epidermal necrolysis*. Toxic epidermal necrolysis is a severe, generalized form of erythema multiforme (see Chapter 17) characterized by intense erythema and extensive blistering that occurs in sheets. Skin biopsy in this disease shows the blister to be subepidermal, rather than intraepidermal.

Group A streptococci are recovered from the pharynx in patients with scarlet fever. Absence of mucous membrane involvement suggests staphylococcal scarlatiniform or scalded skin eruption. Multisystem involvement including hypotension in a menstruating female patient strongly suggests toxic shock syndrome. Striking mucous membrane involvement and lymphadenopathy in a child who appears seriously ill are features of Kawasaki syndrome. The diagnostic criteria for toxic shock syndrome and Kawasaki syndrome are listed in Table 15–3.

Laboratory and Biopsy. Bacterial cultures from potential foci of infection are mandatory. In suspected cases of scarlet fever, a throat culture should be taken. Less often, streptococcal impetigo serves as the focus of infection. For staphylococcal toxic erythemas, a focus of bacterial colonization or infection should be sought and cultured. In women with suspected toxic shock syndrome, vaginal cultures should be obtained. In seriously ill patients, blood cultures also should be drawn because some patients with staphylococcal toxic shock syndrome are septic. The focus of infection in patients with streptococcal toxic shock syndrome most often is a severe, necrotizing cellulitis, which should be cultured. These patients often also have positive blood cultures. Laboratory evaluation of other organ systems is appropriate in toxic shock syndrome and Kawasaki disease. These include tests of hematopoietic, hepatic, cardiac, and renal functions. In toxic shock syndrome, thrombocytopenia occurs early; in Kawasaki disease, thrombocytosis occurs late.

Mucous membrane involvement accompanies all toxic erythemas except staphylococcal scarlatiniform eruption and scalded skin syndrome.

Cultures should be obtained from potential bacterial reservoirs:
1. **Throat**
2. **Skin**
3. **Vagina**
4. **Blood**

TABLE 15–3 ■ DIAGNOSTIC CRITERIA FOR TOXIC SHOCK SYNDROME AND KAWASAKI SYNDROME

Diagnostic Criteria for Toxic Shock Syndrome	Diagnostic Criteria for Kawasaki Syndrome
Fever of 38.9°C or higher	Fever for 5 or more days
Scarlatiniform rash	Red palms and soles with edema, then desquamation
Desquamation of skin 1 to 2 weeks after onset	Exanthem on trunk
Hypotension	Conjunctivitis
Clinical or laboratory abnormalities of at least three organ systems	Mucosal erythema (lips, tongue, or pharynx)
Absence of other causes of the illness	Cervical lymphadenopathy
(All six are required for diagnosis)	(Fever plus 4 of the remaining 5 criteria are required for diagnosis)

The biopsy is nonspecific in toxic erythemas, except in straphylococcal scalded skin syndrome, in which an intraepidermal separation is found.

Initial treatment: Antibiotics for infections Aspirin and γ-globulin for Kawasaki syndrome

Therapy. Streptococcal disease is usually treated with penicillin, although penicillin-resistant strains of streptococci are beginning to be reported. Staphylococcal infections are treated with penicillinase-resistant antibiotics such as oral dicloxacillin or intravenous nafcillin. Intravenous γ-globulin and aspirin are used to treat Kawasaki syndrome.

Course and Complications. Scarlet fever and staphylococcal scarlatiniform eruptions pursue a relatively benign course, with complete recovery usually within 5 to 10 days. Penicillin has dramatically altered the course of scarlet fever in both duration and severity. Complications are uncommon with scarlet fever, although poststreptococcal glomerulonephritis may occur. Death has occurred in patients with toxic shock syndrome as a result of severe hypotension, sepsis, or multisystem organ failure.

Fever is most prolonged in Kawasaki syndrome—it usually lasts for more than 5 days. Death can result from Kawasaki syndrome, usually the result of coronary artery aneurysm and thrombosis, which is striking given the young age of these patients. This complication occurs in up to 20% of patients and can be delayed by 1 year or more after the acute episode. It can often be prevented with the acute-phase therapy mentioned earlier.

For all these disorders, postinflammatory desquamation usually occurs in 1 to 2 weeks. It is most striking on the hands and feet, where stratum corneum often sheds in large sheets.

Pathogenesis. The toxins involved in toxic erythemas act as "superantigens" that directly activate T-cells, thus causing the release of massive amounts of cytokines, especially tumor necrosis factor-α, interleukin-1, and interleukin-6. These cytokines are thought to be responsible for the clinical manifestations. An erythrogenic toxin is produced by a lysogenic bacteriophage found in most strains of group A β-hemolytic streptococci. Although repeated streptococcal infections may occur, scarlet fever usually does not recur because of specific antitoxin antibodies that are formed from the first episode.

Staphylococcal scarlatiniform eruption is probably a forme fruste of staphylococcal scalded skin syndrome. In both instances, the toxins involved are produced by phage group II *S. aureus*. In toxic shock syndrome, several staphylococcal toxins have been isolated, but the one most often implicated is an exoprotein designated toxic shock syndrome toxin-1. This toxin is different from the epidermolytic toxin of scalded skin syndrome. Other toxins, as well as the host responses to the toxins, probably also play a role in the pathogenesis of toxic shock syndrome.

The pathogenesis of Kawasaki syndrome remains unknown. An infectious origin continues to be suspected, and toxin-producing bacteria have been isolated in a few cases. The efficacy of γ-globulin in the treatment of this disease also is unexplained. One theory holds that the γ-globulin may neutralize a microbial toxin.

■ LUPUS ERYTHEMATOSUS

Definition. Systemic lupus erythematosus (SLE) is an "autoimmune" disorder in which virtually any kind of skin lesion can occur, including macules, papules, plaques, bullae, purpura, subcutaneous nodules, and ulcers (Fig. 15–6). The face is frequently involved. Discoid lupus erythematosus and subacute cutaneous

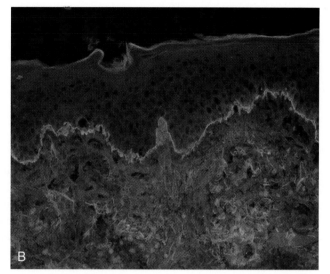
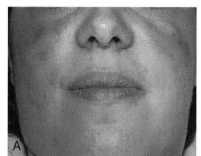

FIGURE 15–6. Systemic lupus erythematosus. **A,** Butterfly rash. Epidermis—normal. Dermis—erythema with or without telangiectasia. **B,** Immunoglobulin G deposition at the dermal-epidermal junction. (From Helm KF, Marks JG Jr: Atlas of Differential Dermatology. New York, Churchill Livingstone, 1998, p. 36.)

lupus erythematosus are scaling disorders and are discussed in Chapter 10. For generalized erythematous eruptions, SLE should be considered a possible (although uncommon) cause, particularly if other signs and symptoms of the disease are present.

Incidence. The prevalence of lupus erythematosus appears to be increasing, but this probably is the result of more widespread recognition of the disease, particularly in its milder forms. In the United States, SLE is estimated to affect approximately 1 in 500 women and 1 in 5,000 men.

History. Mucocutaneous symptoms of SLE include nasal and oral ulcerations, photosensitivity, alopecia, and Raynaud's phenomenon. Arthritis is common. Serositis (with pleuritis or pericarditis) and neurologic manifestations also occur. Renal disease is common but may be asymptomatic. Fatigue is a common complaint that in some patients is a manifestation of anemia.

Because SLE can be drug induced, a careful drug history is important. The drugs most often implicated are procainamide, hydralazine, and isoniazid.

Physical Examination. The erythematous rash of lupus often has a violaceous hue. It is frequently accentuated in sun-exposed areas but in some patients is generalized. The malar area of the face is a common location, where it produces the "butterfly rash." The malar rash in lupus tends to spare the nasolabial folds and is frequently accompanied by telangiectasia.

Differential Diagnosis. The diagnosis of SLE is established by a combination of historical, physical, and laboratory findings. The American Rheumatism Association criteria for lupus are listed in the margin. In this listing, the definitions of the disorders are as follows: persistent heavy proteinuria or cellular casts for renal; seizures or psychosis for neurologic; hemolytic anemia, leukopenia, lymphopenia, or thrombocytopenia for hematologic; and positive LE prep, anti-DNA antibody, anti-Smith (Sm) antibody, or false-positive serologic test for syphilis for immunologic. Patients with four or more of the criteria are diagnosed as having SLE.

American Rheumatism Association criteria for SLE*:
1. Malar rash
2. Discoid rash
3. Photosensitivity
4. Oral ulcers
5. Arthritis
6. Serositis
7. Renal disorder
8. Neurologic disorder
9. Hematologic disorder
10. Immunologic disorder
11. Antinuclear antibody

*SLE is diagnosed if four or more are present.

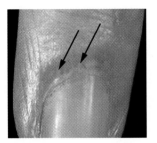

FIGURE 15–7. Periungual telangiectasia in a patient with dermatomyositis.

Other *collagen vascular diseases* may be considered in the differential diagnosis, and sometimes an overlap occurs among several of these disorders; mixed connective tissue disease is an example. In *dermatomyositis*, the characteristic skin findings are violaceous ("heliotrope") edema of the eyelids, flat-topped papules over the knuckles (Gottron's papules), and reticulated patches of pigment, erythema, and telangiectasia (poikiloderma). Periungual erythema with telangiectasia is virtually diagnostic of a collagen vascular disease, most often dermatomyositis (Fig. 15–7). *Scleroderma* is less likely to be confused with SLE, but Raynaud's phenomenon, although less common in SLE, occurs in both conditions, and some patients have features that overlap the two diseases.

In patients with *photosensitivity*, causes other than lupus should be considered. The major causes are drugs, porphyria, and polymorphous light eruption (see Chapter 25).

The most common cause of a butterfly rash is not SLE but rather *seborrheic dermatitis*. Seborrheic dermatitis usually can be distinguished by the presence of the fine, yellowish scale, involvement of the nasolabial folds, and coexistence of a similar scaling rash on the scalp, behind the ears, on the eyebrows, and, often, in the presternal area.

SLE initial screen:
1. **Complete blood count with platelet count**
2. **Urinalysis**
3. **Antinuclear antibody test**

Confirmatory autoantibody tests for lupus:
1. **Double-stranded DNA**
2. **Smith**

Laboratory and Biopsy. The screening tests for SLE are complete blood count, platelet count, urinalysis, and antinuclear antibody (ANA) test. If the ANA is positive, an anti-DNA antibody test is ordered because it is more specific for SLE. Antibodies to the Sm antigen are also highly specific for SLE but are found less frequently than are the antibodies to double-stranded DNA (dsDNA). Serum complement is often depressed in patients with active SLE.

Skin biopsy findings in lupus include vacuolar degeneration of the basal cell layer with a perivascular and periappendageal lymphocytic infiltrate. With immunofluorescence staining, immunoglobulin and complement depositions are found at the dermal-epidermal junction (lupus band test) not only in involved skin but often also in clinically uninvolved skin in patients with SLE. The lupus band test is also positive in involved skin but is negative in clinically uninvolved skin in patients with purely cutaneous lupus. Although still occasionally used, the lupus band test has now been largely replaced by serologic testing (ANA, anti-DNA, anti-Sm).

Initial therapy:
1. **Sun protection**
2. **Topical steroids**

Therapy. Cutaneous involvement can be treated with moderate- to high-potency topical steroids and sunscreens that filter out both short- and long-wave ultraviolet light. An antimalarial such as hydroxychloroquine (Plaquenil) at a dosage of 200 mg daily or twice daily is used for more severe cutaneous disease that is

---

THERAPY OF CUTANEOUS LUPUS

- Sunscreens and protective clothing
- Topical steroids
    Triamcinolone cream 0.1% (medium)
    Fluocinonide cream 0.05% (strong)
- Antimalarials (for more severe disease)
    Hydroxychloroquine: 200 mg BID

unresponsive to topical therapy. Antimalarials are also helpful for fatigue and arthritis. In patients with systemic disease including renal involvement, systemic steroids and other immunosuppressants are used.

Course and Complications. In patients with SLE, 5-year survival rates are now greater than 90%, and more than 80% of patients survive at least 10 years. Patients with nephritis have a worse prognosis than those without the complication. Men do worse than women. Patients less than 16 years of age and who have no renal involvement have an excellent prognosis. In one large series, the most common causes of death were renal disease and sepsis, often secondary to iatrogenic immunosuppression. The improved outlook in patients with SLE in recent years may reflect identification of patients with milder disease or earlier, more effective treatment of patients with potentially severe involvement.

Pathogenesis. The pathogenesis of the skin lesions in lupus is discussed in Chapter 10. Patients with subacute cutaneous lupus erythematosus often have extensive skin disease but limited systemic involvement. These patients frequently are ANA negative but have circulating antibodies to cytoplasmic antigens, designated Ro (Sjögren's syndrome A) and La (Sjögren's syndrome B) antigens. In SLE, autoantibodies are formed to nuclear antigens (ANA and anti-DNA). Autoantibodies are involved in the formation of immune complexes, followed by complement activation, and this process contributes to the inflammatory response in many tissues, including skin and kidney. The degree of complement consumption is reflected by the finding of diminished serum levels of complement in patients with active disease.

In lupus, the autoantibodies are produced by B-cells that appear to be stimulated by activated T-cells that have escaped from the normal mechanisms of tolerance to self-antigens. Increases in some circulating cytokines and decreases in others have also been demonstrated. The significance of these changes is uncertain.

Genetic factors play a role in many patients with lupus. Familial lupus is well documented. Concordant disease is approximately 50% in monozygotic twins compared with 5% in dizygotic twins. In addition, the X chromosome is thought to carry one of the genes involved in the disease; this probably accounts for the much higher incidence rate of lupus in women than in men.

Environmental factors also have been implicated in lupus. Sunlight is definitely involved. As already discussed, some drugs can induce lupus, but patients with "idiopathic" lupus do not have increased risk from these agents. Infections (viral, mycobacterial, and parasitic) have also been implicated but not proven.

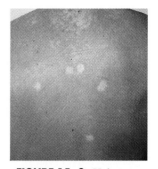

FIGURE 15-8. Unknown.

■ UNKNOWN (Fig. 15-8)

Two days after this patient's coronary artery bypass graft, he developed a pruritic, intensely erythematous eruption that began on his face and trunk, became confluent, and subsequently involved his extremities. He was afebrile and otherwise was recovering uneventfully from his surgical procedure.

He had been taking furosemide and diazepam on a long-term basis. On the day of surgery, he was started on cefazolin, codeine, morphine, and flurazepam.

What is the most likely diagnosis?

A drug eruption is favored by virtue of the intensity of the erythema, the confluence of the rash, the presence of pruritus, and the absence of fever or other constitutional symptoms.

If you suspect a drug reaction, what is the most likely drug?

The most likely drug is one that has been recently administered. From the list of this patient's recent drugs, cefazolin, a cephalosporin antibiotic, is statistically the most likely culprit.

How can you prove it?

No confirmatory tests are available. The diagnosis is purely clinical. Only a rechallenge with the suspected drug (which is rarely done) could confirm your clinical suspicion.

REFERENCES

Drug Eruptions

Bigby M, Jick S, Jick H, Arndt K: Drug-induced cutaneous reactions: a report from the Boston Collaborative Drug Surveillance Program on 15,438 consecutive inpatients, 1975 to 1982. JAMA 256:3358–3363, 1986.

Daoud MS, Schanbacher CF, Dicken CH: Recognizing cutaneous drug eruptions: reaction patterns provide clues to causes. Postgrad Med 104:101–104, 114–115, 1998.

DeShazo RD, Kemp SF: Allergic reactions to drugs and biologic agents. JAMA 278:1895–1906, 1997.

Sharma VK, Sethuraman G: Adverse cutaneous reactions to drugs: an overview. Postgrad Med 42:15–22, 1996.

Wintroub BU, Stern RS, Blacker KL: Cutaneous reactions to drugs. In Fitzpatrick TB, Eisen AZ, Wolff K, et al. (eds.): Dermatology in General Medicine. 4th ed. New York, McGraw-Hill, 1993.

Viral Exanthems

Bialecki C, Feder HM, Grant-Kels JM: The six classic childhood exanthems: a review and update. J Am Acad Dermatol 21:891–903, 1989.

Grossman KL, Rasmussen JE: Recent advances in pediatric infectious disease and their impact on dermatology. J Am Acad Dermatol 24:379–389, 1991.

Hogan PA, Morelli JG, Weston WL: Viral exanthems. Curr Probl Dermatol 4:35–94, 1992.

Mancini AJ: Exanthems in childhood: an update. Pediatr Ann 27:163–170, 1998.

Resnick SD: New aspects of exanthematous diseases of childhood. Dermatol Clin 15:257–266, 1997.

Toxic Erythema

Bell DM, Brink EW, Nitzkin JL, et al.: Kawasaki syndrome: description of two outbreaks in the United States. N Engl J Med 304:1568–1575, 1981.

Manders SM: Toxin-mediated streptococcal and staphylococcal disease. J Am Acad Dermatol 39:383–398, 1998.

Melish ME, Glasgow LA: Staphylococcal scalded skin syndrome: the expanded clinical syndrome. J Pediatr 78:958–967, 1971.

Newburger JW, Takahashi M, Beiser AS, et al.: A single intravenous infusion of gamma globulin as compared with four infusions in the treatment of acute Kawasaki syndrome. N Engl J Med 324:1633–1639, 1991.

Resnick SD: Medical progress. Toxic shock syndrome: recent developments in pathogenesis. J Pediatr 116:321–328, 1990.

Stevens DL, Tanner MH, Winship J, et al.: Severe group A streptococcal infections associated with a toxic shock–like syndrome and scarlet fever toxin A. N Engl J Med 321:1–7, 1989.

Lupus Erythematosus

Boumpas DT, Fessler BJ, Austin HA, et al.: Systemic lupus erythematosus: emerging concepts. Ann Intern Med 123:42–53, 1995.

George R, Kurian S, Jacob M, et al.: Diagnostic evaluation of the lupus band test in discoid and systemic lupus erythematosus. Int J Dermatol 34:170–173, 1995.

Tan EM, Cohen AS, Fries SF, et al.: The 1982 revised criteria for the classification of systemic lupus erythematosus. Arthritis Rheum 25:1271–1277, 1982.

Werth VP, Dutz JP, Sontheimer RD: Pathogenetic mechanisms and treatment of cutaneous lupus erythematosus. Curr Opin Rheumatol 9:400–409, 1997.

Yell JA, Mbuagbaw J, Burge SM: Cutaneous manifestations of systemic lupus erythematosus. Br J Dermatol 135:355–362, 1996.

C H A P T E R

16 LOCALIZED ERYTHEMA

CELLULITIS
ABSCESS AND FURUNCLE
ERYTHEMA NODOSUM

I n the disorders described in this chapter, the erythema is confined to discrete lesions and is localized to a small area of the body surface. The epidermis characteristically is spared, but the dermal inflammation may extend into the subcutaneous fat. The three most common examples of localized erythema are as follows: *cellulitis,* an indurated plaque; *abscess* and *furuncle,* each of which is a fluctuant mass; and *erythema nodosum,* a nodule (Table 16–1).

■ CELLULITIS

Cellulitis is most frequently caused by infection with group A streptococci.

Definition. Cellulitis is a deep infection of the skin resulting in a localized area of erythema (Fig. 16–1). Group A streptococci *(Streptococcus pyogenes)* and *Staphylococcus aureus* are the organisms most often responsible. Before the introduction of the *Haemophilus influenzae* vaccine, facial cellulitis in extremely young children was frequently caused by this bacteria. Streptococcal infection is now the most common cause, even in this age group. Rarely, other aerobic and anaerobic bacteria as well as deep fungi such as *Cryptococcus neoformans* cause cellulitis, particularly in patients who are immunosuppressed.

Erysipelas is sometimes considered separately from cellulitis, but the distinction between the two entities may be a matter of semantics. The border of the involved area is more sharply demarcated in classic erysipelas than in cellulitis, and the surface looks more like an orange peel. However, both disorders are caused by bacteria, most often group A streptococci; for diagnostic and therapeutic purposes, they can be considered the same.

Incidence. Patients with this acute febrile disease are most often seen by their primary physician or an emergency physician. Only 0.1% of our new patients are seen for cellulitis.

Fever is almost always present.

History. Patients usually feel ill and febrile. The fever may precede the physical appearance of the skin involvement. A history of trauma or a preceding infected skin lesion is sometimes elicited. Saphenous venectomy for coronary bypass surgery can predispose patients to recurrent cellulitis of the legs. Buccal cellulitis in children often accompanies otitis media, and symptoms of an ear infection may be present.

TABLE 16-1 ■ LOCALIZED ERYTHEMA

	Frequency*	Etiology	History	Physical Examination	Differential Diagnosis	Laboratory Test
Cellulitis	0.1	Group A streptococci (usually)	Fever	Red, warm, indurated, tender area of skin	Contact dermatitis Superficial thrombophlebitis Erythema infectiosum	Culture 1. Skin aspirate 2. Blood
Abscess and furuncle	0.4	S. aureus (usually)	—	Red, tender, fluctuant mass	Cystic acne Hidradenitis suppurativa	Culture
Erythema nodosum	0.3	Hypersensitivity reaction	Search for associated conditions, including drug history	Red, tender, deep nodules usually on lower legs	Thrombophlebitis Subcutaneous fat necrosis	Chest radiograph Throat culture Antistreptolysin-O titers PPD skin test ± skin biopsy

*Percentage of new dermatology outpatients with this diagnosis seen in the Hershey Medical Center Dermatology Clinic, Hershey, PA.

Physical Examination. The involved skin shows all four cardinal signs of inflammation—redness (rubor), warmth (calor), swelling (tumor), and tenderness and pain (dolor). The epidermis usually is unaltered, although rarely blisters are present. The erythema in *H. influenzae* facial cellulitis characteristically is violaceous.

In adults, cellulitis most often affects the lower legs. In these patients, fissures between the toes owing to tinea pedis often serve as the initial portal of entry of bacteria.

Differential Diagnosis. Contact dermatitis, when severe, can mimic the erythema and swelling of cellulitis, but important distinguishing characteristics of contact dermatitis are the more marked epidermal involvement with vesicles, the symptom of itch rather than of tenderness, and the absence of fever.

Superficial thrombophlebitis of the lower legs can cause redness and tenderness and sometimes is difficult to distinguish from cellulitis. Fever is not present in

The skin shows all four signs of inflammation:
1. Rubor
2. Calor
3. Tumor
4. Dolor

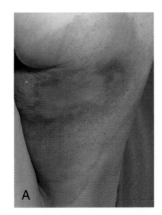 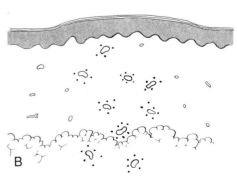

FIGURE 16-1. Cellulitis. **A,** Epidermis—normal. Dermis—erythema, edema, warmth, and tenderness. **B,** Epidermis—normal. Dermis—inflammation diffusely through the dermis, extending into the subcutaneous fat.

superficial thrombophlebitis, however, and the involved vein often can be palpated as a hard cord.

Facial cellulitis in children can be confused with the "slapped cheek" appearance seen in *erythema infectiosum.* In erythema infectiosum, however, the erythema is bilateral and usually not tender, and the patient's condition does not appear toxic.

Skin cultures are often negative.

Laboratory and Biopsy. Skin and blood cultures may be obtained, but the responsible bacterial pathogen is not always recovered. A skin culture is taken from the leading edge of the lesion by injecting and then aspirating 0.5 mL of nonbacteriostatic saline. The aspirate is Gram stained and is cultured. Unfortunately, the highest reported yield from this procedure is only 50%, and in most series it is much less than this. Culture of a skin biopsy increases the yield but not to 100%.

A skin biopsy is usually not needed in ambulatory, immunocompetent patients. However, a biopsy is often done to identify a responsible organism in an immunocompromised patient whose cellulitis has not responded to antibiotic therapy. If a biopsy is performed, the examiner will see an inflammatory infiltrate composed primarily of neutrophils throughout the dermis, occasionally extending into the subcutaneous fat. Edema and dilatation of lymphatics and small blood vessels are also present. Special stains for bacteria may be positive. Fungal stains to search for cryptococcal organisms also should be done, particularly on tissue from immunocompromised patients.

Complete blood count reveals leukocytosis in immunocompetent patients.

Initial therapy: Antibiotics

Therapy. Systemic antibiotics are the mainstay of therapy. Mild cases of cellulitis on an extremity may be treated with an oral antibiotic, warm wet compresses, bed rest, and close outpatient follow-up. Cephalexin (Keflex) or dicloxacillin, in doses of 500 mg four times daily, is prescribed for a 10-day course. Patients who are more seriously ill, particularly those with facial cellulitis, should be hospitalized and administered parenteral antibiotics, such as 2 g nafcillin intravenously every 4 hours. In immunocompromised patients, coverage may be needed for gram-negative bacteria or fungal organisms. In young children with facial cellulitis, antibiotic therapy must include coverage for *H. influenzae*, with amoxicillin combined with trimethoprim-sulfamethoxazole (Bactrim) or amoxicillin-clavulanate (Augmentin) combined with a third-generation cephalosporin such as ceftriaxone.

Cutaneous inflammation is slow to subside.

Course and Complications. With antibiotic therapy, the fever usually resolves within 24 hours. If it persists beyond 48 hours, a change in antimicrobial therapy should be considered, optimally guided by the initial culture results. The skin inflammation resolves more slowly than the fever, sometimes taking 1 or 2 weeks to subside completely. For most patients, complete recovery can be expected.

THERAPY OF CELLULITIS

- Oral antibiotics
    Cephalexin: 500 mg QID
    Dicloxacillin: 500 mg QID
- Intravenous antibiotics (if severe)
    Nafcillin: 2.0 g q4h

Bacterial sepsis frequently accompanies cellulitis and was present in 86% of patients in one pediatric series. Facial cellulitis caused by *H. influenzae* is often accompanied by otitis media and less often by meningitis. Local abscesses and osteomyelitis are rare sequelae.

Cellulitis once was a serious and sometimes life-threatening disease, but the use of antibiotics has reduced mortality to near zero in immunocompetent hosts. In immunosuppressed patients, cellulitis from usual as well as unusual pathogens still may be a serious, sometimes life-threatening infection.

Pathogenesis. In cellulitis, the bacteria may enter the dermis by an external or a hematogenous route. In immunocompetent hosts, the source is usually external. Tissue edema predisposes to bacterial proliferation. Proteolytic enzymes elaborated by bacteria such as group A streptococci contribute to the spread of inflammation. Host defense mechanisms involve cellular infiltrates and elaboration of cytokines, which rapidly kill the bacteria and thereby contribute to the inflammation. Damage to local lymphatics during an acute episode can result in residual lymphedema and may predispose the patient to recurrent episodes.

■ ABSCESS AND FURUNCLE

Definition. Abscesses and furuncles (boils) are pus-filled nodules in the dermis. *S. aureus* is the usual pathogen, but gram-negative organisms and anaerobic bacteria may also be causes. Abscesses often arise from traumatic inoculation of bacteria into the skin, whereas furuncles arise from infected hair follicles. The clinical lesion is a red, tender, fluctuant nodule (Fig. 16–2).

Staphylococcus aureus **is the usual pathogen.**

Incidence. In one survey, cutaneous abscesses accounted for 2% of all patient visits to the emergency department of a large city hospital. Patients with recurrent furuncles are seen more often by a dermatologist.

History. Patients with abscesses may give a history of preceding trauma, including surgery. Some patients with furuncles give a history of recurrent lesions. Immunodeficiency and perhaps diabetes mellitus predispose some patients to bacterial infections, but the usual patient with a furuncle or an abscess has no underlying medical disease.

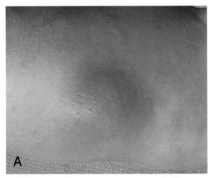
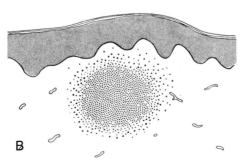

FIGURE 16–2. Abscess. **A,** Abscess. Epidermis—normal. Dermis—fluctuant nodule. **B,** Epidermis—normal. Dermis—dense aggregate of acute inflammatory cells replacing necrotic dermis.

Physical Examination. Furuncles and abscesses often begin as hard, tender, red nodules that become more fluctuant and more painful with time. Abscesses tend to be larger and deeper than furuncles. Regional lymph nodes are sometimes enlarged, but fever is rarely present.

Differential Diagnosis. Abscesses and furuncles are rarely confused with other entities. Acne and hidradenitis suppurativa can cause pus-filled nodules and cysts. In both conditions, the distribution of the lesions usually provides the diagnostic clue. In *cystic acne,* multiple lesions are distributed on the face and upper trunk, and other acne lesions (e.g., comedones, papules, pustules) are usually present. In *hidradenitis suppurativa*, draining nodules are present in the axillary, inguinal, and perineal areas. These nodules are often accompanied by open comedones and scars.

Laboratory and Biopsy. The diagnosis is usually made clinically and is confirmed by routine culture of the purulent material that has been obtained from incision and drainage. In immunocompromised patients, anaerobic cultures may be desired. Blood cultures are rarely positive and are not indicated unless the patient has signs of sepsis.

Biopsy is rarely indicated. If biopsy is performed, a large, dense collection of neutrophils will be found in necrotic dermis.

Therapy. The principal therapy consists of incision and drainage. In a study of 135 cases, this approach resulted in complete healing in all patients, including those who did not receive systemic antibiotics. Systemic antibiotics, however, may result in involution of early lesions, may prevent progression of nodular lesions to fluctuant ones, and may decrease contagiousness. Because *S. aureus* is the usual responsible organism, the antibiotic of choice is cephalexin (Keflex) or dicloxacillin, in doses of 250 to 500 mg four times daily for 1 week. If the clinical response is poor, a change in antibiotic therapy can be considered. For this, culture results are helpful.

Course and Complications. Untreated lesions often spontaneously rupture and drain. After surgical or spontaneous drainage, healing usually occurs. Large lesions may leave scars.

Patients with recurrent furuncles are often staphylococcal carriers.

In patients with recurrent furunculosis, an underlying predisposing systemic defect may be considered but usually is not found. Many such patients, however, harbor *S. aureus* in sequestered mucocutaneous sites, the most common of which is the nose. In such patients, the regular use of antiseptic agents may decrease bacterial colonization and thereby may prevent furuncles from recurring. We recommend a total body scrub every other day with an antiseptic cleansing agent such as chlorhexidine and twice-daily nasal application of an antibiotic ointment such as bacitracin.

THERAPY OF ABSCESSES

- Incision and drainage
- Antibiotics
     Cephalexin: 250 mg QID
     Dicloxacillin: 250 mg QID

Pathogenesis. For abscesses and furuncles, the bacteria usually gain entry to the dermis by an external route. For abscesses, this may be a traumatic inoculation such as a puncture wound, laceration, or surgical incision.

For furuncles, the bacteria enter by a hair follicle, in which they form deep folliculitis and extend into the surrounding dermis. In both instances, the presence of a large number of bacteria in the dermis elicits a vigorous inflammatory response and eventuates in a massive collection of inflammatory cells, primarily neutrophils.

■ ERYTHEMA NODOSUM

Definition. Erythema nodosum is an inflammatory reaction in the subcutaneous fat that, in most cases, represents a hypersensitivity response to a remote focus of infection or inflammation. Clinically, erythema nodosum appears as deep, tender, red nodules that are usually located on the lower legs (Fig. 16–3).

Incidence. Erythema nodosum is an uncommon disorder, representing 0.3% of our new dermatology patients. It occurs most often in young adults, with females outnumbering males by a ratio of 3:1.

History. The history is guided by consideration of the etiologic possibilities. In erythema nodosum precipitated by streptococcal infection, the nodules occur within 3 weeks of pharyngitis. Fever and lower respiratory symptoms may be elicited from patients with pulmonary infections caused by deep fungi or tuberculosis. A history of abdominal pain and diarrhea suggests an inflammatory bowel disorder. Ulcerative colitis is the most common inflammatory bowel disease associated with erythema nodosum. Regional enteritis and *Yersinia* enterocolitis are less frequently encountered. Inquiry should be made regarding pregnancy. A complete drug history should be elicited, although, with the exception of birth control pills, drugs are uncommon causes.

Pain and tenderness are usually associated with the skin nodules. Fever and arthralgias may also be present regardless of the cause. Joint symptoms most often affect the ankles and sometimes the knees and may precede the rash.

Causes:
1. **Poststreptococcal infection**
2. **Sarcoidosis**
3. **Deep fungal infection: coccidioidomycosis, histoplasmosis**
4. **Tuberculosis**
5. **Inflammatory bowel disease**
6. ***Yersinia* enterocolitis**
7. **Pregnancy**
8. **Drugs**
9. **Idiopathic**

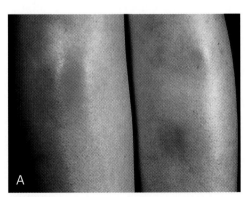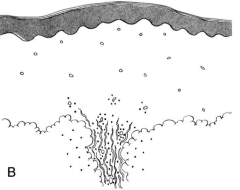

FIGURE 16–3. Erythema nodosum. **A,** Epidermis—normal. Dermis—multiple, deep, tender nodules. **B,** Epidermis—normal. Dermis inflammation in the lower dermis and in widened septa in the subcutaneous fat.

Physical Examination. Lesions of erythema nodosum appear as erythematous, well-localized, extremely tender, deep nodules that are 1 to 5 cm in diameter and have indistinct borders. As lesions evolve, they become yellowish purple and look like bruises. Multiple lesions are usually present, with the typical location being the pretibial areas. Much less often, lesions occur on the thighs and arms. Ulceration rarely occurs.

Differential Diagnosis. The diagnosis is usually evident clinically. Lesions of erythema nodosum may appear as *traumatic bruises*, but the history should discriminate between the two. *Superficial thrombophlebitis* also produces tender lesions on the lower legs, but these lesions usually are more linear and are not multiple. *Subcutaneous fat necrosis* is a rare condition that produces tender nodules on the lower legs and occurs in the setting of pancreatitis or pancreatic carcinoma. Patients with this disorder usually have elevated serum amylase and lipase levels and a diagnostic skin biopsy.

Laboratory and Biopsy. Laboratory testing takes into consideration the possible causes, and a few simple tests can screen for most of these conditions. Appropriate tests include a throat culture, antistreptolysin-O titer, tuberculosis skin test, and chest radiograph. The chest radiograph is used to screen for both pulmonary infection and sarcoidosis. In patients with bowel symptoms, further gastrointestinal tract evaluation should be pursued.

A skin biopsy is usually not required. If biopsy is performed, the changes will be found primarily in the subcutaneous fat, where vascular and perivascular inflammation is present in the fibrous septa separating the fat lobules. The septa become widened by edema and, subsequently, by fibrosis. Acutely, the inflammation shows numerous neutrophils and also involves the lower dermis. Hemorrhage may be present. In older lesions, a granulomatous infiltrate may be found.

Therapy. Therapy is aimed at the underlying disease, if one is identified. Symptomatic therapy may be achieved with aspirin or other nonsteroidal anti-inflammatory drugs (e.g., 25 mg indomethacin three times daily). Bed rest is also helpful. In patients with extensive involvement and marked discomfort, a short course of systemic steroids (e.g., prednisone starting with 40 mg daily and tapered over 2 to 3 weeks) often provides dramatic relief, provided the cause is not infectious. Some patients with chronic idiopathic erythema nodosum have been treated successfully with oral saturated solution of potassium iodide or oral gold. The mechanisms of action for these drugs are not known. Support stockings may be helpful in patients with chronic or recurrent disease.

THERAPY OF ERYTHEMA NODOSUM

- Identification of the precipitating disease, if any
- Bed rest or support stockings
- Nonsteroid anti-inflammatory drugs
    Aspirin: 650 mg QID
    Indomethacin: 25 mg TID
- Prednisone (if severe)

Course and Complications. The course is usually self-limited, typically lasting 3 to 6 weeks. Erythema nodosum associated with inflammatory bowel disease may parallel the course of the underlying disorder, relapsing with the bowel disease. Erythema nodosum in most other settings often does not recur.

Cutaneous complications are infrequent and inconsequential. Although ulceration does not occur, slightly depressed scars may result.

Pathogenesis. Evidence suggests that erythema nodosum is mediated by immune complexes. Deposition of immunoglobulins and complement has been demonstrated in the blood vessels in early lesions of erythema nodosum. In addition, many patients have circulating immune complexes, presumably related to the underlying disorder. The usual localization of the disease to the skin of the lower legs may be related to hemodynamic factors. The relatively sluggish circulation in the dependent lower extremities predisposes patients to the deposition of immune complexes in those blood vessels.

R E F E R E N C E S

Cellulitis

Baddour LM, Bisno AL: Recurrent cellulitis after saphenous venectomy for coronary bypass surgery. Ann Intern Med *97*:493–496, 1982.

Bisno AL, Stevens DL: Streptococcal infections of skin and soft tissues. N Engl J Med *334*: 240–246, 1996.

Carlson KC, Mehlmauer M, Evans S, Chandrasoma P: Cryptococcal cellulitis in renal transplant recipients. J Am Acad Dermatol *17*:469–472, 1987.

Feingold DS: Gangrenous and crepitant cellulitis. J Am Acad Dermatol *6*:289–299, 1982.

Hook EW, Hooton TM, Horton CA, et al.: Microbiologic evaluation of cutaneous cellulitis in adults. Arch Intern Med *146*:295–297, 1986.

Sachs MK: Cutaneous cellulitis. Arch Dermatol *127*:493–496, 1991.

Sadow KB, Chamberlain JM: Blood cultures in the evaluation of children with cellulitis. Pediatrics *101*:E4, 1998.

Abscess and Furuncle

Brook I, Finegold SM: Aerobic and anaerobic bacteriology of cutaneous abscesses in children. Pediatrics *67*:891–895, 1981.

Meislin HW, Lerner SA, Graves MH, et al.: Cutaneous abscesses: anaerobic and aerobic bacteriology and outpatient management. Ann Intern Med *87*:145–149, 1977.

Erythema Nodosum

Blomgren SE: Erythema nodosum. Semin Arthritis Rheum *4*:1–24, 1974.

Labbe L, Perel Y, Maleville J, et al.: Erythema nodosum in children: a study of 27 patients. Pediatr Dermatol *13*:447–450, 1996.

Ozols II, Wheat LJ: Erythema nodosum in an epidemic of histoplasmosis in Indianapolis. Arch Dermatol *117*:709–712, 1981.

Salvatore MA, Lynch PJ: Erythema nodosum, estrogens, and pregnancy. Arch Dermatol *116*:557–561, 1980.

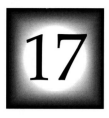

17

SPECIALIZED ERYTHEMA

■

URTICARIA (HIVES)
ERYTHEMA MULTIFORME
ERYTHEMA MIGRANS

Urticaria and erythema multiforme are characterized by lesions that are so distinctive that they are assigned special names. In urticaria, the lesion is a *hive* (or wheal), which is defined in Chapter 4 as a papule or plaque of dermal edema, often with central pallor and an irregular, erythematous border. The *target lesion*, when present, is diagnostic of erythema multiforme and is characterized by three concentric zones of color. The third disease in this chapter is erythema migrans, an expanding annular erythematous skin lesion found in Lyme disease. Additional features of these disorders are outlined in Table 17–1 and in the discussion that follows.

■ URTICARIA (HIVES)

Definition. Urticaria is a condition characterized by transient wheals in the skin resulting from acute dermal edema (Fig. 17–1). Acute urticaria is often caused by drugs. For chronic (lasting more than 6 weeks) urticaria, a cause is usually not found.

Incidence. Urticaria is common, with the highest incidence in young adults. Investigators have reported that 20% of the general population had hives at some point. Two percent of our new clinic patients were seen for this condition.

History. The drug history is the most important but often the most difficult to obtain. Many patients neglect to mention over-the-counter medications because they think that these drugs are unimportant. It is often helpful to ask about specific meditations (e.g., analgesics, vitamins, and laxatives) to jog their memory. For urticaria, a history of aspirin ingestion, for example, is particularly important because salicylates cause hives in some patients and aggravate them in as many as one third of all patients with urticaria, regardless of the cause. Other nonsteroidal anti-inflammatory agents cause similar reactions.

    Although allergy to an external allergen is most often manifested by contact dermatitis, in some patients contact of the skin to certain chemicals can cause an urticarial response, such as contact urticaria. For example, the latex in rubber gloves and other rubber objects is a relatively common cause of contact urticaria in medical and dental personnel.

Ask about over-the-counter medications as well as prescription drugs.

TABLE 17–1 ■ SPECIALIZED ERYTHEMA

	Frequency*	Etiology	History	Physical Examination	Differential Diagnosis	Laboratory Test
Urticaria	2	Ingestants Drugs Foods Infection Physical agents ?Emotions Idiopathic	Lesions last less than 24 hours	Wheals Generalized distribution	Erythema multiforme Juvenile rheumatoid arthritis Erythema marginatum	—
Erythema multiforme	0.3	Drugs Infection Idiopathic	Constitutional prodrome Prior herpes simplex	Erythematous plaques Bullae Target lesions Mucous membrane involvement	Viral exanthem Scalded skin syndrome Pemphigus Pemphigoid	May be indicated: Chest radiograph Skin biopsy
Erythema migrans	< 0.1	Tick-borne spirochete (*B. burgdorferi*)	Constitutional symptoms accompany rash Prior tick bite	One or more *expanding* red, annular macules at least 5 cm in diameter	Cellulitis Tinea corporis Granuloma annulare Fixed-drug reaction Other insect bite reactions	Serology Skin biopsy

* Percentage of new dermatology patients with this diagnosis seen in the Hershey Medical Center Dermatology Clinic, Hershey, PA.

Other causes of urticaria that should be sought include infections, physical modalities (e.g., cold, pressure, sunlight), possibly emotions, and, rarely, foods. A history of associated symptoms may also be important. Itching is nearly always present. A history of obstructive airway or other anaphylactic symptoms imparts greater seriousness to the problem. Urticaria accompanied by fever and arthralgias occurs in serum sickness reactions and in prodromal viral hepatitis.

Itching is a prominent symptom.

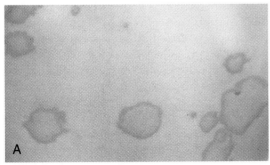
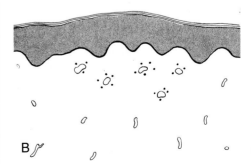

FIGURE 17–1. Urticaria (hives). **A,** Epidermis—normal. Dermis—erythema and edema. **B,** Epidermis—normal. Dermis—papillary dermal edema; sparse inflammatory cell infiltrate around dilated vessels; eosinophils sometimes present.

**An individual hive lasts
less than 24 hours.**

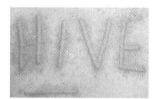

FIGURE 17–2. Dermo-
graphism.

**Initial therapy:
Antihistamines**

Physical Findings. Hives are skin lesions that are easily recognized. They appear as edematous plaques, often with pale centers and red borders. They frequently assume geographic shapes and sometimes are confluent. The lesions may be scattered but usually are generalized. By definition, an individual hive is transient, lasting less than 24 hours, although new hives may develop continuously. Serum sickness reactions include lymphadenopathy, fever, and arthralgias.

Dermographism can be elicited in many patients with urticaria, including patients who have no visible hives at the time. This "writing with wheals" reaction represents a wheal and flare response to scratching the skin (Fig. 17–2). It indicates that the cutaneous mast cells are unstable and are easily provoked to release their histamine content. Many healthy patients develop erythema after stroking the skin, but wheal formation is mainly limited to patients with urticaria. In eliciting this reaction, one should realize that it takes several minutes for the wheal to develop after the skin has been scratched.

Differential Diagnosis. Lesions sometimes mistaken for urticaria include those seen in erythema multiforme, juvenile rheumatoid arthritis, and erythema marginatum. In *erythema multiforme,* erythematous plaques are often seen, but they last much longer than 24 hours. The individual lesions in *juvenile rheumatoid arthritis* are transient, like hives, but they differ in size (only 2 to 3 mm), color (typically salmon), and timing (usually appearing with fever spikes). *Erythema marginatum* is associated with acute rheumatic fever. The skin lesions are erythematous, annular, and either macular or papular. They are also often transient but rarely itch.

Laboratory and Biopsy. Drug-induced urticaria may be accompanied by a blood eosinophilia. Liver function tests are appropriate in patients with urticaria and fever to rule out hepatitis. However, for most patients, the laboratory is rarely helpful in eliciting a cause. A biopsy is rarely required. If biopsy is performed, the pathologic findings are minimal, with vasodilation, dermal edema, and a sparse perivascular inflammatory infiltrate composed mainly of lymphocytes, sometimes admixed with eosinophils.

For penicillin-induced hives, skin testing can be performed, but it should be done with resuscitation support readily available. This testing is recommended only in a patient with a history of penicillin allergy who requires penicillin therapy. Skin test results are usually, but not always, predictive of a potential anaphylactic reaction. Both false-positive and false-negative responses can occur.

Therapy. Any suspected medication, including aspirin, should be discontinued. Avoidance may be helpful for some of the physical urticarias, such as solar and cold urticaria. Symptomatic therapy is usually achieved with H_1 antihistamines given on a regular, rather than an intermittent, as-necessary, basis. Taking an antihistamine after the hives break out, as in the as-necessary schedule, is analogous to closing the barn door after the horses have escaped. Hydroxyzine (Atarax) is often used in doses of 10 to 25 mg four times daily for 1 to 2 weeks in acute urticaria. For chronic disease, long-term therapy (months to years) may be required, with frequent attempts to taper the dose. Patients who are bothered by sedation from hydroxyzine can be treated with the nonsedating (but more expensive) antihistamines—10 mg daily of loratadine (Claritin) or 60 mg twice daily of fexofenadine (Allegra).

The tricyclic antidepressant doxepin (Sinequan), in doses of 25 mg once or twice daily, is also effective and has been shown to have both H_1 and H_2 antihis-

---

THERAPY OF URTICARIA

- Discontinue drugs suspected to be responsible
- Avoid aspirin and other nonsteroidal anti-inflammatory drugs
- Antihistamines:
    Hydroxyzine: 10–25 mg QID
    Loratadine: 10 mg daily
    Fexofenadine: 60 mg BID
- Tricyclic drugs:
    Doxepin: 25 mg BID
- Less frequently used agents:
    Terbutaline
    Nifedipine
    Prednisone

---

tamine activity. The β-adrenergic agonist terbutaline has occasionally been used as adjunctive therapy in patients with refractory disease. The calcium channel blocker nifedipine has also been reported to be helpful. Prednisone is effective but not usually needed and is to be avoided in long-term therapy.

Course and Complications. Drug-induced urticaria usually clears within several days of discontinuation of the responsible medication. Physical urticarias often have a prolonged course. Idiopathic hives may be acute or chronic. They usually resolve eventually, although resolution sometimes takes years. Hives have no complications other than discomfort from intense itching. Hives, however, may precede or accompany a potentially life-threatening anaphylactic response in patients with severe reactions.

Chronic urticaria may last for years.

Pathogenesis. As summarized in Table 17–2, hives can be mediated immunologically or nonimmunologically. Immunoglobulin E (IgE) mediation is the most common immunologic mechanism. In this pathway, a sensitized individual possesses IgE antibodies against a specific antigen, such as penicillin. These IgE antibodies are attached to the surface of mast cells and, when rechallenged, are bridged by the antigen. This results in a sequence of reactions leading ultimately to the release of numerous biologically active products from the mast cells, the most important of which appears to be histamine.

Autoantibodies to the high-infinity IgE receptor or to IgE itself have been identified in some patients with chronic idiopathic urticaria. These autoantibodies possess histamine releasing activity, and this activity may play a role in this disorder.

Complement-mediated urticaria occurs in several settings, the most spectacular of which is the syndrome of hereditary or acquired *angioedema*, in which patients have a deficiency of the inhibitor of the activated first component of the complement system. Trauma often precipitates attacks that result clinically in massive local swelling and, occasionally, fatal laryngeal edema. The complement system also participates in the hives that occur in *serum sickness*. The postulated mechanism is deposition of immune complexes in blood vessel walls, with fixation of complement and ensuing inflammation. Several drugs can cause direct release of

---

TABLE 17-2 ■ MECHANISMS FOR THE PRODUCTION OF HIVES

Immunologic
Immunoglobulin E mediated
Complement mediated
Nonimmunologic
Agents that directly cause mast cell degranulation (e.g., opiates and radiocontrast media)
Agents that cause alteration in arachidonic acid metabolism (e.g., aspirin and other non-
    steroidal anti-inflammatory agents)
Idiopathic

---

histamine from mast cells. The most commonly encountered are opiates and radiocontrast media.

The mechanism by which aspirin and other nonsteroidal anti-inflammatory agents cause hives is thought to be their effect on arachidonic acid metabolism. By blocking the production of prostaglandins from arachidonic acid, the pathway is shifted to the production of other metabolites, including the leukotrienes, a family of compounds that includes the previously designated slow-reacting substance of anaphylaxis. As that name suggests, this chemical has the ability to induce urticarial reactions. All the foregoing pathways ultimately result in the release of vasoactive substances (e.g., histamine) that alter vascular permeability and produce dermal edema, which appears clinically as a hive.

■ ERYTHEMA MULTIFORME

Definition. Erythema multiforme is an immunologic reaction in the skin possibly triggered by circulating immune complexes. Innumerable etiologic agents have been implicated. Most of these are poorly substantiated, with the exception of drugs and infection, particularly recurrent herpes simplex. As its name suggests, the eruption is characterized clinically by a *variety* of lesions, including erythematous plaques, blisters, and "target" lesions (Fig. 17–3). Mucous membrane involvement also occurs in the severe form of the disease—*Stevens-Johnson syndrome.*

The most common causes of erythema multiforme:
1. Drugs
2. Infection

Incidence. Erythema multiforme, although not rare, is uncommon. Fewer than 1% of our new dermatology patients are seen for this condition. The disorder most often affects older children and young adults.

History. A complete drug history should be elicited. Penicillins, barbiturates, hydantoin, and especially sulfonamides have been most often implicated. *Mycoplasma pneumoniae* infection is the precipitating event in some patients; a history of fever and cough is usually found. *Mycoplasma*-related and drug-induced erythema multiforme reactions are often severe (Stevens-Johnson syndrome), but they do not usually recur.

Recurrent herpes simplex is the most common cause of recurrent disease.

Recurrent herpes simplex infection is the precipitating event in the majority of patients with *recurrent* erythema multiforme. The herpetic lesion usually precedes the erythema multiforme by a few days to 1 week or more. For the most extended intervals, the herpetic lesions may have healed by the time the patient presents for treatment, so the history is important.

A cause is not always identifiable, particularly in patients with a single episode of erythema multiforme. In some patients, a febrile prodrome with upper

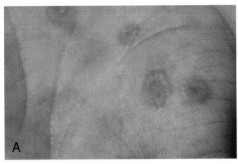 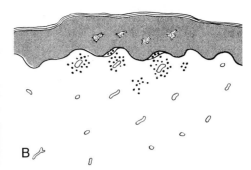

FIGURE 17–3. Erythema multiforme. **A,** Target lesions with *three zones* of color. Epidermis—normal or blistered. Dermis—erythema. **B,** Epidermis—normal or may have individual cell necrosis or exocytosis of mononuclear cells. Dermis—subepidermal separation (center of target lesion); inflammation in the papillary dermis.

respiratory symptoms precedes the cutaneous eruption by 1 to 14 days. Treatment of the prodrome with antibiotics probably led in the past to a falsely high rate of incrimination of these drugs as etiologic agents.

Physical Findings. The disorder ranges in severity from mild to severe. In the mild form of the disease *(erythema multiforme minor)*, erythematous papules and plaques predominate. Characteristically, the distribution of the lesions favors the extremities and is strikingly symmetric (Fig. 17–4). Target lesions are often present and are diagnostic. To meet the criteria for a target lesion, *three* zones of color must be present: (1) a central dark area or a blister surrounded by (2) a pale edematous zone surrounded by (3) a peripheral rim of erythema. Target lesions are most often seen on the palms and soles but may occur anywhere. Patients with erythema multiforme minor are not usually systemically ill. In the severe form of erythema multiforme *(erythema multiforme major* or *Stevens-Johnson syndrome)*, the skin disease is more widespread, blisters develop frequently, and mucous membrane involvement is characteristic. The oral mucosa, lips, and conjunctivae are usually the most severely affected. Blisters inside the mouth cause painful erosions that make eating difficult or even impossible when involvement is extensive. Purulent conjunctivitis may become so severe that the eyes swell shut. Patients with Stevens-Johnson syndrome look and feel systemically ill, with fever and prostration.

Target lesions have three zones of color and are diagnostic for erythema multiforme.

Differential Diagnosis. For the minor form of erythema multiforme, the usual differential diagnosis includes urticaria and viral exanthems. *Hives* may be confused with target lesions, but hives have only two zones of color (a central pale area surrounded by erythema), and individual lesions last less than 24 hours. *Viral exanthems* are usually monomorphous, less red, more confluent, and more centrally distributed than erythema multiforme. Conditions to be considered in the differential diagnosis of the major form of erythema multiforme are the other blistering disorders, including the *staphylococcal scalded skin syndrome*, in which the skin is diffusely red and the superficial epidermis strips off easily, pemphigus, in which histologically shows an intraepidermal blister, and *pemphigoid*, in which blisters often arise on clinically uninflamed skin and mucous membrane involvement is uncommon. As in erythema multiforme, the blister in bullous pemphigoid is subepidermal, but immunofluorescent studies of a skin biopsy specimen enable one to distinguish between the two. IgG is present at the dermal-epidermal interface in pemphigoid but not in erythema multiforme.

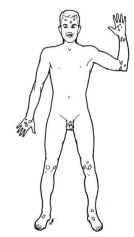

FIGURE 17–4. Distribution of erythema multiforme is symmetric and favors the extremities.

Laboratory and Biopsy. A chest radiograph is appropriate to screen for pulmonary infection. *Mycoplasma* infection can be further confirmed with acute and convalescent cold agglutinin titers. For herpes simplex–precipitated disease, if the responsible vesicular lesion is still present, a Tzanck preparation or viral culture can be obtained. For drug-induced cases, the laboratory is not helpful.

The disease is so clinically distinctive, particularly when target lesions are present, that a skin biopsy is usually not required for diagnosis. Biopsy of an erythematous plaque shows dermal changes with a lymphohistiocytic perivascular infiltrate and edema in the papillary dermis. Histologically, the epidermis may also be involved, with changes ranging from spongiosis and individual cell necrosis to full-thickness epidermal necrosis. Subepidermal separation is found in blisters and in the center of target lesions.

Therapy. No convincing evidence indicates that medical therapy favorably alters the course of this disease once the disease is established. Treatment of a precipitating infection is appropriate—erythromycin, azithromycin, or clarithromycin is recommended for *M. pneumoniae* and a 5-day course of oral valacyclovir (Valtrex) 500 mg twice daily or famciclovir (Famvir) 125 mg twice daily for herpes simplex infection. Recurrent herpes-associated erythema multiforme can be prevented with maintenance antiviral therapy. This is expensive and is reserved for patients with frequently recurring disease.

For the Stevens-Johnson syndrome, systemic steroids often have been used, but their value remains controversial; one retrospective study found that steroid treatment of children with the Stevens-Johnson syndrome resulted in longer hospitalization and more frequent complications than no treatment. Nevertheless, systemic prednisone in doses ranging from 40 to 80 mg/m^2 is still frequently used in patients with severe erythema multiforme. A prospective study is needed to evaluate the wisdom of this approach more thoroughly. For patients with Stevens-Johnson syndrome, supportive measures are also important. These are directed toward restoring and maintaining hydration, preventing secondary infection, and providing pain relief. Intravenous fluids are required in patients with severe oral involvement. Local therapy with antiseptics and dressings may help to prevent secondary infections, and systemic analgesics are used for pain. The intraoral use of topical anesthetics helps to provide temporary relief for patients with painful mouth lesions; viscous lidocaine or dyclonine liquid can be used.

Initial therapy: Treat infection, if present.

Systemic steroids are controversial but are frequently used.

THERAPY OF ERYTHEMA MULTIFORME

- Treat infection, if present
    For *Mycoplasma pneumoniae:* erythromycin, azithromycin, or clarithromycin
    For recurrent herpes simplex: valacyclovir: 500 mg BID; or famciclovir: 125 mg BID
- Discontinue responsible drug, if any
- For Stevens-Johnson syndrome:
    Supportive care
    Systemic steroids

Course and Complications. The mild form of erythema multiforme usually resolves spontaneously within 2 to 3 weeks. The time course is longer in patients with more severe involvement, lasting up to 6 weeks.

Death occasionally occurs in patients with Stevens-Johnson syndrome; reported mortality rates range from 0% to 15%. Pneumonia and renal involvement can complicate the cutaneous picture but are uncommon. The major complications result from infection and fluid loss. The entire skin surface can become involved, resulting in a clinical presentation that resembles an extensive burn; this process is called *toxic epidermal necrolysis*. Dehydration results from both decreased oral intake and increased transcutaneous fluid loss. Conjunctivitis can be complicated by secondary bacterial infection and may result in corneal scarring.

Spontaneous resolution occurs in 2 to 6 weeks.

Pathogenesis. Circulating immune complexes have been found in patients with erythema multiforme. The antigen is presumed to be derived from the implicated drug or infectious agent. Evidence supporting a pathogenetic role for immune complexes includes the localization of IgM deposits around dermal blood vessels in affected skin and the finding of immune complexes containing herpes antigen in the serum in patients with herpes-associated recurrent erythema multiforme but not in patients with recurrent herpes simplex alone or in patients with drug-induced erythema multiforme.

Some investigators favor a cellular immune mechanism. The predominance of mononuclear cells and the absence of leukocytoclastic vasculitis in the skin biopsy favor this mechanism.

■ ERYTHEMA MIGRANS

Definition. Erythema migrans represents the skin lesion associated with Lyme disease. Erythema migrans begins as a small, erythematous macule or papule and expands slowly over days to weeks. It must achieve a diameter of at least 5 cm to qualify as erythema migrans. The border usually is macular but sometimes is elevated, and central clearing often, but not always, develops as the lesion expands (Fig. 17–5).

The size criterion for erythema migrans is a 5-cm diameter.

Erythema migrans is the most diagnostic manifestation of *Lyme disease*, a tick-borne illness caused by the spirochete *Borrelia burgdorferi*. The case definition of Lyme disease has been established as a person with erythema migrans or a person

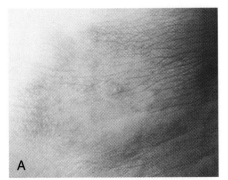
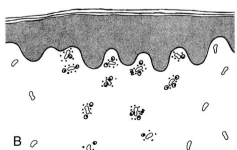

FIGURE 17–5. Erythema migrans. **A,** Epidermis—normal; central punctum may be present. Dermis—erythema. **B,** Epidermis—normal. Dermis—superficial and deep perivascular infiltrate with lymphocytes, histiocytes, and plasma cells. Spirochetes are occasionally seen with silver stain.

Erythema migrans occurs in 60% to 80% of patients with Lyme disease.

with at least one late manifestation and laboratory confirmation of infection. Erythema migrans occurs in 60% to 80% of patients with Lyme disease. The late manifestations include involvement of the musculoskeletal, nervous, or cardiovascular system.

Incidence. Lyme disease was first described in 1977 when it was diagnosed in a cluster of children living near Lyme, Connecticut, who were initially thought to have juvenile rheumatoid arthritis. Since then, the number of reported cases and their geographic distribution have increased steadily. Although still most often found in northeastern United States, cases have been reported from nearly every state in the country. Many thousands of cases are reported annually. Lyme disease is the most frequently reported arthropod-borne disease in the United States.

Lyme disease is the most frequent arthropod-borne disease in the United States.

History. Erythema migrans begins 3 to 30 days after a tick bite. Because the tick is so small, many patients do not recall having received a bite. Most patients, however, do have a history of recent exposure to potential tick habitats such as woodlands or grassy areas. Many patients with erythema migrans have accompanying systemic symptoms such as fever, myalgias, arthralgias, headache, malaise, or fatigue. The skin lesion itself is usually asymptomatic but is noted by the patient to expand slowly over time.

A history of tick bite is often lacking.

Physical Findings. The erythema migrans lesion is located at a body site favored by a feeding tick, such as the waistband and intertriginous areas, as well as the extremities. The diameter of the lesion must be at least 5 cm to qualify as erythema migrans. From reported cases, the average diameter has been found to be 15 cm, but diameters of 68 cm have been reported.

A central punctum from the tick bite may be evident but often is not. Typical erythema migrans has a macular border and a clearing center, but less classic features are common and include a papular border, alternating rings of erythema and clearing, and a center that is intensely erythematous, vesicular, purpuric, necrotic, or even ulcerated. However, all erythema migrans lesions have in common an expanding border.

Erythema migrans lesions expand slowly over days to weeks.

Differential Diagnosis. The differential diagnosis includes cellulitis, tinea corporis, granuloma annulare, fixed-drug reaction, and other insect bite reactions. Except for cellulitis, these conditions are not accompanied by systemic symptoms. In addition, compared with erythema migrans, cellulitis is more tender and usually more acute, warmer, and redder; *tinea corporis* has a scaling border that is potassium hydroxide–positive for fungal elements and is more chronic; granuloma annulare, an idiopathic dermal granulomatous process, has a firm, elevated border and persists for months to years; *fixed-drug eruption* has no central clearing, is violaceous, and characteristically recurs in the same spot within hours of ingestion of the offending agent (Fig. 17–6); and other insect bite reactions often have more prominent central puncta, are smaller, and usually are more transient than erythema migrans.

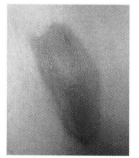

FIGURE 17–6. Fixed drug eruption.

Laboratory and Biopsy. With routine staining, skin biopsy findings are nonspecific, showing a superficial and deep perivascular lymphocytic infiltrate that may also contain histiocytes and plasma cells. With a silver stain, spirochetes can occasionally be demonstrated in the dermis. Although this finding obviously is important, it usually is absent. Accordingly, skin biopsies are usually not performed, especially if the clinical picture is highly suggestive of erythema migrans.

B. burgdorferi has been cultured from skin specimens, but this technique is not readily available, and the yield is low. Detection of *B. burgdorferi* DNA by polymerase chain reaction amplification can increase the sensitivity, but this test is also not widely available. Serologic tests for IgM and IgG anti-*B. burgdorferi* antibodies are commonly used, but results remain questionable because of the following: (1) the antibodies do not appear until after the first 2 to 4 weeks of illness, and early antibiotic therapy may prevent their development; (2) late false-negative results also occur in some infected patients who had not been treated; and (3) false-positive results occur in a variety of settings, including systemic lupus erythematosus, rheumatoid arthritis, infectious mononucleosis, and syphilis. Additionally, because the serology remains positive for years after treatment, a positive antibody test does not distinguish active from inactive disease.

Serologic tests have limited usefulness.

Therapy. All patients with erythema migrans are defined as having Lyme disease and thus require antibiotic therapy. The preferred agent is doxycycline, 100 mg twice daily for 10 to 21 days. Alternatively, 500 mg amoxicillin three times daily for 10 to 21 days can be used. Erythromycin, 250 mg four times daily for 10 to 21 days, is a third but less preferable alternative. Manifestations and therapy of early disseminated infection and late persistent infection are discussed later. A new vaccine for Lyme disease (LYMErix) may be applicable for patients who are at high risk of tick bite.

Course and Complications. The course and manifestations of Lyme disease share many similarities with syphilis. In Lyme disease, even without therapy, the erythema migrans lesion usually resolves spontaneously within a month. However, without treatment of early localized infection (stage 1), the disease may progress to stage 2 or stage 3.

Stages:
1. **Localized**
2. **Early disseminated**
3. **Late persistent**

In stage 2 (early disseminated infection), the *B. burgdorferi* spirochete is spread hematogenously to distant sites. The skin is affected in approximately 50% of patients with annular lesions that usually are smaller than the primary one. Patients are systemically ill with fever, chills, headache, arthralgias, and fatigue. Infection of other organ systems can result in a variety of symptoms, including arthritis, meningitis, cranial neuritis (particularly Bell's palsy), lymphadenopathy, carditis, and atrioventricular conduction defects. After inoculation, neurologic involvement occurs after weeks to months and affects approximately 15% to 20% of patients; cardiac involvement occurs within weeks and affects 4% to 8%. Arthritis is the most common manifestation and occurs at a mean of 6 months, with a range of 2 weeks to 2 years. It affects 60% of patients with intermittent asymmetric arthritis that primarily affects large joints, especially the knee.

Arthritis is the most common manifestation of disseminated disease.

THERAPY OF ERYTHEMA MIGRANS

- Antibiotics for 14–21 days:
    - Doxycycline: 100 mg BID, or
    - Amoxicillin: 500 mg TID
- For children < 12 years:
    - Amoxicillin: 50 mg/kg/day

Without treatment, the disease may enter stage 3, with late persistent infection. The major manifestation of this stage is *continual* arthritis, lasting more than 1 year. Chronic central nervous system involvement also may occur with manifestations that include ataxia and mental disorders.

Cardiac and neurologic manifestations require parenteral antibiotic therapy.

Treatment of cardiac and neurologic manifestations requires parenteral therapy with 2 g ceftriaxone intravenously daily for 14 to 21 days. Lyme arthritis can be treated orally with 100 mg doxycycline twice daily for 30 days or amoxicillin 500 mg orally four times daily for 30 days.

Pathogenesis. The disease is caused by *B. burgdorferi,* a spirochete carried by *Ixodes* ticks. In the northeastern and midwestern United States, the tick species is *I. dammini* (deer tick). In the western United States, the species is *I. pacificus,* and in Europe, it is *I. ricinus.* These ticks have a 2-year life cycle, and their preferred host in North America is the white-footed mouse, which asymptomatically carries the *Borrelia* infection and transmits it to a feeding larval tick. The white-tailed deer is the preferred host for the infected adult tick, hence the name deer tick. Deer, however, are not involved in the life cycle of the spirochete. The *Borrelia* infection is transmitted to humans when an infected tick feeds, thereby injecting the spirochete from its salivary glands into the skin. Once injected, the spirochete produces a local infection with an inflammatory reaction that produces a visible skin lesion—erythema migrans. Untreated, the infection often disseminates, spreading hematogenously to internal organs. One report has implicated the Lone Star tick (*Amblyomma americanum*) as another possible vector for erythema migrans. Confirmation is needed.

R E F E R E N C E S

Urticaria

Matthews KP: Urticaria and angioedema. J Allergy Clin Immunol 72:1–14, 1983.
Monroe EW: The role of antihistamines in the treatment of chronic urticaria. J Allergy Clin Immunol 86:662–665, 1990.
Sabroe RA, Seed PT, Stat C, et al.: Chronic idiopathic urticaria. J Am Acad Dermatol 40: 443–450, 1999.
Soter NA: Urticaria: current therapy. J Allergy Clin Immunol 86:1009–1014, 1990.

Erythema Multiforme

Howland WW, Golitz LE, Weston WL, et al.: Erythema multiforme: clinical, histopathologic, and immunologic study. J Am Acad Dermatol 10:438–446, 1984.
Kazmierowski JA, Peizner DS, Wuepper KD: Herpes simplex antigen in immune complexes of patients with erythema multiforme: presence following recurrent herpes simplex infection. JAMA 247:2547–2550, 1982.
Lemak MA, Duvic M, Bean SF: Oral acyclovir for the prevention of herpes-associated erythema multiforme. J Am Acad Dermatol 15:50–54, 1986.
Rasmussen JE: Erythema multiforme in children: response to treatment with systemic corticosteroids. Br J Dermatol 9:181–185, 1976.
Roujeau J-C, Kelly JP, Naldi L, et al.: Medication use and the risk of Stevens-Johnson syndrome or toxic epidermal neurolysis. N Engl J Med 333:1600–1607, 1995.
Tay Y-K, Huff JC, Weston WL: *Mycoplasma pneumoniae* infection is associated with Stevens-Johnson syndrome, not erythema multiforme (von Hebra). J Am Acad Dermatol 35: 757–760, 1996.

Erythema Migrans

Malane MS, Grant-Kels JM, Feder HM, Luger SW: Diagnosis of Lyme disease based on dermatologic manifestations. Ann Intern Med 114:490–498, 1991.

Masters E, Granter S, Duray P, Cordes P: Physician-diagnosed erythema migrans and erythema migrans–like rashes following Lone Star tick bites. Arch Dermatol *134*:955–960, 1998.

Nadelman RB, Wormsen GP: Erythema migrans and early Lyme disease. Am J Med *98:*155–238, 1995.

Rahn DW, Malawista SE: Lyme disease: recommendations for diagnosis and treatment. Ann Intern Med *114*:472–481, 1991.

Steere AC: Lyme disease. N Engl J Med *321*:586–596, 1989.

CHAPTER

18

PURPURA

THROMBOCYTOPENIC PURPURA
ACTINIC PURPURA
DISSEMINATED INTRAVASCULAR COAGULATION
VASCULITIS

Purpura is purple and nonblanchable.

The word *purpura* is derived from the Latin word for purple, a clinical characteristic that helps to differentiate the lesion from erythema, which is red. Blanchability is the clinical sign that best distinguishes the two. Purpura is nonblanchable because the blood is extravasated outside the vessel walls.

Purpura is divided into two major categories: nonpalpable (macular) and palpable (papular). Nonpalpable purpura results from bleeding into the skin without inflammation of the vessels and is due to either a bleeding disorder or blood vessel fragility. Nonpalpable purpura is divided further according to the size of the lesions. Purpuric macules smaller than 3 mm are called *petechiae*; those larger than 3 mm are called *ecchymoses*. Thrombocytopenia is manifested by petechiae. Ecchymoses are due to blood vessel fragility. *Necrotic ecchymoses* are found in disseminated intravascular coagulation (DIC), in which thrombi in dermal vessels lead to infarction and hemorrhage.

Nonpalpable purpura:
1. **Petechiae are found in thrombocytopenia.**
2. **Ecchymoses result from fragile blood vessels.**
3. **Necrotic ecchymoses occur in DIC.**

Palpable purpura results from inflammatory damage of blood vessels (vasculitis). The inflammation accounts for the elevation of the lesions and allows leakage of blood through the vessel wall. Features of these disorders are outlined in Table 18–1.

Palpable purpura represents vasculitis in the skin.

■ THROMBOCYTOPENIC PURPURA

Definition. Petechiae are purpuric macules less than 3 mm (Fig. 18–1). They frequently are caused by thrombocytopenia, which can result from drugs, preceding viral infections, AIDS, collagen vascular disease, hematologic malignancies, idiopathic (or immune) thrombocytopenic purpura (ITP), and thrombotic thrombocytopenic purpura (TTP).

Causes of thrombocytopenic purpura:
1. **Drugs**
2. **Viral infections**
3. **AIDS**
4. **Collagen vascular disease**
5. **Hematologic malignancies**
6. **ITP**
7. **TTP**

Incidence. Of the causes listed, drugs most often cause thrombocytopenic purpura in adults. In children, *acute* thrombocytopenic purpura most often is precipitated by a viral infection and has an annual incidence of 4 per 100,000 children. About 15,000 new cases of ITP are diagnosed in the United States each year. TTP is uncommon.

TABLE 18–1 ■ PURPURA

	Frequency*	Etiology	History	Physical Examination	Differential Diagnosis	Laboratory Test
Thrombocytopenic purpura	Uncommon	Drugs Malignancy "Autoimmune"	Drugs Fever	Petechiae, often on legs Mucosal bleeding	Valsalva maneuver Schamberg's disease Hypergamma-globulinemic purpura Venous stasis	Complete blood count with platelet count
Actinic purpura	Uncommon	Blood vessel fragility from sun and aging	Sun exposure Steroid use	Ecchymoses confined to the hands and arms	Steroid purpura Amyloidosis	Skin biopsy if amyloid is suspected
Disseminated intravascular coagulation (DIC)	Rare	Sepsis Malignancy Obstetric complications Idiopathic Warfarin	Fever (sepsis) Antecedent viral or streptococcal infection	Necrotic ecchymoses and/or: Petechiae Acral cyanosis Palpable purpura Mucosal bleeding Bleeding from venipuncture sites	Vasculitis	Coagulation studies Protein C levels
Vasculitis	0.3*	Sepsis Collagen vascular disease Cryoglobulinemia Drugs Malignancy		Purpuric papules, nodules, or bullae Legs most commonly affected	DIC	Skin biopsy Screening tests for systemic involvement

* Percentage of new dermatology outpatients with this diagnosis seen in the Hershey Medical Center Dermatology Clinic, Hershey, PA; 2% of inpatient dermatology consultations are for vasculitis.

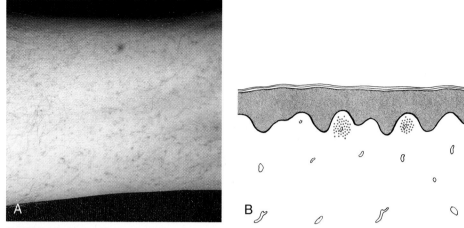

FIGURE 18–1. Petechiae. **A,** Epidermis—normal. Dermis—small (less than 3 mm) purpuric macules. **B,** Epidermis—normal. Dermis—hemorrhage around superficial vessels.

History. In patients with petechiae, a drug history is important. Systemic symptoms also should be sought. For example, children with acute thrombocytopenic purpura usually have a history of a viral infection within the preceding 1 to 3 weeks. TTP is accompanied by fever, hemolytic anemia, and neurologic symptoms.

Physical Findings. Petechiae may be generalized but are usually most pronounced in areas of dependency. Easy bruising may be noted, and mucosal bleeding may also be present, so the conjunctivae and oral cavity should be examined carefully. Splenomegaly is frequent in patients with hematologic malignancies or chronic ITP.

Differential Diagnosis. Petechiae can also result from increased intravascular pressure with forceful retching or coughing. This *Valsalva maneuver* results in petechiae on the face, neck, and upper trunk. Leakage of blood from capillaries also occurs in *Schamberg's disease,* an idiopathic capillaritis, in which inflammation (although not sufficient to cause elevation of the lesion) weakens the capillaries so they leak. This causes petechial lesions of the lower legs that have been likened in appearance to cayenne pepper. Petechiae of the legs also occur in *hypergammaglobulinemic purpura,* a syndrome characterized by episodes of fever, arthralgias, and petechiae, which appear to be the result of immune complex–mediated damage to small blood vessels. Petechiae in the lower extremities can also occur in the setting of *venous stasis,* particularly if the patient also has dermatitis.

Laboratory and Biopsy. In patients with petechiae, a complete blood cell count and platelet count should be ordered. Bleeding from thrombocytopenia usually does not occur unless the platelet count is less than $50,000/mm^3$. Platelet counts of less than $20,000/mm^3$ result in bleeding from even minor trauma, and platelet counts of less than $10,000/mm^3$ predispose the patient to internal bleeding.

Urinalysis and guaiac testing of the stool help to screen for bleeding from the urinary and gastrointestinal tracts. Skin biopsy enables one to distinguish noninflammatory petechiae from vasculitis, but the clinical picture is usually so distinctive that a biopsy is not required.

Screening tests:
1. **Complete blood cell count**
2. **Platelet count**
3. **Urinalysis**
4. **Stool guaiac**

Therapy. Therapy is aimed at the underlying disorder. If a drug is the cause, its discontinuation solves the problem usually within several days. Therapy is not always needed in children with acute thrombocytopenic purpura, although both prednisone and intravenous γ-globulin have been used with good effect. These agents also are useful in AIDS-associated thrombocytopenic purpura. Adults with ITP are treated initially with prednisone to increase platelet production. Chronic ITP (defined by a platelet count of less than 100,000 cells/mm³ for more than 6 months) often is treated with splenectomy. Intravenous γ-globulin is often used to prepare patients for this surgery. Splenectomy prolongs platelet survival and results in sustained remission in 85% of patients with chronic ITP. Treatment failure may require immunosuppressant therapy. Plasmapheresis with plasma replacement is used, with good success, in the treatment of TTP.

Therapy:
1. **Discontinue drug (if drug-induced)**
2. **Prednisone (for ITP)**
3. **Plasmapheresis (for TTP)**

Course and Complications. The course and complications depend on the nature of the underlying disease. Drug-induced thrombocytopenia can produce bleeding at other sites, particularly in the gastrointestinal tract. Virus-induced acute thrombocytopenia resolves without therapy and without complications in 90% of children. ITP in adults may resolve spontaneously but more often becomes chronic with a waxing and waning course that requires splenectomy in many patients. ITP is the presenting problem in some patients with underlying "autoimmune" diseases such as systemic lupus erythematosus. TTP is the most severe disorder and had been associated with a 75% mortality rate. With plasma exchange and infusion therapy, this rate has been reduced to 25%.

Pathogenesis. Platelets normally plug small defects in capillary walls and also help to initiate the clotting mechanism. Deficiency or dysfunction of platelets leads to "leaky" vessels.

Drugs can cause both thrombocytopenia and platelet dysfunction. Drug-induced thrombocytopenia results from either a toxic or an antibody-mediated mechanism. Drugs causing immunologic platelet destruction include quinidine, quinine, sulfonamides, heparin, digitoxin, phenytoin (Dilantin), and methyldopa.

Drugs that can cause thrombocytopenia:
1. **Quinidine**
2. **Quinine**
3. **Sulfonamides**
4. **Heparin**
5. **Digitoxin**
6. **Phenytoin**
7. **Methyldopa**

Cancer chemotherapy causes thrombocytopenia through inhibition of marrow production. Aspirin causes platelet dysfunction through inhibition of thromboxane production. Decreased platelet production occurs in hematologic malignancies as a result of bone marrow replacement with malignant cells.

An autoimmune mechanism is operative in viral-induced acute childhood thrombocytopenia, AIDS-associated thrombocytopenia, and chronic ITP. In these disorders, immunoglobulin G (IgG) antiplatelet antibodies bind to specific platelet membrane glycoproteins. The immunoglobulin-coated platelets are then recognized and are removed by the reticuloendothelial system, especially the spleen. Splenectomy often leads to improvement in platelet survival in this setting.

In TTP, the process appears to start with damage to endothelial cells, which release clotting factors and thereby cause platelet aggregation and platelet (not fibrin) thrombi. Most recently, von Willebrand factor has been implicated as the most likely aggregating agent.

■ ACTINIC PURPURA

Definition. Purpura resulting from blood vessel fragility clinically appears as ecchymoses, that is, purpuric macules of more than 3 mm (Fig. 18–2). Dermal tissue atrophy resulting from sun exposure and aging is the most common cause.

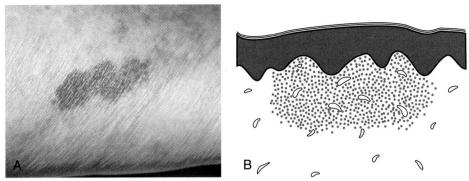

FIGURE 18–2. Actinic purpura. **A,** Epidermis—normal. Dermis—macular purpura with a regular border (ecchymosis). **B,** Epidermis—normal. Dermis—confluent hemorrhage in the superficial dermis; damaged collagen.

Incidence. Actinic purpura is extremely common in elderly people, in whom it is usually noted only as an incidental finding.

History. The trauma that induces the purpura is often so minor that it is not remembered by the patient. The patient has no symptoms, and health is unaffected.

Actinic purpura occurs on only the hands and forearms.

Physical Findings. Ecchymoses are usually round or oval macules. In actinic purpura, they are characteristically confined to the dorsa of the hands and forearms. The skin itself in these areas may also be more fragile and may tear easily.

Differential Diagnosis. Other causes of blood vessel fragility, in declining order of frequency, are corticosteroid use, amyloidosis, and Ehlers-Danlos syndrome. *Steroid purpura* with skin atrophy can result from topically or systemically administered corticosteroids. Patients with excessive systemic steroids also have a moon facies, a "buffalo hump" on the upper back, purple striae, and, in younger patients, steroid acne.

Causes of blood vessel fragility:
1. **Actinic damage**
2. **Steroid use**
3. **Amyloidosis**
4. **Ehlers-Danlos syndrome**

In patients with *amyloidosis*, the amyloid may infiltrate the skin and may result in papules and nodules, which are most often present on the face, particularly the eyelids. These characteristically bleed easily. Purpura also occurs in the absence of papules and can be precipitated by trauma, including pinching ("pinch" purpura). The tongue may also be enlarged.

Ehlers-Danlos syndrome is the least common cause of blood vessel fragility. Several variants of this syndrome are known, in which joint hyperextensibility, skin hyperelasticity, increased fragility of the skin, and increased tendency to bruise occur in varying combinations. Ecchymoses resulting from blood vessel fragility are distinguished from *vasculitis* by being macular and from the ecchymoses in *DIC* by their usually smooth rather than ragged contour and by the absence of necrosis.

Ecchymoses resulting from fragile blood vessels have a smooth border and are not necrotic.

Laboratory and Biopsy. Because the diagnosis of actinic purpura is clinically obvious, a biopsy is not required. If a biopsy is done, hemorrhage without inflammation will be noted in the dermis along with actinically damaged collagen, which appears disorganized, smudged, fragmented, and more basophilic than normal collagen on routine hematoxylin and eosin stain.

Therapy. No therapy exists for actinic purpura. Protection against sun exposure with sunscreens is advisable to prevent further damage.

Course and Complications. Ecchymoses slowly fade, leaving brown macules from residual hemosiderin. New ecchymoses, however, continue to develop. Scars frequently occur after tearing of the skin.

Pathogenesis. The diseases of blood vessel fragility have in common the problem of defective collagen, which weakens the vessels and makes them more susceptible to bleeding from minor trauma. In actinic purpura, blood vessel fragility results from both aging and the damaging effect of sunlight on connective tissue support to blood vessels in sun-exposed skin. Steroid purpura results from inhibition of collagen metabolism by high-dose corticosteroids. In amyloidosis, amyloid material infiltrates and weakens the vessel walls. In Ehlers-Danlos syndrome, fragility of blood vessels results from an intrinsic abnormality in collagen biosynthesis.

■ DISSEMINATED INTRAVASCULAR COAGULATION

Definition. DIC is a condition in which uncontrolled clotting results in diffuse thrombus formation. The skin is frequently affected, with thrombosed vessels causing skin necrosis. Hemorrhage from these vessels appears as ecchymoses (Fig. 18–3). Petechiae also occur as a result of the thrombocytopenia from platelet consumption.

Incidence. DIC is an uncommon, life-threatening disease. It usually occurs in the setting of bacterial sepsis (particularly meningococcemia). DIC may also be associated with malignancies, particularly prostatic carcinoma and acute promyelocytic leukemia. It can also be precipitated by massive trauma. Occasionally, it may result from amniotic fluid embolism, or it may occur as an idiopathic or "post-infection" phenomenon *(purpura fulminans)*. Localized intravascular coagulation occurs in patients with protein C deficiency who are given warfarin *(Coumadin necrosis)*.

Causes of DIC:
1. **Bacterial sepsis**
2. **Malignancy**
3. **Amniotic fluid embolism**
4. **Trauma**
5. **Idiopathic (purpura fulminans)**

History. Patients with DIC are usually systemically ill, often severely so. Fever and shock are frequently present. Symptoms of infection (e.g., headache and stiff neck with meningococcal meningitis) should be sought. A history of a malignancy may be important. Patients with purpura fulminans often have a prodrome of upper respiratory tract symptoms from viral or streptococcal infection. Patients with

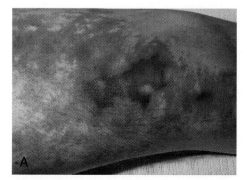
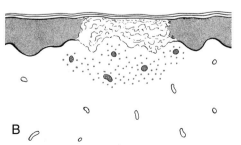

FIGURE 18–3. Disseminated intravascular coagulation. **A,** Epidermis—normal or necrotic. Dermis—stellate ecchymosis: Dark gray areas are necrotic and eventually slough; petechiae are also present. **B,** Epidermis—central necrosis. Dermis—fibrin thrombi in the capillaries in the middle to upper dermis; hemorrhage from necrotic vessels; no inflammation.

Coumadin necrosis are not systemically affected, but rather develop localized areas of skin hemorrhage and necrosis approximately 1 week after starting warfarin.

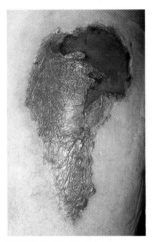

Stellate purpura with dark gray central areas indicates thrombosis and infarction.

FIGURE 18–4. Warfarin (Coumadin) necrosis.

Physical Findings. Various hemorrhagic skin lesions may be present. The most distinctive is a purpuric, stellate ecchymosis, which often appears to be necrotic in the center. The stellate shape is characteristic of blood vessel thrombosis with infarction. Dark gray central areas indicate necrosis and impending slough. Most lesions are flat, but palpable purpura occurs in approximately 20% of patients as a result of edema associated with skin infarction. Petechiae are common, and hemorrhagic bullae, acral cyanosis, mucosal bleeding, dissecting hematomas, and prolonged bleeding from wound sites can also occur. Coumadin necrosis is usually limited to one or a few localized areas, but the skin involvement is severe and results in a full-thickness slough (Fig. 18–4).

Differential Diagnosis. Ecchymoses from *fragile blood vessels* are round or oval, have smooth borders, and are not necrotic; DIC-related ecchymoses are irregular (stellate) in outline and often become necrotic. In addition, patients with DIC are usually severely systemically ill. In contrast to *vasculitis* lesions, the purpura in DIC is usually flat but can occasionally be palpable. Elevated lesions in DIC can be distinguished from those of vasculitis by a skin biopsy. In bacterial sepsis, vasculitis and DIC can coexist.

Laboratory and Biopsy. The laboratory findings characteristic for DIC are thrombocytopenia, prolonged prothrombin time, hypofibrinogenemia, and the presence of fibrin and fibrinogen degradation products. Of these tests, the platelet count and fibrinogen levels are the most useful for diagnosing and following patients with DIC.

Skin biopsy reveals the presence of intravascular thrombi, blood vessel necrosis, and extravasated red blood cells with little or no associated inflammation. Epidermal and dermal necrosis may result from infarction.

Therapy:
1. **Treatment of underlying condition**
2. **Repletion of clotting factors**
3. **Heparin (in patients with thromboses)**

Therapy. In DIC, the most important principle is to treat the underlying condition. Clotting factors should be repleted with infusions of platelets, cryoprecipitate (for fibrinogen and factor VIII), and fresh plasma (for factor V). Clinical thromboses, which occur particularly in patients with malignancy-associated DIC, are additionally treated with heparin to help control the clotting. Patients with Coumadin necrosis are also treated with heparin. Full-thickness skin necrosis may occur, particularly in Coumadin necrosis, and requires skin grafting for repair.

Course and Complications. DIC is a serious disorder, with an overall mortality of about 50%. Early diagnosis and prompt therapy improve survival rates. Cutaneous complications result from infarction, causing necrosis of skin and the tips of digits.

Pathogenesis. The primary process appears to be widespread thrombus formation in which coagulation factors are consumed. Fibrinogen, the target protein, is acted on by thrombin and plasmin, and fibrin clots are formed. In DIC associated with gram-negative bacterial sepsis, bacterial endotoxins are thought to induce this process. Cytokines such as tumor necrosis factor may also play a role. The clotting process also produces fibrinogen and fibrin degradation products that act as anticoagulants. These anticoagulants compound the bleeding diathesis produced by consumption of clotting factors.

Patients with inherited or acquired protein C deficiency are also susceptible to intravascular coagulation. Protein C is a vitamin K–dependent anticoagulant.

Patients with congenital absence of protein C die early in life from purpura fulminans with internal thromboses. Patients who have inherited or acquired protein C deficiency are susceptible to recurrent venous thromboses and to skin necrosis if warfarin is administered. Warfarin causes necrosis in these patients by depleting their marginal reserves of protein C before depleting the vitamin K–dependent clotting factors. The resultant imbalance in the anticoagulation-to-coagulation ratio allows the formation of clots with subsequent skin necrosis.

■ VASCULITIS

Definition. Strictly speaking, any inflammation of blood vessels could be called "vasculitis," but the term is generally used to describe a necrotizing reaction in blood vessels. Numerous vasculitis disorders have been described, classified, and reclassified, and this has led to much confusion. When the skin is affected by vasculitis, the result is purpuric papules *(palpable purpura)* (Fig. 18–5). The lesions are elevated (palpable) because of inflammation and edema and purpuric because of extravasation of blood from damaged blood vessels.

Palpable purpura indicates vasculitis.

Most often, cutaneous vasculitis affects only small vessels and results in purpuric papules. This process is mediated by neutrophils and is often termed *leukocytoclastic vasculitis*. Leukocytoclastic vasculitis can occur in a variety of settings, including sepsis, collagen vascular disease (particularly systemic lupus erythematosus and rheumatoid arthritis), cryoglobulinemia, drug reactions, and, occasionally, malignant lymphoma and myeloma. Henoch-Schönlein purpura is an idiopathic syndrome of cutaneous vasculitis associated with arthritis and abdominal pain and accompanied by gastrointestinal and renal vasculitis. Vasculitis confined to the skin in which an underlying cause cannot be found has been called *allergic cutaneous vasculitis* or *hypersensitivity vasculitis*. This is a common type of vasculitis, but a diagnosis of exclusion.

Causes of cutaneous vasculitis:
1. **Sepsis**
   Bacterial
   Rickettsial
   Viral
2. **Collagen vascular diseases**
   Systemic lupus erythematosus
   Rheumatoid arthritis
3. **Cryoglobulinemia**
4. **Drugs**
5. **Lymphoma and myeloma**
6. **Idiopathic**
   Henoch-Schönlein purpura
   "Hypersensitivity"

Incidence. Cutaneous vasculitis is uncommon. Of new patients seen in our dermatology clinic, 0.3% had cutaneous vasculitis. It was more common in our hospital practice, in which 2% of the dermatology consultations were for vasculitis.

History. Systemic disease must be ruled out, and the history is the first step in doing so. In patients with a history of fever and cutaneous vasculitis, sepsis must be considered. Bacteria causing septic vasculitis include *Neisseria meningitidis, Neis-*

First rule out sepsis as the cause of vasculitis.

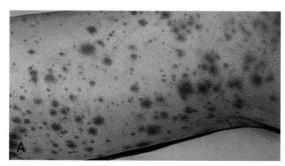 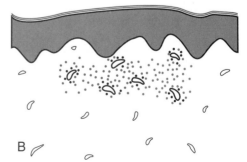

FIGURE 18–5. Vasculitis. **A,** Epidermis—elevated. Dermis—purpuric papules. **B,** Epidermis—normal. Dermis—neutrophils and nuclear debris in and around blood vessels; endothelial swelling and necrosis of blood vessel walls; hemorrhage.

seria gonorrhoeae, Staphylococcus aureus, Streptococcus pneumoniae, viridans streptococci, and *Pseudomonas aeruginosa.* Fever may also occur in patients with viral infections, collagen vascular diseases, and even drug reactions, but the first responsibility is to rule out sepsis. This includes rickettsial sepsis *(Rocky Mountain spotted fever),* in which the abrupt onset of fever is accompanied by headache and myalgias and is followed in several days by an erythematous rash, which characteristically begins on the wrists and ankles and then involves the palms and soles as it becomes generalized and purpuric. The history and appearance of the rash permit an early clinical diagnosis of this disease, which is fatal if not treated promptly.

The rash in Rocky Mountain spotted fever starts on the wrists and ankles.

Symptoms of multisystem involvement in vasculitis may include arthritis, hematuria, abdominal pain and melena, cough and hemoptysis, and neurologic involvement with headaches and peripheral neuropathy. Although drug-induced vasculitis is uncommon, drug history is important. The drugs most frequently implicated include aspirin, gold, phenothiazines, penicillin, sulfonamides, and thiazides.

Physical Examination. The primary lesion in cutaneous vasculitis is a purpuric papule (palpable purpura). Necrosis sometimes follows; it is heralded by the appearance of a dark gray color in the center of a lesion, which is followed by slough. In the absence of necrosis, lesions evolve by flattening and fading. The flattening may occur surprisingly quickly, so a lesion that is palpable the first day may be flat by the second. As lesions fade, hemosiderin remains, leaving the affected skin brown. In gonococcemia, lesions are distinctive in that they are pustular as well as purpuric, sparse, and distributed distally on the extremities. Lesions of vasculitis are most often located on the lower extremities, but they may be generalized in patients with extensive disease.

Gonococcemia is characterized by purpuric pustules in acral distribution.

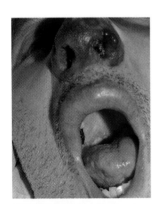

FIGURE 18–6. Wegener's granulomatosis. Necrotic lesions of the nose and ulcerations in the mouth are due to vasculitis of larger vessels.

Differential Diagnosis. For purpuric lesions, the first step is to determine whether they are palpable. The causes of nonpalpable purpura are listed in the previous section. Lesions in DIC may be flat or elevated. Those that are elevated are so because of edema that acutely accompanies necrosis. Vasculitis may coexist with DIC in some patients who have bacterial sepsis (e.g., meningococcemia)—bacterial emboli cause the vasculitis, and endotoxin initiates the DIC. *Candidal sepsis* produces papular skin lesions that usually are erythematous but also may be purpuric when they are accompanied by thrombocytopenia. Patients with *large vessel vasculitis* (e.g., *polyarteritis nodosa and Wegener's granulomatosis*) frequently experience ulcerations of the skin as a manifestation of obliterative necrosis of vessels that are larger than those involved in the vasculitis lesions discussed earlier (Fig. 18–6).

Laboratory and Biopsy. The diagnosis of necrotizing vasculitis is confirmed by skin biopsy. The histologic features are (1) presence in and around the blood vessel walls of neutrophils with leukocytoclasis (i.e., destruction of neutrophils leaving nuclear debris), (2) hemorrhage, (3) endothelial cell swelling, and (4) fibrinoid necrosis of the vessel wall. Immunofluorescent stains may show immunoglobulin deposition in the vessel walls in early lesions, but this is not diagnostically helpful except in Henoch-Schönlein purpura, in which the immunoglobulin deposited is characteristically IgA rather than the IgG or IgM seen in all other types of vasculitis.

Laboratory tests are used to rule out systemic involvement or specific systemic diseases. Blood cultures should be obtained in all patients with vasculitis and fever. Acute and convalescent serologic titers confirm (posthumously, if treatment is not instituted early in the disease) a diagnosis of Rocky Mountain spotted fever. Other laboratory work includes a complete urinalysis, guaiac test of stool, complete blood count with differential and platelet count, sedimentation rate, serum creatinine, serum protein electrophoresis, cryoglobulins, antinuclear antibody test, rheumatoid factor, hepatitis-associated antigen, and chest radiograph.

Obtain blood cultures in patients with vasculitis and fever.

Therapy. Treatment is of the underlying disease, if one is found. In patients with suspected bacterial sepsis, treatment should be instituted *immediately*, not after culture results are returned. Meningococcemia is a dramatic example in which a treatment delay of a few hours can mean the difference between a favorable and a fatal outcome. The same is true for Rocky Mountain spotted fever, in which early treatment (with tetracycline) is lifesaving and must be instituted on the basis of clinical suspicion.

If a drug reaction is suspected, the drug should be discontinued. Most other forms of vasculitis are treated with prednisone or immunosuppressant therapy. Patients with idiopathic vasculitis limited to the skin respond well to prednisone, but dapsone also frequently controls the process and is safer for long-term administration. Colchicine has also been used with success in some patients. One should not be overzealous in the treatment of cutaneous vasculitis because this condition is chronic and often does not affect the viscera.

Course and Complications. The course and complications depend on the underlying disease and extent of organ involvement by the vasculitis. Vasculitis associated with bacterial or rickettsial sepsis responds promptly to antibiotic therapy. If a drug is responsible, its withdrawal solves the problem. Purpuric lesions associated with viral diseases (e.g., enterovirus infections and atypical measles) resolve spontaneously. The skin disease in Henoch-Schönlein purpura is usually self-limited, but renal impairment persists in nearly 30% of these patients. Rheumatoid vasculitis is usually associated with a high titer of rheumatoid factor; usually, a reduction in rheumatoid factor is accompanied by improvement in the vasculitis. Idiopathic cutaneous vasculitis has a tendency to wax and wane, frequently over a period of years, and is not usually a harbinger of serious internal involvement.

Serious complications are related less to the skin than to internal organ involvement, with the kidney most often and usually most seriously affected.

Kidneys are the most frequently involved internal organ.

THERAPY OF VASCULITIS

- Treat infection if suspected
- Discontinue implicated drugs, if any
- For acute noninfectious vasculitis: prednisone
- For chronic cutaneous vasculitis
    Dapsone
    Colchicine
    Immunosuppressants

Pathogenesis. Vasculitis is thought to be an immune complex–mediated disease. The antigen in the immune complex may be exogenous (e.g., bacterial, drug) or endogenous (e.g., another antibody, as in the rheumatoid factor, or nuclear antigens, as in lupus). These circulating immune complexes lodge in the walls of blood vessels; in the skin, small venules are most often involved. The propensity for involvement in the lower legs may relate to hydrostatic forces that predispose to sluggish blood flow and immune complex deposition. The complement cascade is then activated, producing chemotactic factors that attract polymorphonuclear leukocytes into the vessel wall. Lysosomes are released from the leukocytes and cause sufficient damage to the vessel wall to permit extravasation of red blood cells.

Vasculitis is a type III immune complex reaction.

The antibodies in the immune complexes are usually of the IgG or IgM class, with the exception of Henoch-Schönlein purpura, in which they are characteristically IgA. Vasoactive substances such as histamine have also been found to be important mediators early in the reaction. These substances cause vasodilation, which presumably results in gaps between endothelial cells and predisposes to the lodging and trapping of immune complexes in the vessel wall.

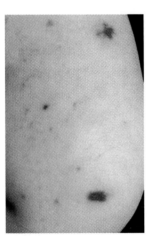

FIGURE 18–7. Unknown.

■ UNKNOWN (Fig. 18–7)

This 4-month-old infant was brought to the emergency room because of sudden onset of fever and irritability that progressed within hours to obtundation. On physical examination, hypotension, nuchal rigidity, and the skin lesions shown in Figure 18–7 were noted.

What do you see?

The lesions (shown here on the thigh) are palpable and purpuric. Petechiae are also present.

What is the most likely diagnosis?

In a patient with fever and palpable purpura, sepsis is the first and most important diagnosis to consider. In an infant or young child, meningococcemia is the most likely diagnosis, particularly if the child has signs of meningeal irritation or altered consciousness.

How would you prove it?

Blood for bacterial cultures and cerebral spinal fluid (CSF) should be immediately obtained. In addition to culturing the CSF, a Gram stain should be done. This often demonstrates the organism. A latex agglutination test of the CSF often also rapidly confirms the diagnosis.

How would you treat it?

This is a medical emergency, and antibiotic therapy must be promptly administered. If the patient's condition is unstable, immediate treatment may require deferral of the lumbar puncture. High-dose intravenous aqueous penicillin G remains the treatment of choice. Chloramphenicol and third-generation cephalosporins have been used in patients allergic to penicillin.

Important Points

1. In a patient with fever and palpable purpura, sepsis must be considered first.

2. If bacterial sepsis is *suspected*, antibiotic treatment should be initiated immediately.

R E F E R E N C E S

Thrombocytopenic Purpura

Lord RV, Coleman MJ, Milliken ST: Splenectomy for HIV-related immune thrombocytopenia: comparison with results of splenectomy for non-HIV immune thrombocytopenia purpura. Arch Surg *133*:205–210, 1998.

McMillan R: Therapy for adults with refractory chronic immune thrombocytopenic purpura. Ann Intern Med *126*:307–314, 1997.

Moake JL, Chow TW: Thrombotic thrombocytopenic purpura: understanding a disease no longer rare. Am J Med Sci *316*:105–119, 1998.

Myers TJ, Wakem CJ, Ball ED, et al.: Thrombotic thrombocytopenic purpura: combined treatment with plasmapheresis and antiplatelet agents. Ann Intern Med *92*:149–155, 1980.

Warrier I, Bussel JB, Valdez L, et al.: Safety and efficacy of low-dose intravenous immune globulin (IVIG) treatment for infants and children with immune thrombocytopenic purpura: Low-dose IVIG Study Group. J Pediatr Hematol Oncol *19*:197–201, 1997.

Actinic Purpura

Rubinow A, Cohen AS: Skin involvement in generalized amyloidosis: a study of clinically involved and uninvolved skin in 50 patients with primary and secondary amyloidosis. Ann Intern Med *88*:781–785, 1978.

Disseminated Intravascular Coagulation

Auletta MJ, Headington JT: Purpura fulminans. Arch Dermatol *124*:1387–1391, 1988.

Carey MJ, Rogers GM: Disseminated intravascular coagulation: clinical and laboratory aspects. Am J Hematol *59*:65–73, 1998.

Levi M, ten Cate H: Disseminated intravascular coagulation. N Engl J Med *341*:586–592, 1999.

Robboy S J, Mihm MC, Colman RW, et al.: The skin in disseminated intravascular coagulation: prospective analysis of thirty-six cases. Br J Dermatol *88*:221–229, 1973.

Spicer TE, Rau JM: Purpura fulminans. Am J Med *61*:566–571, 1976.

Vasculitis

Fauci AS, Haynes BF, Katz P: The spectrum of vasculitis: clinical, pathologic, immunologic, and therapeutic considerations. Ann Intern Med *89*:660–676, 1978.

Gilliam JN, Smiley JD: Cutaneous necrotizing vasculitis and related disorders. Ann Allergy *37*:328–339, 1976.

Jennette CJ, Milling DN, Falk RJ: Vasculitis affecting the skin: a review. Arch Dermatol *130*: 899–906, 1994.

Lott T, Ghersetich I, Comacchi C, et al.: Cutaneous small-vessel vasculitis. J Am Acad Dermatol *39*:667–687, 1998.

Sais G, Vidallen A, Jucgla A, et al.: Prognostic factors in leukocytoclastic vasculitis: a clinicopathologic study of 160 patients. Arch Dermatol *134*:309–315, 1998.

CHAPTER

DERMAL INDURATION

19

■

Induration represents dermal thickening resulting in skin that feels thicker or firmer than normal. Scleroderma is the disease that best exemplifies this process.

■ SCLERODERMA

Definition. In scleroderma, an increase in the number and activity of fibroblasts produces excessive collagen, which results in thickening of the dermis (Fig. 19–1). Localized scleroderma is confined to the skin and is called *morphea*. It is distinct from systemic scleroderma, which is also called *progressive systemic sclerosis* (PSS). In PSS, fibrosis more diffusely affects the skin and also affects some internal organs. Blood vessels are also involved in some organs, with endothelial thickening resulting in luminal narrowing. Scleroderma is classified as an "autoimmune" collagen vascular disease, but the origin of the increased collagen and the vascular alterations remains unknown.

Incidence. Both forms of scleroderma are uncommon. The annual incidence of PSS has been estimated at fewer than 3 new patients per 1 million population. A linear variant of morphea affects children. Otherwise, morphea and PSS are diseases of adults, with women affected 3 times more often than men.

History. Morphea is usually asymptomatic; patients present for treatment because of concern over the appearance of their lesions.

Morphea is localized scleroderma, confined to the skin; systemic scleroderma affects skin and viscera.

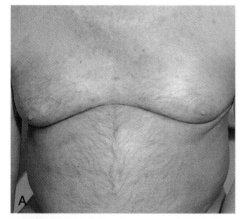
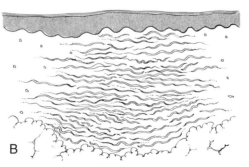

FIGURE 19–1. Scleroderma. **A,** Epidermis—normal or hyperpigmented. Dermis—thickened, feels indurated. **B,** Epidermis—normal. Dermis—thickened; fibroblasts are increased in number; collagen bundles are increased in thickness and number.

White is the most diagnostic color in Raynaud's phenomenon.

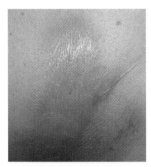

FIGURE 19–2. Morphea is sharply demarcated.

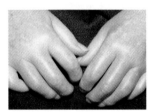

FIGURE 19–3. Sclerodactyly in a patient with systemic scleroderma.

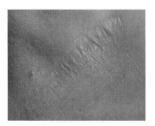

FIGURE 19–4. Lichen sclerosus et atrophicus.

Patients with PSS frequently have symptoms. Early in the disease, the most common symptom is Raynaud's phenomenon, which is characterized by pain and color change of the digits on exposure to cold. The classic color changes are, in sequence, white, purple, and red, but the most important is white, which is caused by cold-induced vasoconstriction. Patients with more advanced disease also notice tightening of the skin, manifested by an inability to open the mouth widely (their dentist may comment on this) and contractures of fingers causing decreased manual dexterity. Ulcerations of the fingertips also occur frequently. Systemic symptoms include difficulty in swallowing, joint pain, and shortness of breath.

Physical Examination. Morphea appears as a sharply demarcated plaque, which may be flat, slightly elevated, or slightly depressed (Fig. 19–2). Most important, it *feels* indurated. Early lesions have a violaceous hue. Mature lesions are brown or yellow brown. Lesions of morphea most often affect the trunk, except for the linear variant, which usually involves the head or an extremity.

The thickened skin in PSS is *not* sharply separated from normal skin, although some areas, such as the hands and face (acrosclerosis), may be more thickened than others. Thickened facial skin appears unusually smooth, except around the mouth, where it is furrowed and has a purse-string appearance. Involvement of the digits produces thickened, sausage-shaped digits (sclerodactyly: Fig. 19–3). Ulcerations followed by pitted scars occur on the fingertips. In generalized involvement, the skin is often hyperpigmented and may have areas that are speckled light and dark ("salt and pepper"). Patients with marked generalized thickening of the skin (see Fig. 19–1) appear to have the worst prognosis.

Telangiectasia is prominent in some patients with scleroderma. It appears as multiple, small, punctate macules that are particularly prominent on the face and hands. Cutaneous calcinosis and impaired esophageal motility also occur in patients with the CREST syndrome (calcinosis, Raynaud's phenomenon, esophageal dysfunction, sclerodactyly, and telangiectasia).

Differential Diagnosis. The differential diagnosis of morphea includes two uncommon disorders. *Lichen sclerosus et atrophicus* is an idiopathic disorder that appears as a porcelain-white, dermal, indurated plaque with an atrophic, slightly wrinkled epidermis (Fig. 19–4). It most often affects the vulvar area but sometimes occurs in scattered patches on the trunk. Occasionally, lichen sclerosus et atrophicus and morphea coexist. *Necrobiosis lipoidica diabeticorum* most often (but not always) occurs on the lower legs in diabetic patients as an orange-red, indurated plaque with an atrophic epidermis through which large telangiectatic blood vessels are seen.

The generalized thickened skin in PSS may be confused with several uncommon disorders. In *myxedema* from hypothyroidism, the skin may be markedly thickened, but it feels more doughy than hard (Fig. 19–5). Scleromyxedema is a rare disease characterized by mucin deposition in the skin. It can mimic scleroderma clinically, but the biopsy is diagnostic, and the skin involvement is accompanied by a serum monoclonal immunoglobulin G (IgG) protein. *Mixed connective tissue disease* is an "overlap" syndrome with features of several collagen vascular diseases—scleroderma, dermatomyositis, and lupus erythematosus. This syndrome is characterized serologically by high levels of antibodies against ribonuclear protein in extractable nuclear antigen. In chronic *graft-versus-host disease*, skin manifestations are prominent and may be strikingly similar to those of generalized scleroderma. *Porphyria cutanea tarda* occasionally is accompanied by diffusely thickened, hyperpigmented, "sclerodermoid" skin. The more usual manifestations, however, are blisters and fragility of the skin on the dorsa of the hands and hyperpigmentation and hypertrichosis of the upper lateral cheeks. The anticancer drug *bleomycin* can cause sclerodermatous skin changes that are indistinguishable from those of systemic sclerosis.

Patients with CREST syndrome and prominent telangiectasia are sometimes misdiagnosed as having *hereditary hemorrhagic telangiectasia* (Osler-Weber-Rendu disease). Hereditary hemorrhagic telangiectasia is an uncommon, dominantly inherited syndrome characterized by telangiectasia on the hands, lips, and oral mucosa and bleeding of telangiectasia in the nose and gastrointestinal tract.

Sclerodermatous skin changes also occur as a late manifestation in the *eosinophilia-myalgia syndrome*. This disorder was first recognized in 1989. The syndrome is defined by the presence of myalgias sufficient to affect daily activity and an otherwise unexplained blood eosinophil count of more than $1,000/mm^3$. Other early manifestations include a diffuse erythematous skin rash, edema, and fever. Approximately 40% of patients also develop sclerotic induration of the skin, primarily affecting the extremities, face, and neck and characteristically sparing the hands. Histologic examination reveals fibrosis and eosinophils in the deep dermis and underlying fascia. The clinical and histologic features are similar to those found in *eosinophilia fasciitis*, an idiopathic process. The cause of the eosinophilia-myalgia syndrome, however, was found to be ingestion of contaminated L-tryptophan. When this product was taken off the market, the incidence of eosinophilia-myalgia syndrome dropped dramatically.

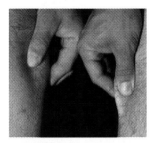

FIGURE 19–5. Thickened skin in myxedema (left) compared with normal skin (right).

Laboratory and Biopsy. Laboratory tests are not needed in patients with morphea, except for a skin biopsy if the diagnosis is in question. Patients with generalized scleroderma require laboratory and radiographic evaluation for systemic involvement that includes a complete blood count, urinalysis, renal function tests, chest radiograph, pulmonary function testing, and barium swallow. An antinuclear antibody test is positive in 95% of patients with systemic scleroderma. Human epithelial (HEp-2) cells are used as the substrate for the antinuclear antibody test. The pattern of positive staining on these cells correlates with the type of systemic scleroderma as follows: Nucleolar staining is associated with mixed connective tissue disease; anticentromere staining is associated with CREST syndrome; and a pattern of diffuse fine speckles is associated with a positive Scl-70 antibody found in diffuse scleroderma.

Laboratory and radiologic tests for systemic scleroderma:
1. **Complete blood count**
2. **Urinalysis**
3. **Renal function tests**
4. **Chest radiograph**
5. **Antinuclear antibody test**
6. **Pulmonary function tests**
7. **Barium swallow**

Morphea and PSS show the same histologic changes in the skin. Collagen bundles are increased in number and thickness and appear more eosinophilic on hematoxylin and eosin stain. These changes are most marked in the lower two thirds of the dermis and extend into the subcutaneous fat. Inflammation is present in the early stages, when the diagnosis is easily missed histologically because the collagen changes may not be appreciated. In later stages, the sclerotic process entraps, and finally obliterates, the dermal appendages, with an end result that may resemble a scar. Also in the late stages, blood vessels appear thickened, hyalinized, and decreased in number.

Therapy. Therapy of scleroderma is frustrating. Topical, intralesional, and even systemic steroids have been used for morphea, usually with disappointing results. Long lists of drugs have been used in PSS, most with little or no proven effect. These include D-penicillamine, which prevents cross-linking of collagen fibers, and immunosuppressant agents such as prednisone and azathioprine or methotrexate. D-Penicillamine is the agent of first choice for systemic scleroderma, but monitoring (e.g., monthly complete blood counts and urinalyses) must be done

---

THERAPY OF SCLERODERMA

- Morphea
    - Steroids
        - Topical
        - Intralesional
        - Systemic (for widespread disease)
- Systemic sclerosis
    - Penicillamine
    - Prednisone
    - Immunosuppressants
    - Physical therapy (for contractures)
    - Nifedipine (for Raynaud's phenomenon)

---

because of potential resulting toxicity. For patients with sclerodactyly, physical therapy should not be overlooked. Daily range-of-motion exercises are important to help limit the flexion contractures that often develop over time.

Raynaud's phenomenon associated with scleroderma also is difficult to treat. Many patients achieve some benefit from calcium channel blockers such as nifedipine (Procardia) in doses of 30 to 60 mg daily. Prevention of exposure to cold, including the use of insulated or electrically heated gloves, also is extremely important.

Course and Complications. Morphea is usually limited to a few plaques, although it may be more widespread. Linear morphea in children may be accompanied by involvement of underlying muscle and even bone, with resulting atrophy of these tissues. Morphea often "burns out" over time (usually years), with subsequent softening of the affected skin. Residual hypopigmentation or hyperpigmentation is common. Although rare cases of progression to systemic scleroderma have been reported, in most patients morphea is a benign disease.

Systemic scleroderma is frequently progressive, and death from systemic involvement is not uncommon. Reported 5-year survival rates range from 50% to 90%, depending on the type and extent of visceral involvement. Renal failure, often accompanied by severe hypertension, is a frequent cause of death. Cardiac complications include conduction detects, pericarditis, and heart failure. Pulmonary fibrosis is another serious complication. Involvement of the smooth muscle of the lower part of the esophagus produces impaired esophageal motility with reflux, causing strictures. Weight loss and malnutrition can result.

The skin thickening often begins with an early, edematous phase followed by hardening and increasing thickening. Cutaneous complications include ulcerations of the ischemic fingers, sometimes complicated by infection with osteomyelitis. Flexion contractures of the hands and fingers can result from sclerosis.

Pathogenesis. Patients with scleroderma have increased numbers of fibroblasts and an increased rate of collagen biosynthesis in the skin. Although the primary causes are unknown, increasing evidence suggests that the process is immunologically mediated.

Cellular immunity to collagen has been demonstrated with increased collagen production stimulated by lymphokines. A vicious circle may then occur, with increased fibroblasts and collagen synthesis provoking a cellular immune response with the elaboration of lymphokines, a process that further stimulates fibroblast activity. Transforming growth factor-β is one cytokine that has been implicated in the process. It has been shown to upregulate collagen gene expression and has been found to be present in markedly increased concentrations in involved sclerodermatous skin.

Several European studies have implicated the spirochete *Borrelia burgdorferi* in the pathogenesis of morphea and have reported success with penicillin treatment in some patients. These results have not been duplicated in the United States.

Although they have not been clearly defined, immune processes may also play a role in the vascular disease inherent in PSS. Damage to endothelial cells and endothelial basement membranes leads to thickening of vessel walls, and this results in luminal narrowing and ischemic effects. Vessels in the fingers, kidneys, and heart appear to be particularly prone to these effects.

The role, if any, of the antinuclear antibodies in the pathogenesis of scleroderma is unknown. They may be a result, rather than a cause, of the disease.

REFERENCES

Aberer E, Stanek G, Ertl M, Neumann R: Evidence for spirochetal origin of circumscribed scleroderma (morphea). Acta Derm Venereol 67:225–231, 1987.

Chosidow O, Bagot M, Vernant JP, et al.: Sclerodermatous chronic graft-versus-host disease: analysis of seven cases. J Am Acad Dermatol 26:49–55, 1992.

Falanga V, Medsger TA, Reichlin M, Rodnan GP: Linear scleroderma: clinical spectrum, prognosis, and laboratory abnormalities. Ann Intern Med 104:849–857, 1986.

Perez MI, Kohn SR: Systemic sclerosis. J Am Acad Dermatol 28:525–547, 1993.

Steen VD: Clinical manifestations of systemic sclerosis. Semin Cutan Med Surg 17:48–54, 1998.

Steen VD, Medsger TA Jr, Rodnan GP: D-Penicillamine therapy in progressive systemic sclerosis (scleroderma): a retrospective analysis. Ann Intern Med 97:652–659, 1982.

ULCERS

∎

ULCERS 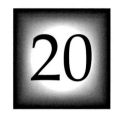 20

Definition. An *ulcer* is an open sore that results from loss of the epidermis and part or all of the dermis (Fig. 20–1). Ulcers have numerous causes (Table 20–1). A detailed history and physical examination are often sufficient to establish a diagnosis; however, laboratory tests may be necessary to confirm the initial clinical impression.

Incidence. An ulcer is the chief complaint in 0.5% of our new patients. The frequency of different types of ulcers depends in part on the circumstances of the patient population. For example, decubitus ulcers are a common problem in bedridden patients, whereas leprosy should be considered in a patient from a tropical environment.

History. The history begins with the mode of onset. Is the ulcer acute or chronic? The sudden appearance of severe pain associated with numbness in an extremity suggests *arterial occlusion* due to an embolus or a thrombus. The gradual onset of pain with exertion relieved by rest is characteristic of intermittent claudication due to *arteriolosclerosis*. A history of lower leg heaviness, aching, and swelling, particularly after periods of inactive standing or sitting, is typical of *venous stasis*.

Patients with *neoplastic* ulcers often have a history of a growth that preceded the ulceration. A family history is important in the diagnosis of ulcers caused by *hemoglobinopathies* such as thalassemia and sickle cell anemia.

Factitial ulcers are suspected in patients with a history of emotional disorders and overly dramatic and reactive behavior or indifference. If an ulcer is painless, sensory neuropathy should be suspected.

Various *infectious agents* cause ulceration. Acute onset after wildlife exposure in a patient with fever, chills, and malaise suggests a diagnosis of tularemia, plague, or anthrax. Travel history is particularly important in considering tropical diseases such as amebiasis or leishmaniasis. Sexual history is important if a venereal cause is suspected.

The *drug* history should not be overlooked. Medications alone, however, are a rare cause of ulcers. More often, ulcers are secondary to drug-induced epidermal necrolysis or vasculitis. Allopurinol, barbiturates, anticonvulsants, and antibiotics may cause these eruptions. The cause of a *physical* ulcer usually is not a diagnostic problem because it is readily apparent to the patient.

Physical Examination. The physical examination should include characteristics of the ulcer (e.g., size, shape, color), its location (e.g., leg, genitals, buttock), and associated physical findings (e.g., surrounding skin, pulses, neurologic findings). Changes in skin color, skin temperature, and pulse pattern suggest *arteriosclerotic*

History:
1. Onset
2. Symptoms
3. Neoplasm
4. Family history
5. Social history
6. Travel
7. Medications

Physical examination:
1. Size, shape, and color of ulcer
2. Location
3. Associated physical findings

295

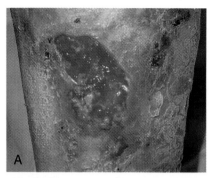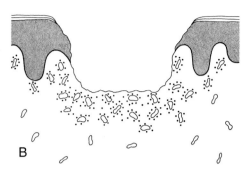

FIGURE 20–1. Stasis ulcer. **A,** Epidermis—absent. Dermis—granulation tissue. **B,** Epidermis—absent. Dermis—chronic inflammation, dilated capillaries.

TABLE 20–1 ■ ETIOLOGY OF ULCERS

Vascular

Venous stasis*
Arteriosclerosis*
Thromboangiitis obliterans
Vasculitis*
Embolic—tumor, infections (SBE)
Hypertension

Neoplastic

Carcinoma—cutaneous or metastatic*
Lymphoma—mycosis fungoides
Sarcoma—Kaposi's

Hematologic

Hemoglobinopathy—sickle cell anemia,
　　spherocytosis, thalassemia*
Dysglobulinemia—cryoglobulinemia,
　　macroglobulinemia

Drug-Related

Methotrexate
Bleomycin
Ergots
Coumarin
Heparin
Iodine
Bromide

Connective Tissue Disease

Rheumatoid arthritis
Lupus erythematosus
Scleroderma
Dermatomyositis

Neurologic

Neurotrophic—diabetes, syringomyelia,
　　tabes dorsalis, leprosy, trigeminal
　　trophic syndrome*
Factitial*

Infectious

Bacteria—tuberculosis, diphtheria, an-
　　thrax, tularemia, chancroid, granuloma
　　inguinale, syphilis
Fungus—blastomycosis, histoplasmosis,
　　chromomycosis, sporotrichosis, crypto-
　　coccosis
Protozoa—leishmaniasis, amebiasis
Virus—herpes*

Physical

Chrome
Coral
Beryllium
Radiographs
Trauma
Cold
Heat
Pressure (decubitus)*
Bites (brown recluse spider)

Unknown

Pyoderma gangrenosum
Necrobiosis lipoidica

* Most common causes.

SBE, subacute bacterial endocarditis.

peripheral vascular disease. The skin is purplish red with dependency but changes to pallor when the extremity is elevated. In chronic severe ischemia, the skin and muscles become atrophic in association with hair loss and brittle, opaque nails. The skin is cool, and peripheral pulses are lost. Patients with ischemic leg or ankle ulcers may also have ulceration of the toes.

Lower leg edema, brawny induration, brownish discoloration, petechiae, and dermatitis are typical of *venous insufficiency*. Stasis ulcers rarely occur below the level of the malleolus. Varicose veins may or may not be prominent.

Multiple small ulcers (0.5 to 2 cm) occurring predominantly on the lower legs suggest *vasculitis*. The ulcer borders are usually purpuric, hemorrhagic, and necrotic, and crusted purpuric papules and nodules also occur.

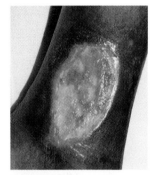

FIGURE 20–2. Sickle cell anemia.

The development of individual or multiple cutaneous nodules that become ulcerated is characteristic of an underlying *neoplasm*. However, a preceding nodule is not always present in a malignant ulcer. Ulceration of the lower third of the leg above the ankle in an adult black patient is a major manifestation of homozygous *sickle cell disease* (Fig. 20–2).

Areas of pressure and trauma, particularly the foot, are susceptible to developing a *neurotrophic ulcer* (mal perforans), which occurs mainly in patients with diabetes or leprosy. The skin surrounding the ulcer is anesthetic and is invariably callused.

Geometric, bizarre-shaped angular ulcers are characteristic of a self-inflicted *factitial* cause. Genital ulceration is highly suggestive of a venereal cause, which may be *herpes simplex*, *syphilis*, *chancroid*, or *granuloma inguinale*.

The most common physical ulcer (3% of hospitalized patients) is the *pressure sore* or *decubitus ulcer*. Shearing forces, friction, moisture, and pressure contribute to the development of these sores. Bedridden or wheelchair-bound patients unable to ambulate are most at risk. These patients usually are elderly and frequently are incontinent. The most frequent sites are the sacral and coccygeal areas, ischial tuberosities, and greater trochanter. These ulcers begin as irregular, ill-defined, reddish, indurated areas that resemble abrasions. A full-thickness skin defect develops with extension into the subcutaneous tissue and ultimate penetration into the deep fascia and muscle.

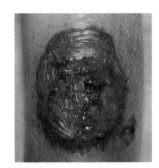

FIGURE 20–3. Pyoderma gangrenosum.

A rapidly developing, painful ulcer with an undetermined edge and gangrenous border is characteristic of *pyoderma gangrenosum* (Fig. 20–3). These ulcers usually occur on the lower legs. Pyoderma gangrenosum is frequently associated with ulcerative and granulomatous colitis, rheumatoid arthritis, and myeloproliferative diseases.

Laboratory and Biopsy. Laboratory tests are necessary to confirm the origin of some ulcers after the history and physical examination. Several *vascular studies* can be used to assess for peripheral vascular disease. Indirect and direct noninvasive testing is used initially to determine arterial competence. When limb savage is indicated, selective arteriography can locate and define the extent of arterial obstruction. Photoplethysmography is performed in patients to delineate venous pathologic and physiologic abnormalities. In addition, photoplethysmography can be used to determine cutaneous blood perfusion at ulcer margins and thus help to predict the potential for healing. Venous duplex scanning is used to rule out deep vein thrombosis and superficial thrombophlebitis.

Several *blood tests* can be helpful in the workup of ulcers. Connective tissue diseases are diagnosed clinically with supportive serologic tests, including tests for antinuclear antibody, rheumatoid factor, and anti-DNA antibody. Patients

Laboratory tests:
1. **Vascular studies**
2. **Blood tests**
3. **Cultures**
4. **Biopsy**

with suspected hematologic disorders can be easily diagnosed with the appropriate tests for sickle cell anemia, spherocytosis, thalassemia, and dysglobulinemias.

Cultures are necessary for diagnosing tropical or unusual infections. Routine cultures of chronic ulcers generally grow out a mixture of organisms. When the quantitative bacterial counts are more than 10^5 organisms per gram of tissue or per square centimeter of surface area, healing is impeded. However, antibiotic therapy for secondarily infected ulcers without treatment of the underlying cause does not result in healing. Diagnostic radiographs are indicated when underlying osteomyelitis is a potential complication.

A *biopsy* is indicated in all chronic ulcers of unknown origin; it is particularly helpful in ruling out neoplasms (Fig. 20–4). Vascular causes of ulcers, including venous stasis and vasculitis, have characteristic histologic changes. Infectious ulcers are diagnosed by skin biopsy, with special stains used to demonstrate the causative organism. In addition, a portion of the biopsy specimen is sent to the microbiology laboratory for culture (Fig. 20–5).

Therapy. Appropriate treatment depends on correctly identifying and removing the cause. Venous or arterial insufficiency is the most common cause of ulceration in the ambulatory patient, and correcting the underlying vascular abnormality, if possible, is paramount. For example, *stasis ulcers* are unlikely to heal in a patient with persistent edema caused by incompetent veins. External compression of venous diseased legs is the most effective therapy. Initially, stasis ulcers and edema are treated with a compressive boot (Dome-Paste) that is changed weekly or a polyurethane dressing pad covered by an inner liner stocking and outer zippered compression stockings (Jobst UlcerCare System). After healing, knee-high, medium-pressure elastic compression stockings (Jobst) are used to prevent recurrent stasis ulcers.

Surgery, chemotherapy, and radiotherapy are used to treat *neoplastic ulcers*. The most important treatment of *neurotrophic* ulcers and *pressure sores* is prevention

Biopsy of chronic ulcers of unknown origin is indicated to rule out cancer.

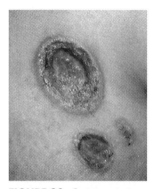

FIGURE 20–4. Mycosis fungoides.

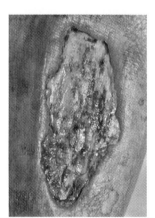

FIGURE 20–5. Cryptococcosis.

THERAPY OF ULCERS

- Correct or treat the underlying cause
  - Venous insufficiency—compression boot or stocking
  - Arterial insufficiency—surgery
  - Neoplasm—surgery, chemotherapy, radiotherapy
  - Infection—antibiotics
  - Neurotrophic or decubitus ulcer—relief of pressure
  - Vasculitis or pyoderma gangrenosum—prednisone, treatment of associated disease
- Promote wound healing
  - Debridement—whirlpool, surgical, enzymes
  - Dressings—nonadherent, occlusive, or wet-to-dry
  - Infection control—antibiotics
  - Growth factors—platelet derived
  - Skin grafting

of friction and trauma. Pressure is relieved with mechanical devices, such as soft, comfortable shoes for a diabetic patient with a foot ulcer. Adjunct treatment with platelet-derived growth factor (becaplermin [Regranex]) helps to promote healing in patients with diabetic neuropathic foot ulcers. *Infection* requires appropriate antibiotic selection for treatment. Removal of the offending *drug* is the obvious remedy for ulcers caused by drugs.

The general management of ulcers includes measures that promote wound healing, such as medical or surgical debridement, occlusive dressings, treatment of infection, and good nutrition. Numerous agents are used to remove devitalized and purulent tissue from wounds, including wet-to-dry dressings with normal saline or antiseptics such as povidone-iodine (Betadine). Enzyme preparations are used to liquefy necrotic wound debris. Dextran polymer beads (Debrisan) have been used with good results and are particularly helpful in patients who are allergic to components of topical preparations.

Occlusive dressings made of various polymers (e.g., polyethylene, polyurethane) have made a significant contribution to ulcer therapy. These dressings keep the ulcer moist, a feature that promotes epidermal repair through migration of epithelial cells over the ulcer. Initially, large amounts of exudate form under the occlusive dressing and remove crust and necrotic debris through a process of autolytic digestion. The dressing must be changed every 2 to 3 days because of exudate buildup, but with healing the dressing may be changed less frequently (i.e., every 5 to 7 days). Another characteristic of occlusive dressings (e.g., Op-site, Vigilon, DuoDerm) is significant pain relief.

The use of oral and topical antibiotics is often ineffective because of the development of resistant bacteria. Antibiotics should be reserved for ulcers that are complicated by cellulitis, lymphangitis, and septicemia or for when a single organism is cultured.

Surgical intervention (bypass graft or thromboendarterectomy) is required in patients with peripheral vascular disease. In venous ulcers that have failed to respond to more conservative therapy, skin grafting often is necessary with the patient's own skin or with an in vitro living skin construct (Apligraf).

Course and Complications. The healing rate of ulcers is directly related to successful treatment of the cause and aggravating factors as well as prevention of complications. For example, a venous stasis ulcer may persist for years if it is inadequately treated. Removal of aggravating factors such as secondary infection and necrotic debris promotes ulcer healing. Complications such as cellulitis, lymphangitis, septicemia, and osteomyelitis affect many patients and prolong the duration of the ulcer.

Complications:
1. **Cellulitis**
2. **Lymphangitis**
3. **Septicemia**
4. **Osteomyelitis**

Pathogenesis. Infectious agents, toxic chemicals, physical injury, and loss of nutrition from interruption of the cutaneous vasculature cause cell death, tissue loss, and ulceration. As long as cell death continues, the ulcer will persist.

Ulcer healing is a complex biologic process that requires an intact vascular supply and proliferation of fibroblasts, endothelial cells, and keratinocytes. Dermal integrity depends on the synthesis of collagen, elastin, and proteoglycans (ground substance) by fibroblasts. Epidermal repair requires the proliferation and migration of keratinocytes over a fibrin-fibronectin support matrix. Inflammation always accompanies the wound healing process, in which the macrophage is the essential and most important cell. Various growth factors (e.g., epidermal, platelet-derived, fibroblast, and transforming growth factor-β) appear to have a role in wound healing by enhancing re-epithelialization and granulation tissue.

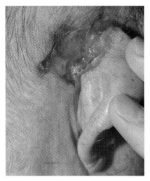

FIGURE 20-6. Unknown.

■ UNKNOWN (Fig. 20–6)

This 60-year-old man had a 1-year history of a nonhealing ulcer. He had otherwise been in excellent health and had no previous history of ulcers. The general physical examination was normal. The skin examination revealed a fair-skinned Caucasian man with a 6-cm shallow ulcer behind his ear. The base of the ulcer was clean, and the surrounding skin appeared normal. He had used a number of topical preparations and had been treated with systemic antibiotics without success.

What is your differential diagnosis of this ulcer?

The differential diagnosis of ulcer is extensive. Neither the history nor the physical examination gives us a clue to its origin. However, a negative history and normal general physical examination make a vascular, hematologic, neurologic, drug, connective tissue disease, or physical cause of this ulcer less likely. This leaves a neoplastic, infectious, or unknown origin.

What would you do now?

The next step is a biopsy of the ulcer for routine and special stains.

What is the best treatment?

The biopsy revealed a basal cell carcinoma. Treatment was excision of the tumor with the Mohs' technique.

Important Points

1. Ulcers of unknown origin must be examined by biopsy to rule out neoplasm.
2. Appropriate therapy is dictated by correct identification of the cause.

REFERENCES

Falanga V, Zitelli JA, Eaglstein WH: Wound healing. J Am Acad Dermatol 19:559–563, 1988.

Kitachama A, Elliott LF, Kerstein MD, et al.: Leg ulcer: conservative management or surgical treatment? JAMA 274:197–199, 1982.

Lookingbill DP, Miller SH, Knowles RC: Bacteriology of chronic leg ulcers. Arch Dermatol 114:1765–1768, 1978.

Phillips TJ: Chronic cutaneous ulcers: etiology and epidemiology. J Invest Dermatol 102: 38S–41S, 1994.

Reuler JB, Cooney TG: The pressure sore: pathophysiology and principles of management. Ann Intern Med 94:661–666, 1981.

Samson RH, Showalter DP: Stockings and the prevention of recurrent venous ulcers. Dermatol Surg 22:373–376, 1996.

Witkowski JA, Parish LC: Cutaneous ulcer therapy. Int J Dermatol 25:420–426, 1986.

6

HAIR

AND

NAILS

■

HAIR LOSS

21

STRESS-INDUCED ALOPECIA
ANDROGENIC ALOPECIA
TRICHOTILLOMANIA
ALOPECIA AREATA
LUPUS ERYTHEMATOSUS
TINEA CAPITIS

The evaluation of a patient with hair loss requires a detailed history, physical examination, and, in some cases, laboratory tests and biopsy (Table 21–1). Important elements of the history include the age of onset, medications taken, recent emotional or physical stress, diet, grooming techniques, and family history of baldness or hair disorders.

The physical examination is helpful in making an accurate diagnosis by observing the pattern (patchy or diffuse) of hair loss and whether scarring is present. Patchy hair loss is readily apparent. However, diffuse hair loss may not be noticeable until the patient has more than 50% hair loss. The presence or absence of scarring is important diagnostically and prognostically. In nonscarring alopecia, the diagnosis is usually made without biopsy. In scarring alopecia, a biopsy is useful in establishing the diagnosis and should be performed. Nonscarring alopecia may be a temporary phenomenon, whereas scarring indicates permanent hair loss. Except for discoid lupus, the disorders discussed in this chapter are nonscarring.

Observe the pattern of hair loss and whether scarring is present.

■ STRESS-INDUCED ALOPECIA

Definition. Marked emotionally or physiologically stressful events may result in an alteration of the normal hair cycle and diffuse hair loss. The scalp is made up of a mosaic of anagen (growing) and telogen (resting) hairs. Stress-induced alopecia is characterized by excessive and early entry of hairs into the telogen phase *(telogen effluvium)* (Fig. 21–1). Causes of stress-induced alopecia include high fever, childbirth, chronic illness, major surgery, severe emotional disorders, crash diets, hypothyroidism, and drugs (e.g., heparin, warfarin, boric acid, indomethacin, nitrofurantoin, sulfasalazine, and vitamin A).

Incidence. The incidence of stress-induced alopecia is probably greater than that seen by the dermatologist because most episodes are transient and minor.

Stress-induced alopecia occurs most often post partum.

TABLE 21–1 ■ ALOPECIA

	Incidence*	History	Physical Examination	Scarring	Pattern	Differential Diagnosis	Laboratory Test (Biopsy)
Stress-induced (telogen effluvium)	1.0	Physical or emotional stress 2–3 months prior	Positive hair pull >25% telogen hair	–	Diffuse	Thyroid dysfunction Drug-induced Nutritional deficiency	None
Androgenic	0.6	Family history of baldness	Normal scalp	–	Male pattern	Androgen excess in women	None
Trichotillomania	0.1	Emotional problems	Broken hair	–	Patchy	Alopecia areata Fungus infection	None
Alopecia areata	0.9	Acute onset	Exclamation point hairs	–	Circular patches	Trichotillomania Secondary syphilis Fungal infection	None
Discoid lupus erythematosus	<0.1	Photosensitivity Other symptoms of lupus	Erythema Follicular plugs	+	Patchy	Fungal infection Lichen planus Neoplasm	Biopsy
Fungal	0.1	Schoolmates with hair loss	Scaling, erythema, pustules	–	Patchy	Seborrheic dermatitis Alopecia areata Bacterial infection Trichotillomania	KOH preparation, culture

*Percentage of new dermatology patients with this diagnosis seen in the Hershey Medical Center Dermatology Clinic, Hershey, PA.
>, More than; <, Less than; –, absent; +, present.

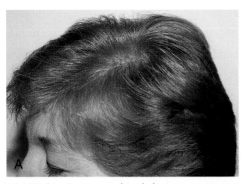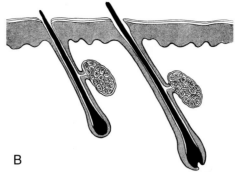

FIGURE 21-1. Stress-induced alopecia. **A,** Thinning of hair not readily apparent to a casual observer. **B,** More than 25% of the hairs are telogen (left). Anagen hair (right) is shown for comparison.

History. Hair loss occurs 2 to 3 months after the physical or mental stress. Most of our patients are women who have diffuse hair thinning post partum. They are concerned about going bald and characterize their hair loss as coming out by "handfuls" after combing and shampooing. If the patient has not recently given birth, a history of other physical or emotional stress, dietary habits, and medications should be sought.

Physical Examination. The patient has diffuse thinning of the hair that at first is not readily apparent to the examiner. The scalp is normal, with no scarring or erythema. The remainder of the skin examination, including hair elsewhere on the body, nails, and teeth, is normal. Gentle pulling of the hair (hair pull test) verifies excessive hair shedding. The hair pull is done by grasping a group of two to three dozen hairs and applying gentle traction. Normally, fewer than three hairs are pulled out with this maneuver. Pulling out more than five hairs confirms that excessive shedding is present.

> **The excessive loss of telogen hairs is characteristic and manifested by the positive hair pull test.**

In stress-induced alopecia, the number of telogen hairs is increased from a normal percentage of 10% to 20% to more than 25%. This results in as many as 400 to 500 lost hairs daily. Normally, fewer than 100 hairs are lost daily.

Differential Diagnosis. Metabolic causes of diffuse, nonscarring alopecia must be differentiated from stress. *Abnormal thyroid function*, particularly hypothyroidism, produces hair that is dry and sparse diffusely, often with loss of the lateral third of each eyebrow. *Nutritional deficiencies* (e.g., lack of an essential fatty acid, biotin, or zinc) also cause diffuse alopecia. *Toxic drugs,* particularly alkylating agents, cause loss of hair in the anagen phase.

Laboratory and Biopsy. The history and clinical examination usually are diagnostic of stress-induced alopecia.

Therapy. In most patients, the stressful event has passed, and reassurance is all that is required.

Course and Complications. This condition is usually a self-limited reversible problem that resolves within 2 to 6 months. It may be prolonged for years if the underlying stress continues or in some patients, particularly middle-aged women, without a recognizable initiating factor.

Pathogenesis. The normal hair cycle is disturbed in stress-induced alopecia. Growing anagen hairs are prematurely converted to resting telogen hairs, which are

THERAPY OF STRESS-INDUCED ALOPECIA

- Reassurance

subsequently shed. The mechanism for this alteration of the normal hair cycle is unknown.

■ ANDROGENIC ALOPECIA

Definition. Androgenic alopecia (common baldness) represents postpubertal replacement of terminal hairs by vellus hairs and eventually completely atrophic follicles (Fig. 21–2). It occurs in individuals, both male and female, who are genetically predisposed. Clinically, the disorder is nonscarring and involves the vertex and frontotemporal regions of the scalp.

Incidence. The prevalence of common baldness varies with the population studied. Among male Caucasians, it approximates 100%, but age at onset is highly variable. In Native American, Japanese, and Chinese populations, baldness is uncommon.

History. The process begins at any age after puberty, but temporal recession often is noticed between the ages of 20 and 30 years. The onset and progression are gradual. The patient usually has a family history of baldness.

Vellus hairs replace terminal hairs in androgenic alopecia.

Physical Examination. In areas of baldness, the coarse, dark terminal hairs are replaced by finer, depigmented (vellus) hairs, which then become atrophic, leaving a smooth, shiny scalp with barely visible follicular orifices. The number of hair follicles remains unchanged. Baldness characteristically occurs in a distinctive pattern that spares the posterior and lateral margins of the scalp. In men, the process begins with bitemporal recession, followed by balding of the vertex. In women, androgenic alopecia most often is manifested by diffuse thinning over the top of the scalp and an intact frontal hairline. Total hair loss in women is rare.

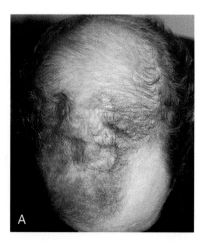

A

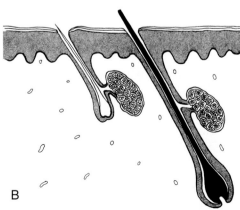

B

FIGURE 21–2. Androgenic alopecia. **A,** Frontal and vertex alopecia. **B,** Vellus hair (left) is found in areas of baldness. Terminal hair (right) is shown for comparison.

In areas of baldness, the scalp appears completely normal, with no evidence of scarring or inflammation.

Differential Diagnosis. In men, the diagnosis is usually straightforward. In women, the diagnosis of androgenic alopecia may be more difficult. In most women, it is simply an inherited trait. *Hormonal abnormality* should be considered in women with baldness, particularly if it is accompanied by acne or hirsutism. They should be asked about menstrual irregularities and infertility. In some women, hypothyroidism may also be present.

Laboratory and Biopsy. Ordinarily, no laboratory examination or biopsy is done. Androgen excess in women can be screened for with measurements of serum-free and total testosterone and dehydroepiandrosterone sulfate.

Therapy. *Minoxidil*, 2% solution (Rogaine) and 5% solution (Rogaine Extra Strength for Men) applied twice daily, is a moderately effective treatment for men with androgenic alopecia, but it appears to be less effective in women. It stops or reduces the rate of hair loss and restores lost hair in some individuals. After 1 year of treatment, 20% to 40% of men achieve moderate-to-dense regrowth of terminal hairs with the 2% solution and some increased effectiveness with the 5% solution. This new hair growth is not permanent. Cessation of treatment results in loss of hair within a few months. Even with continued therapy, hair regrowth plateaus after 1 year and slowly declines over subsequent years. The vertex of the scalp responds, but the frontal region generally does not.

Finasteride, 1 mg (Propecia), a type II 5α-reductase inhibitor, is given once daily. Eighty-three percent of men maintained their hair after 2 years, and 36% had moderate-to-dense regrowth. Finasteride is contraindicated in women of childbearing potential because of its teratogenic effects on male offspring.

Extensive areas of baldness can be covered with a hairpiece or wig. For selected patients, surgical treatment with hair transplantation or scalp reduction is successful.

Course and Complications. The balding process is usually gradual and is most evident between the ages of 30 and 50 years. Thereafter, it is much slower, although hair thinning continues into later life.

Pathogenesis. The development of common baldness is genetically predetermined and androgen dependent. Castration of males before puberty prevents the development of baldness. However, when testosterone is administered, a predisposed eunuch becomes bald. It seems contradictory that androgens cause scalp baldness but stimulate hair growth on the chest, face, and genital regions. This phenomenon

Common baldness is androgen dependent.

THERAPY OF ANDROGENIC ALOPECIA

- Minoxidil 5% solution BID
- Finasteride: 1 mg daily
- Surgery—hair transplant, scalp reduction
- Wig

may be explained by regional differences in androgen metabolism. Hair follicles in bald areas of the scalp have increased levels and activity of 5α-reductase, which causes increased levels of dihydrotestosterone that shortens the hair cycle and miniaturizes scalp follicles.

■ TRICHOTILLOMANIA

Definition. Trichotillomania is traumatic, self-induced alopecia. It results from compulsive plucking, twisting, and rubbing, which causes broken or epilated hair shafts (Fig. 21–3).

Incidence. Trichotillomania occurs in both children and adults. In children, it affects both sexes equally, and patients usually have no significant underlying emotional problem. In adults, it occurs predominantly among women and is usually a sign of a personality disorder.

History. A history of emotional problems may be elicited, often with difficulty.

Physical Examination. The scalp is affected most often; much less often, the eyebrows and eyelashes are plucked. Ill-marginated, irregular patchy areas of alopecia characterize trichotillomania. The scalp is normal, without inflammation or scarring. The patient has numerous twisted and broken hairs, which have a characteristic feel of coarse stubble.

> **Coarse-feeling, broken hairs are characteristic of trichotillomania.**

Differential Diagnosis. *Alopecia areata* and *tinea capitis* should be considered in the differential diagnosis of trichotillomania. Exclamation point hairs, if present, are diagnostic of alopecia areata. Biopsy findings are also discriminating. Potassium hydroxide (KOH) examination and fungal culture enable one to diagnose fungal infection.

Laboratory and Biopsy. The biopsy (usually not required) reveals normally growing hairs, empty hair follicles in a noninflammatory dermis, and traumatized follicles that have broken hair matrixes and perifollicular hemorrhage.

Therapy. Treatment is based on the degree of underlying emotional disturbance. In children, the condition is usually self-limited. When insight and reassurance are given to the child and the parents, the process often resolves. In adults, this habit may be much more difficult to stop. Gentle probing into the stresses and anxieties that have led to the hair pulling can be explored. Referral for psychiatric

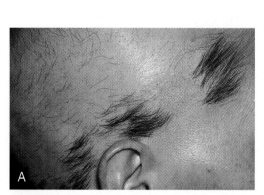
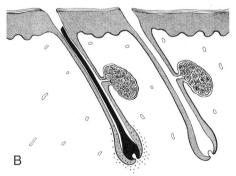

FIGURE 21–3. Trichotillomania. **A,** Patch of broken hairs. **B,** Broken hair. Empty follicle. Dermis—perifollicular hemorrhage.

THERAPY OF TRICHOTILLOMANIA

- Emotional support
- Clomipramine: 25–250 mg daily

evaluation should be considered in severely disturbed patients. Clomipramine (Anafranil), a tricyclic antidepressant with antiobsessional effects, appears to be effective in the short-term treatment of trichotillomania.

Course and Complications. Trichotillomania is generally chronic and may be resistant to treatment, especially in adults, in whom it can be a serious problem. Symptoms may be severe enough to interfere with daily life; a patient's appearance may be sufficiently embarrassing to result in social isolation. Follow-up is required to establish rapport and to determine whether trichotillomania is a symptom of a serious underlying psychiatric disorder.

Pathogenesis. The obsessive urge to pull out one's own hair has been attributed to various psychodynamic conflicts. In children, problems at home or at school, sibling rivalry, mental retardation, and hospitalization have been associated with trichotillomania.

■ ALOPECIA AREATA

Definition. Alopecia areata is an idiopathic disorder characterized by well-circumscribed, round or oval patches of nonscarring hair loss (Fig. 21–4).

Incidence. Alopecia areata affects both sexes equally, with onset occurring most often in early adulthood. Almost 1% of our new patients had this diagnosis. The incidence in Olmsted County, Minnesota was 20.2 per 100,000 person-years.

History. Alopecia areata has an acute onset. It is sometimes associated with emotional stress, but in most patients it seems that the emotional stress is caused by the hair loss. Patients are generally healthy otherwise. From 20% to 25% of patients have a family history of alopecia areata.

Physical Examination. The disorder is characterized by well-circumscribed, round or oval patches of hair loss, leaving a smooth, normal-appearing scalp. Erythema and slight tenderness may be present early in the course. Subsequently, the scalp may become slightly depressed. Characteristically, the periphery of the patches of hair loss is studded with *exclamation point hairs*, which are so named because of their resemblance to that punctuation mark. These fractured hairs are 2 to 3 mm long and are tapered at the base.

Alopecia areata is characterized by nonscarring circular patches of alopecia with exclamation point hairs.

Alopecia areata most often affects the scalp, frequently with several 2- to 3-cm patches of hair loss. The eyebrows, eyelashes, and beard may also be affected, as may hair elsewhere on the body. Approximately 1% to 2% of patients develop loss of all scalp hair *(alopecia totalis)* or loss of all body hair *(alopecia universalis)*. Fine stippling and pitting of the nails are an infrequent associated finding.

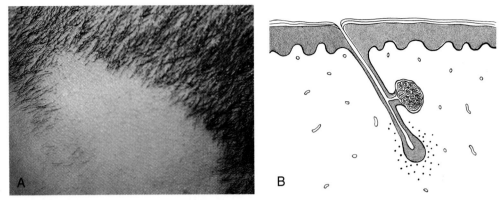

FIGURE 21-4. Alopecia areata. **A,** Alopecia, normal scalp. **B,** Dystrophic follicle without a hair shaft. Dermis—lymphocytes surrounding the hair bulb.

Differential Diagnosis. Other nonscarring forms of alopecia need to be considered in the differential diagnosis. *Secondary syphilis* can be ruled out by appropriate serologic examination. *Trichotillomania* and *fungal infection* should also be considered. Ill-marginated, irregular patches of alopecia containing the stubble of broken hairs are typical of trichotillomania. If doubt exists, a biopsy helps to differentiate trichotillomania from alopecia areata. A KOH preparation and culture enable one to diagnose a fungal infection.

Laboratory and Biopsy. Histopathologic examination of alopecia areata reveals the presence of small, dystrophic hair structures. A lymphocytic infiltrate surrounds the early anagen hair bulbs like a "swarm of bees."

Therapy. The treatment of alopecia areata depends on the extent of involvement and the patient's emotional need for regrowth of hair. Topical, intralesional, and oral corticosteroids are used most often. In localized disease, topical potent steroids (clobetasol [Temovate] gel) or intralesional injections of triamcinolone (Kenalog-10) are sometimes effective. In widespread disease, systemic steroids are sometimes used, but their hazards must be considered before starting treatment. Prompt hair loss after discontinuation of oral steroids is discouraging. Other modes of therapy include immunotherapy by induction of allergic contact dermatitis, photochemotherapy with PUVA (psoralen plus ultraviolet light A), topical minoxidil, and oral cyclosporine. Patients with alopecia areata need psychologic support. A wig is recommended when the hair loss is extensive.

Course and Complications. Alopecia areata has a variable, unpredictable course. Most patients have spontaneous recovery. However, relapses are not uncommon. Duration of more than 1 year and extensive hair loss are poor prognostic signs. Spontaneous regrowth of hair in alopecia totalis (scalp) and alopecia universalis (total body) may occur but is uncommon; fewer than 5% of patients show any tendency toward hair regrowth.

Poor prognosis:
1. **Long duration**
2. **Large areas of alopecia**

Pathogenesis. The pathogenesis of alopecia areata remains poorly understood, although an immunologic process is favored. A lymphocytic inflammatory infiltrate surrounds the affected bulbs and presumably has a role in the disease. In response to this autoimmune process, the hair matrixes become arrested but retain the capacity for normal hair regrowth after months or years.

THERAPY OF ALOPECIA AREATA

- Steroids
    Topical—clobetasol BID
    Intralesional—triamcinolone every 4–6 weeks
    Systemic—prednisone
- PUVA
- Immunotherapy

Alopecia areata is occasionally associated with autoimmune diseases such as Hashimoto's thyroiditis and pernicious anemia. However, autoantibody studies have been inconsistent, and the presence of autoantibodies is heterogeneous targeting multiple structures in the anagen hair follicles.

■ LUPUS ERYTHEMATOSUS

Definition. Lupus erythematosus is an autoimmune disorder that often affects the scalp and causes alopecia. The loss of hair may be diffuse and nonscarring (systemic lupus erythematosus [SLE]) or patchy and scarring (discoid lupus erythematosus [DLE]) (Fig. 21–5). A general discussion of lupus erythematosus is found in Chapters 10 and 15.

Physical Examination. Diffuse nonscarring alopecia of the scalp accompanies the acute phases of SLE in more than 20% of patients. In addition, short, broken hairs ("lupus hair") may be present, particularly in the frontal margin.

SLE—nonscarring

DLE is characterized by oval, scarring areas of alopecia. A typical plaque has an active erythematous margin and a white, atrophic, inactive center. Within the plaques, telangiectasia and dilated keratin-filled follicles are present. Similar discoid lesions may be found on the ears, face, trunk, and extremities.

DLE—scarring

Differential Diagnosis. For the nonscarring alopecia caused by SLE, other causes of diffuse alopecia, such as *stress, thyroid disease, drugs,* and *nutritional defi-*

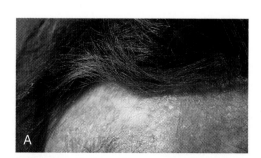
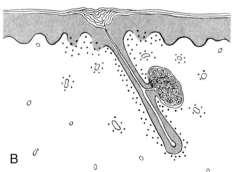

FIGURE 21–5. Discoid lupus erythematosus. **A,** Epidermis—alopecia, scarring. Dermis—erythema. **B,** Epidermis—dystrophic follicle without a hair shaft, hyperkeratosis. Dermis—lymphocytic infiltrate at the dermal-epidermal junction and around hair follicles and blood vessels.

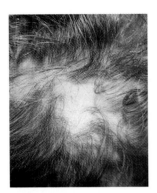

FIGURE 21-6. Lichen planus.

ciency, may be considered. However, in most patients with SLE, other manifestations of the disease are almost always evident.

Scarring alopecia caused by DLE must be differentiated from alopecia caused by *lichen planus* (Fig. 21–6), *fungal infection,* or *neoplasm.* A biopsy helps to differentiate DLE from lichen planus and a neoplasm. A KOH preparation and culture enable one to diagnose a fungal infection.

Laboratory and Biopsy. A biopsy of the scalp for routine histologic examination is usually diagnostic of DLE. Atrophic epidermis, keratotic plugging of the follicles, hydropic degeneration of the basal cells, and patchy perivascular and perifollicular lymphocytic infiltrate are characteristic. The lupus band test (direct immunofluorescence) is positive but is usually not necessary to make the diagnosis. Appropriate laboratory tests, starting with a complete blood count, platelet count, antinuclear antibody test, and urinalysis, should be ordered to rule out SLE.

Therapy. The goal of treatment in DLE is to prevent the follicular destruction that results in permanent alopecia. In many cases, the process can be arrested by the use of a potent topical (clobetasol [Temovate] gel) or intralesional corticosteroids (triamcinolone [Kenalog-10]). When this therapy fails, the addition of an antimalarial agent (hydroxychloroquine [Plaquenil]) is indicated.

Course and Complications. Chronic scarring DLE causes permanent alopecia, whereas the diffuse alopecia associated with SLE is temporary and improves when the condition improves.

Pathogenesis. The pathogenesis of lupus erythematosus is discussed in Chapters 10 and 15.

■ TINEA CAPITIS

Definition. Tinea capitis is a superficial fungal infection of the scalp (Fig. 21–7). The three most common dermatophytes that cause tinea capitis are *Trichophyton tonsurans, Microsporum canis,* and *M. audouinii.* The disease varies from noninflamed scaling patches to inflamed, pustule-studded plaques (kerion) that may leave scars.

Incidence. Epidemic tinea capitis occurs worldwide, mostly in school-age children. Males and females are equally affected. *T. tonsurans* is the predominant cause of tinea capitis in blacks. *M. audouinii* and *M. canis* cause tinea capitis in Caucasians.

History. Often, the patient has a history of a family member, friend, or pet with hair loss.

THERAPY OF DISCOID LUPUS ERYTHEMATOSUS

- Steroids
    - Topical—clobetasol BID
    - Intralesional—triamcinolone every 4–6 weeks
- Hydroxychloroquine: 200 mg BID

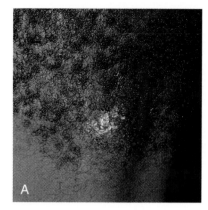

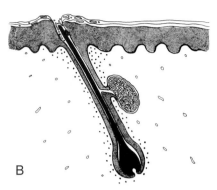

FIGURE 21–7. Tinea capitis. **A,** Epidermis—lost and broken hair, scaling. Dermis—erythema. **B,** Epidermis—hyperkeratosis, broken hair; spores and hyphae in the stratum corneum and hair shaft. Dermis—perifollicular inflammation.

Physical Examination. Tinea capitis can appear as seborrheic-like dermatitis with minimal inflammation, patchy alopecia with broken hair shafts leaving residual black stumps ("black dot" ringworm), or a severe infection with indurated, boggy plaques (kerion) covered with pustules and crusting accompanied by lymphadenopathy and resulting in scarring.

Tinea capitis causes:
1. **Seborrheic-like dermatitis**
2. **"Black dot" ringworm**
3. **Kerion**

Differential Diagnosis. *Alopecia areata, seborrheic dermatitis, bacterial scalp infection,* and *trichotillomania* should be considered in the differential diagnosis of tinea capitis. A KOH preparation or fungal culture confirms the diagnosis of tinea capitis.

Laboratory and Biopsy. Until recently, the Wood's lamp examination was a simple method to screen for tinea capitis. Hairs infected with *M. audouinii* and *M. canis* fluoresce bright green with this long-wave ultraviolet light. The Wood's lamp, however, has become much less useful because most cases of tinea capitis are now caused by nonfluorescing *T. tonsurans.*

Diagnosis is made by KOH microscopic examination and culture of broken hairs. The KOH preparation reveals spores surrounding the hair shaft (ectothrix), characteristic of *Microsporum sp.,* or within the shaft (endothrix), characteristic of *T. tonsurans.* Although biopsy is not usually performed, histopathologic sections that are stained with periodic acid–Schiff or silver reveal spores and hyphae in the stratum corneum and the hair shaft.

Therapy. Topical agents are ineffective in treating tinea capitis. For children, microsize griseofulvin (Grifulvin V tablets or suspension), 20 mg/kg daily for 6 to 8 weeks,, is the treatment of choice. In addition, shampooing with 2.5% selenium sulfide (Selsun) twice a week helps to reduce viable fungal spores and probably should be used by asymptomatic family members to reduce the carrier state. Oral terbinafine (Lamisil) or itraconazole (Sporanox) are alternative drugs if treatment with griseofulvin fails.

Course and Complications. With treatment, tinea capitis is cured in 1 to 3 months in most cases. Without treatment, the course is variable. In some children, particularly those with inflammatory tinea capitis, the course is self-limited, with resolution within several few months. In others, the disease lasts for years, with resolution at puberty. Scarring and permanent hair loss may be the sequelae of a kerion, but often the permanent damage is surprisingly little given the intense inflammation.

THERAPY OF TINEA CAPITIS

- Griseofulvin—microsize: 20 mg/kg daily
- Terbinafine
    - <20 kg: 62.5 mg daily
    - 20–40 kg: 125 mg daily
    - >40 kg: 250 mg daily
- Itraconazole
    - <20 kg: 5 mg/kg daily
    - 20–40 kg: 100 mg daily
    - >40 kg: 200 mg daily

Pathogenesis. Epidemic tinea capitis is transmitted by human-to-human spread of the dermatophytes *M. audouinii* and *T. tonsurans*. Fungi have been cultured from fallen hairs, scales, and shared combs, hats, and brushes. *M. canis* is spread from animals (cats and dogs) to humans.

After an incubation period of several days, the fungal hyphae grow into the hair shaft and follicle. This growth causes broken hair, scaling, and a host inflammatory response. The infection spreads centrifugally for 8 to 10 weeks, involving an area of scalp up to 7 cm in diameter. Spontaneous cure ensues, or a host-parasite equilibrium is maintained that results in a smoldering infection.

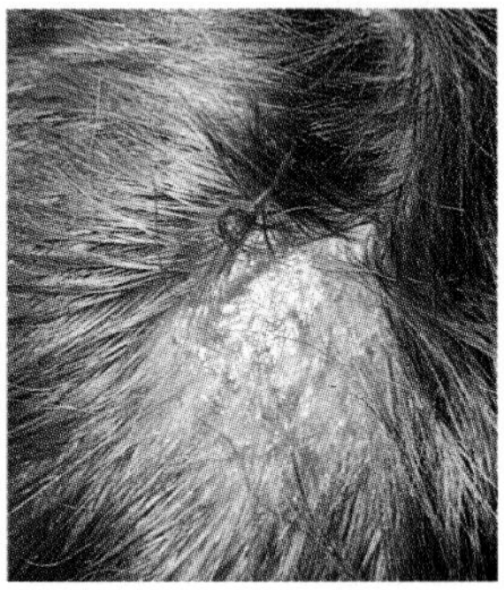

FIGURE 21–8. Unknown.

■ UNKNOWN (Fig. 21–8)

This 7-year-old boy developed itching of the scalp and progressive areas of hair loss 6 weeks before he was seen in the dermatology clinic. The use of an antiseborrheic shampoo, oral erythromycin, and a topical antifungal agent had not helped. The physical examination revealed a circular area of nonscarring alopecia. The scalp was erythematous, crusted, and scaling in the patches of hair loss.

What is your differential diagnosis?

The differential diagnosis of nonscarring alopecia includes stress-induced alopecia, androgenic alopecia, trichotillomania, alopecia areata, lupus erythematosus, and fungal infection. The patchy nature of the hair loss ruled out stress-induced and androgenic alopecia and SLE. This was not DLE because the patient had no scarring or follicular plugging. Alopecia areata and trichotillomania do not scale. The inflammation and scaling of the scalp favored a fungal infection.

What would you do now?

A KOH preparation of several plucked broken hairs was positive for spores and hyphae. If the KOH preparation had been negative or equivocal, a fungal culture would have been done. A biopsy with special stains also enables one to diagnose a fungal infection but usually is not needed.

How would you treat the patient?

The patient should be treated with oral griseofulvin for at least 6 weeks. Treatment is continued until the scalp appears normal, new hair regrowth appears, and the KOH preparation is negative.

Important Points

1. KOH preparations of tinea capitis require plucked hairs. The scale may be negative. When in doubt, do a fungal culture.

2. Treatment of tinea capitis requires oral preparations; topical antifungals are ineffective.

R E F E R E N C E S

Stress-Induced Alopecia

Headington JT: Telogen effluvium. Arch Dermatol 129:356–363, 1993.
Whiting DA: Chronic telogen effluvium: increased scalp hair shedding in middle-aged women. J Am Acad Dermatol 35:899–906, 1996.

Androgenic Alopecia

Burton JL, Halim MMB, Meyrick G, et al.: Male-pattern alopecia and masculinity. Br J Dermatol 100:567–571, 1979.
Drake LA, Dinehart SM, Farmer ER, et al.: Guidelines of care for androgenetic alopecia. J Am Acad Dermatol 35:465–469, 1996.
Kaufman KD, Olsen EA, Whiting D et al.: Finasteride in the treatment of men with androgenetic alopecia. J Am Acad Dermatol 39:578–589, 1998.
Medical Letter: Propecia and Rogaine extra strength for alopecia. Med Lett Drugs Ther 40:25–27, 1998.
Olsen EA, Weiner MS, Amara IA, DeLong ER: Five-year follow-up of men with androgenetic alopecia treated with topical minoxidil. J Am Acad Dermatol 22:643–646, 1990.
Price VH: Testosterone metabolism in the skin. Arch Dermatol 111:1496–1502, 1975.

Trichotillomania

Oranje AP, Peereboom-Wynia JDR, DeRaeymaecker DMJ: Trichotillomania in childhood. J Am Acad Dermatol 15:614–619, 1986.
Sticher M, Abramovits W, Newcomer VD: Trichotillomania in adults. Cutis 26:100–101, 1980.
Swedo SE, Leonard HL, Rapoport JL, et al.: A double-blind comparison of clomipramine and desipramine in the treatment of trichotillomania (hair pulling). N Engl J Med 321:497–501, 1989.

Alopecia Areata

Claudy AL, Gagnaire D: PUVA treatment of alopecia areata. Arch Dermatol 119:975–978, 1983.
Drake LA, Ceilley RI, Cornelison RL, et al.: Guidelines of care for alopecia areata. J Am Acad Dermatol 26:247–250,1992.
Mitchell AJ, Krull EA: Alopecia areata: pathogenesis and treatment. J Am Acad Dermatol 11:763–765, 1984.
Price VH, Khoury EL: Alopecia areata. Prog Dermatol 25:1–7, 1991.
Safavi KH, Muller SA, Suman VJ, et al.: Incidence of alopecia areata in Olmsted County, Minnesota, 1975 through 1989. Mayo Clin Proc 70:628–633, 1995.
Tobin DJ, Hann SK, Song MS, et al.: Hair follicle structures targeted by antibodies in patients with alopecia areata. Arch Dermatol 133:57–61, 1997.
Tobin DJ, Orentreich N, Fenton DA, et al.: Antibodies to hair follicles in alopecia areata. J Invest Dermatol 102:721–724, 1994.

Tosti A, Guidetti MS, Bardazzi F, et al.: Long-term results of topical immunotherapy in children with alopecia totalis or alopecia universalis. J Am Acad Dermatol 35:199–201, 1996.

Unger WP, Schemmer RJ: Corticosteroids in the treatment of alopecia totalis: systemic effects. Arch Dermatol 114:1486–1490, 1978.

Lupus Erythematosus

Tuffanelli DL, Duboid EL: Cutaneous manifestations of systemic lupus erythematosus. Arch Dermatol 90:377–385, 1964.

Tinea Capitis

Drake LA, Dinehart SM, Farmer ER, et al: Guidelines of care for superficial mycotic infections of the skin: tinea capitis and tinea barbae. J Am Acad Dermatol 34:290–294, 1996.

Gupta AK, Hofstader SLR, Adam P, et al.: Tinea capitis: an overview with emphasis on management. Pediatr Dermatol 16:171–189, 1999.

Herbert A: Tinea capitis: current concepts. Arch Dermatol 124:1554–1557, 1988.

Krowchuk DP, Lucky AW, Primmer SI, et al.: Current status of the identification and management of tinea capitis. Pediatrics 72:625–631, 1983.

Laude TA, Shah BR, Lynfield Y: Tinea capitis in Brooklyn. Am J Dis Child 136:1047–1050, 1982.

Prevost E: Nonfluorescent tinea capitis in Charleston, SC: a diagnostic problem. JAMA 242:1765–1767, 1979.

NAIL DISORDERS

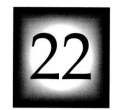

22

FUNGAL INFECTION
PSORIASIS
PARONYCHIA

The nail is a specialized keratinized appendage found on the dorsum of each finger and toe. It protects the distal phalanx against trauma, is used for fine grasping and scratching, and has aesthetic value. The diagnosis of nail diseases can be difficult because a single disease can cause widely varying changes of the nail and, conversely, because a given nail malformation can be the expression of a variety of diseases. Numerous disorders may affect the nail, including cutaneous and systemic diseases, tumors, infections, hereditary disorders, physical factors, and drugs. In this chapter, the three most common causes of nail disease are discussed: fungal infection, psoriasis, and paronychia (Table 22–1).

The physical appearance of the nail cannot reliably be used to make a diagnosis. History, skin examination, and laboratory tests are necessary.

■ FUNGAL INFECTION

Definition. *Onychomycosis* and *tinea unguium* are synonyms for infection of the nail with dermatophytic fungi (Fig. 22–1). The most common etiologic dermatophytes are *Trichophyton rubrum* and *T. mentagrophytes*.

Incidence. The prevalence of onychomycosis is 22 per 1,000 population. Twenty percent of persons in the United States between 40 and 60 years old have onychomycosis. The most common sites of infection are the toenails, especially in the elderly.

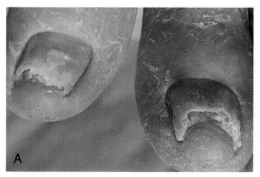
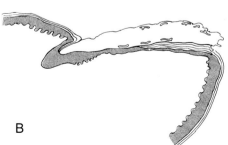

FIGURE 22-1. Fungal infection. **A,** Nail plate—white, thick, and crumbly. **B,** Nail plate—thick, hyphae.

TABLE 22–1 ■ NAIL DISORDERS

		Physical Examination		Differential Diagnosis	Laboratory Test	
	Frequency*	Pits	Brown Stains		KOH	Culture
Fungal infection	0.4	−	+	Psoriasis Trauma Aging Secondary to eczema	+	+
Psoriasis	<0.1	+	+	Fungus Trauma Aging Secondary to eczema Alopecia areata	−	−
Paronychia	0.3	−	−	Herpes simplex	− +	Bacterial Candida albicans

*Percentage of new dermatology patients with this diagnosis seen in the Hershey Medical Center Dermatology Clinic, Hershey, PA.

<, Less than; −, negative; +, positive.

Onychomycosis is associated with tinea pedis and tinea manuum.

History. The onset of onychomycosis is slow and insidious. The condition is often asymptomatic, but it can also cause pain in the affected toe, nail-trimming problems, discomfort when wearing shoes, and embarrassment because of the nails' distorted appearance.

Physical Examination. Infection of toenails is more frequent than infection of fingernails, and it is uncommon for all 10 nails to be involved. Dermatophytes most often infect the distal nail bed and undersurface of the distal nail, with resulting discoloration (white, yellow, or brown) of the nail plate and accumulation of subungual debris with separation of the plate from the nail bed. Less often, dermatophytes infect the top surface of the nail plate and cause a white, crumbly surface (superficial white onychomycosis) to develop. Neither type of infection produces much inflammatory reaction. Proximal white subungual onychomycosis, infection of the proximal nail plate, is a marker of HIV infection.

Differential Diagnosis. Often, the nail changes of onychomycosis cannot be distinguished clinically from nail dystrophy caused by *psoriasis, eczema of the digits, trauma* (Fig. 22–2), and *aging*. Associated skin findings and fungal studies differentiate these entities.

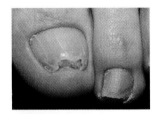

FIGURE 22–2. Traumatic nail dystrophy.

Laboratory and Biopsy. Documentation of nail fungal infection with a potassium hydroxide (KOH) preparation or fungal culture should be done because therapy is expensive and may have unwanted side effects. Compared with skin scrapings, more time must be allowed for the KOH to dissolve thin nail specimens before microscopic examination. If the infection is in the nail bed or the deeper portion of the nail plate, scrapings should be obtained from as far back under the nail as possible. Occasionally, a nail biopsy is needed to obtain a positive result.

Asymptomatic onychomycosis of toenails is often not treated.

Therapy. Topical antifungal agents are ineffective in treating onychomycosis because of their poor penetration of the nail plate. Oral therapy with terbinafine (Lamisil) or itraconazole (Sporanox) should be given. Studies suggest that terbinafine is the most effective agent. The nail will not look completely normal at the

---

THERAPY OF ONYCHOMYCOSIS

- Terbinafine: 6 weeks for fingernails, 12 weeks for toenails
    - <20 kg: 62.5 mg daily
    - 20–40 kg: 125 mg daily
    - >40 kg: 250 mg daily
- Itraconazole: 2 pulses for fingernails, 3 pulses for toenails
    - <20 kg: 5-mg/kg daily 1 week/month
    - 20–40 kg: 100-mg daily 1 week/month
    - >40–50 kg: 200-mg daily 1 week/month
    - >50 kg: 200 mg twice daily 1 week/month

---

end of treatment. Because terbinafine and itraconazole remain in the nail for months after therapy, retreatment should not be considered for approximately 6 months for fingernails and 12 months for toenails. Periodic monitoring of hepatic and hematopoietic functions is recommended. In many individuals with asymptomatic onychomycosis of the toenails, systemic therapy is neither requested nor suggested. The risks and cost may outweigh any possible benefit.

Course and Complications. Onychomycosis is a chronic infection that is difficult to eradicate permanently. Even with oral therapy, failure rates for treating toenail infections are 20% to 30%. Residual fungal spores present in the patient's shoes and environment are probably responsible for recurrence of the infection. For this reason, a topical antifungal (e.g., tolnaftate [Tinactin], miconazole [Micatin], or terbinafine [Lamisil]) applied to the feet every week may be helpful for long-term prophylaxis.

Pathogenesis. Superficial fungal infection of the nail is probably a direct extension of involvement of the surrounding digital skin. Invasion and deformity of the nail are facilitated by fungal keratinases, which disrupt the keratin structure of the plate.

■ PSORIASIS

Definition. Nail dystrophy caused by psoriasis is the result of abnormal keratinization of the nail matrix and bed secondary to involvement of these structures with psoriasis (Fig. 22–3).

Incidence. Nail involvement in patients with psoriasis is common. Reported incidences range from 10% to 50%.

History. Psoriasis of the nail is usually asymptomatic. However, involvement of fingernails may be a significant cosmetic liability, and deformity of the toenails may cause pain secondary to pressure from shoes.

Examination:
1. Pits
2. Oil stain
3. Onycholysis
4. Thickening

Physical Examination. In psoriasis, fingernails are affected more often than toenails. All or a few nails may be involved. It is unusual for psoriasis to involve only the nails; fewer than 5% of patients have involvement of the nails alone without cutaneous disease. The examiner should look elsewhere to confirm the diagnosis, especially other areas frequently affected by psoriasis—the scalp, el-

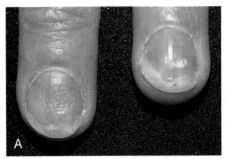 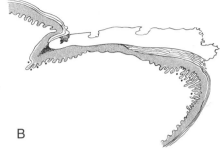

FIGURE 22-3. Psoriasis. **A,** Nail plate—rough and pitted, brown discoloration, distal separation. **B,** Nail plate—thick and pitted. Epidermis—thick, hyperkeratosis.

bows, knees, and intergluteal fold. In the nails, the most characteristic lesions are small, multiple pits produced by punctate psoriatic lesions in the nail matrix. Involvement of the nail bed produces brownish discoloration (oil stain), thickening of the nail plate, separation of the nail plate from the nail bed (onycholysis), distal crumbling, and splinter hemorrhages.

Differential Diagnosis. The differential diagnosis of psoriasis of the nails includes *onychomycosis, trauma, aging,* and *dystrophy secondary to eczema* or some other inflammatory process in the nail fold area. Fungal infections of the nail can be ruled out by a KOH preparation and culture. Otherwise, psoriatic nails can be diagnosed with confidence only when other typical lesions of psoriasis are found elsewhere. Although nail pitting is the finding most characteristic for psoriasis, it is also occasionally associated with *alopecia areata.*

Laboratory and Biopsy. Nails are rarely examined by biopsy to confirm the diagnosis of psoriasis.

Therapy. Treatment of psoriasis of the nails is difficult and usually unsatisfactory. Consequently, therapy is often not recommended. Injection of steroids into the proximal nail fold is painful, and the results are often disappointing. Topical preparations are ineffective.

Systemic medications used for psoriasis often help the nail involvement, but nail disease alone does not justify the use of these potent therapies. Trimming and paring of deformed nails reduce discomfort caused by pressure. Fingernails may be cosmetically improved by the use of sculptured plastic nails and the application of fingernail polish.

Course and Complications. Psoriasis of the nail is a chronic condition and has a waxing and waning course. Frequently, distal interphalangeal joint arthritis is associated with nail involvement. The nail is sometimes secondarily infected with *Candida albicans* or *Pseudomonas aeruginosa. Pseudomonas* infection is easily recog-

---

THERAPY OF NAIL PSORIASIS

- Trimming
- Cosmetics

nized by green discoloration and is treated with 2% thymol in alcohol, one to two drops three times daily.

Pathogenesis. Psoriasis is characterized by a marked acceleration of the rate of epidermal cell replication resulting in proliferation of keratinocytes. When this occurs in the nail bed, excess keratin is trapped under the nail plate, and onycholysis results. The "oil stain" appearance is produced by keratinous debris and inflammation in the nail bed. The nail pits result from involvement of the nail matrix, in which the psoriasis presumably produces small defective foci in the nail plate. As the nail plate advances, these defective portions fall out, leaving behind the characteristic pits.

■ PARONYCHIA

Definition. Paronychia is an inflammatory process of the nail fold (Fig. 22–4). Acute paronychia is most often the result of bacterial infection, commonly from *Staphylococcus aureus*. Chronic paronychia is usually caused by *C. albicans*. The predisposing factor in the production of chronic paronychia is trauma or maceration producing a break in the seal (cuticle) between the nail fold and the nail plate. This break produces a pocket that holds moisture and promotes the growth of microorganisms.

Acute paronychia is usually caused by *Staphylococcus aureus*; chronic paronychia is caused by *Candida albicans*.

Incidence. Chronic paronychia occurs in children who habitually suck their thumbs and in adults who do "wet" work. Particularly vulnerable are adults (nondiabetic, 3.4%; diabetic, 9.6%) who are exposed to a wet environment while they perform the chores of child rearing and housework. Bartenders, janitors, and other workers in wet occupations are also at risk.

History. Acute paronychia develops rapidly, leading to marked tenderness of the nail fold. Chronic paronychia develops insidiously and often initially goes unnoticed by the patient. A history of manicuring or wet work in adults or of finger sucking in children is common.

Physical Examination. Although any finger may be involved with paronychia, the second and third digits are the most commonly affected. Acute paronychia is painful, red, and swollen and may be accompanied by an abscess or cellulitis.

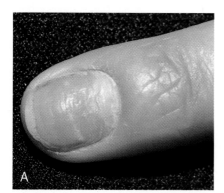
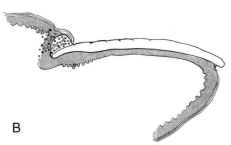

FIGURE 22–4. Chronic paronychia. **A,** Nail fold—loss of cuticle, erythematous, swollen. **B,** Nail fold—no cuticle, edema and inflammation, pocket with pus and candidal hyphae.

Chronic paronychia is characterized by loss of the cuticle, slight tenderness, swelling, erythema, and, sometimes, separation of the nail fold from the plate. One frequently sees a purulent or "cheesy" discharge and deformity of the nail plate.

Differential Diagnosis. Acute bacterial paronychia can be confused with *herpetic whitlow*. Tzanck preparation and cultures help distinguish the two. Chronic paronychia is a distinctive clinical entity and should not be confused with other inflammatory processes.

Laboratory and Biopsy. Acute paronychia that does not respond to appropriate antibiotic therapy should be cultured and possibly radiographed, to rule out osteomyelitis. For chronic paronychia, a candidal origin can be confirmed with a KOH examination of debris taken from under the cuticle. Culture, if taken, often reveals mixed flora, including bacteria and *Candida species*.

Therapy. Acute paronychia should be incised and drained when it is fluctuant. Appropriate antibiotic therapy for the causative agent should be instituted. In most cases, this therapy consists of cephalexin (Keflex), erythromycin (Ilosone), or dicloxacillin (Dynapen).

Chronic paronychia requires the avoidance of prolonged exposure to wetness. Wearing gloves is mandatory, preferably cotton under rubber or vinyl gloves. Frequent washings and manicuring should be avoided. Broad-spectrum topical preparations, such as Lotrisone (clotrimazole and betamethasone dipropionate) applied twice daily, are helpful.

Course and Complications. Acute paronychia is usually not a precursor of chronic paronychia. It resolves after appropriate antibiotic therapy and incision and drainage.

By definition, chronic paronychia continues for a long time because repeated mechanical trauma and exposure to water predispose to the chronic infectious and inflammatory process.

Trauma and exposure to water must be stopped to cure chronic paronychia.

Pathogenesis. Chronic paronychia is caused by microorganisms that produce swelling and inflammation of the nail fold. Interruption of the cuticle and wetness create an environment that fosters the growth of yeast and bacteria. These microorganisms also cause inflammation of the nail matrix, resulting in abnormal nail formation and subsequent nail dystrophy.

THERAPY OF PARONYCHIA

- Acute
    Cephalexin: 25–50 mg/kg/day in oral suspension, 500 mg BID
    Erythromycin: 30–50 mg/kg/day in oral suspension, 500 mg BID
    Dicloxacillin: 500 mg BID
- Chronic
    Avoidance of trauma and exposure to water, irritants
    Lotrisone BID

REFERENCES

General

Drake LA, Dinehart SM, Farmer ER, et al.: Guidelines of care for nail disorders. J Am Acad Dermatol 34:529–533, 1996.

Scher RK, Daniel CR: Nails: Therapy, Diagnosis, Surgery. Philadelphia, WB Saunders, 1990.

Fungal Infection

Angello JT, Voytovich RM, Jan SA: A cost/efficacy analysis of oral antifungals indicated for the treatment of onychomycosis: griseofulvin, itraconazole, and terbinafine. Am J Manage Care 3:443–450, 1997.

Daniel CR: The diagnosis of nail fungal infection. Arch Dermatol 127:1566–1567, 1991.

Drake LA, Scher RK, Smith EB, et al.: Effect of onychomycosis on quality of life. J Am Acad Dermatol 38:702–704, 1998.

Gupta AK, Sibbald RG, Lynde CW, et al.: Onychomycosis in children: prevalence and treatment strategies. J Am Acad Dermatol 36:395–402, 1997.

Korting HC, Schafer-Korting M: Is tinea unguium still widely incurable? A review three decades after the introduction of griseofulvin. Arch Dermatol 128:243–248, 1992.

Scher RK: Onychomycosis: therapeutic update. J Am Acad Dermatol 40:521–26, 1999.

Zaias N: Onychomycosis. Arch Dermatol 105:263–274, 1972.

Paronychia

Daniel CR III, Daniel MP, Daniel CM, et al.: Chronic paronychia and onycholysis: a thirteen year experience. Cutis 58:397–401, 1996.

Stone OJ, Mullins JF: Incidence of chronic paronychia. JAMA 186:71–73, 1963.

7

MUCOUS

MEMBRANE

DISORDERS

■

MUCOUS MEMBRANE DISORDERS

23

■

APHTHOUS STOMATITIS
ORAL ULCERS—UNCOMMON CAUSES
   Autoimmune Diseases
   Infections
   Cancer
THRUSH (ORAL CANDIDIASIS)
LICHEN PLANUS
LEUKOPLAKIA

The examination of the oral cavity can provide important diagnostic information for dermatologic diagnosis and therefore should be included in every skin examination. A variety of skin disorders can be accompanied by mucous membrane involvement. For example, erythema multiforme and systemic lupus erythematosus can cause erosions in the mouth, nose, or eyes. However, this chapter focuses on disorders either exclusively or predominantly confined to mucous membranes, usually of the oral cavity.

Mucous membrane disorders are divided into two broad categories: (1) erosions and ulcerations and (2) white lesions (Table 23–1). Erosions are lesions in which the mucosal epithelium is partly denuded. Ulcerations extend through the epidermis into the underlying tissue, which in mucous membranes is called lamina propria rather than dermis. Erosive and ulcerative diseases range in frequency from common (aphthous stomatitis) to rare (pemphigus), and their causes are idiopathic, immunologic, infectious, and malignant.

White spots are hyperkeratotic lesions of the oral mucosa. Thickened stratum corneum of mucous membranes appears white because of maceration from continuous wetness. Malignancy must be ruled out as a cause.

Mucous membrane disorders:
1. **Erosions and ulcerations**
2. **White lesions**

White lesions represent hyperkeratosis.

■ APHTHOUS STOMATITIS

Definition. Aphthous stomatitis is a common, recurrent, idiopathic disorder of the mouth most often manifested by multiple small, "punched-out" ulcers (minor form) (Fig. 23–1). Two less common variants may occur: major aphthous ulcers, characterized by large ulcers that heal slowly and sometimes scar, and herpetiform ulcers, which are small and grouped.

Incidence. Recurrent aphthous stomatitis is a common disease, occurring in 20% to 60% of the general population. It is most common in young adults; the 60%

Aphthous stomatitis is the most common cause of oral ulcerations.

TABLE 23–1 ■ MUCOUS MEMBRANE DISORDERS

	Etiology	History	Physical Examination	Differential Diagnosis	Laboratory Test
Ulcers					
Common cause:					
Aphthous stomatitis	Unknown	Recurrent disease	Sharply demarcated, round, yellowish erosions surrounded by erythema	Herpes simplex Behçet's syndrome Inflammatory bowel disease	—
Uncommon causes:					
Pemphigus and pemphigoid	Autoimmune	May have associated skin lesions	Ragged erosions and ulcerations; intact blisters rarely present	Erythema multiforme	Biopsy with immunofluorescence
Viral infections	Primary herpes simplex	Fever, malaise	Gingivitis; blisters also on lips	Aphthous stomatitis Erythema multiforme	Tzanck smear or culture
	Coxsackie	Fever	Vesicles in *posterior* oral cavity	Aphthous stomatitis	—
Syphilis	*Treponema pallidum*	Sexual contact	*Indurated,* painless ulcer	Malignancy	Serologic test for syphilis
Deep fungal infection	Histoplasmosis	Immunosuppressed	Systemically ill; indurated ulcer	Malignancy	Biopsy with culture
Malignancy		Nonhealing ulcer	Indurated ulcer	Major aphthous ulcer	Biopsy
White Lesions					
Thrush	*Candida albicans*	Found in newborns and immunosuppressed patients	"Curd-like" papules easily scraped off	Lichen planus	KOH preparation
Lichen planus	Unknown	Chronic disease May have associated skin lesions	Reticulated white lines Sometimes erosions are present	Candidiasis Leukoplakia Secondary syphilis	Biopsy
Leukoplakia	Chronic irritation	Smoking Denture trauma	White patches and plaques	Lichen planus Secondary syphilis White sponge nevus Leukokeratosis	Biopsy
Squamous cell carcinoma		Smoking Alcohol Prior leukoplakia	*Indurated or ulcerated* plaque	Leukoplakia Major aphthous ulcer Erosive lichen planus Chancre Deep fungal infection	Biopsy

328

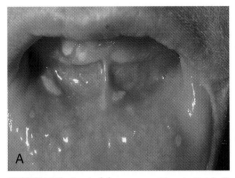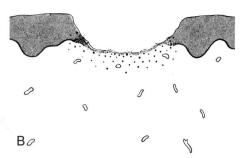

FIGURE 23-1. Aphthous stomatitis. **A,** Epithelium—round, punched-out ulcer with a white-yellow necrotic surface. Lamina propria—surrounding inflammation (the lamina propria is the mucous membrane equivalent of the dermis). **B,** Epithelium—ulcerated. Lamina propria—surrounding inflammation.

prevalence was found in a survey of students attending professional schools. The minor form of the disease represents 80% of all cases.

History. A history of previous episodes is invariable. Recurrences are sometimes precipitated by trauma from biting or misguided toothbrushes. Some patients correlate outbreaks with emotional stress. Lesions are usually preceded by a 1-day prodrome of discomfort in the area of involvement. The ulcers are painful and sometimes interfere with eating.

Physical Examination. Lesions in minor aphthous stomatitis appear as 2- to 5-mm, round, punched-out ulcers with a yellowish necrotic surface and surrounding erythema. Lesions may be single but more often are multiple. The buccal and labial mucosae are the most common locations. Major aphthous ulcers are larger (1 to 3 cm), deeper, and more necrotic. The herpetiform variant, as the name suggests, appears as multiple small erosions that are grouped.

Differential Diagnosis. Recurrent aphthous stomatitis is most often confused with *herpes simplex infection*. Except for the herpetiform variant, however, the two diseases appear quite different. Recurrent herpes simplex rarely occurs inside the mouth. When it does, it appears as grouped small vesicles or erosions on an erythematous base. A Tzanck preparation or culture proves the diagnosis of herpes infection.

> **Herpes simplex rarely recurs inside the mouth.**

The oral ulcerations in *Behçet's syndrome* are indistinguishable from those of aphthous stomatitis. However, Behçet's syndrome is distinguished by its extraoral manifestations. The classic triad consists of oral ulcerations, genital ulcerations, and ocular inflammation (iridocyclitis). Erythema nodosum, thrombophlebitis, arthritis, and neurologic and intestinal involvement may also occur. Patients with inflammatory bowel disease, particularly *ulcerative colitis*, occasionally have oral ulcerations that resemble aphthous stomatitis.

> **Oral ulcerations in Behçet's syndrome look like aphthous stomatitis.**

Laboratory and Biopsy. Usually, a biopsy is not required. If a biopsy is performed, the findings will not be diagnostic and will show only ulceration and nonspecific inflammation primarily composed of lymphocytes. The only other laboratory test to consider is a complete blood count, to screen for the questionable association of iron or folate deficiency anemia in some patients with aphthous stomatitis.

THERAPY OF APHTHOUS STOMATITIS

- Topical steroids
    Fluocinonide gel 0.05%
    Triamcinolone in Orabase
- Tetracycline "swish and swallow"
- Intralesional triamcinolone
- Topical anesthetics
    Dyclonine hydrochloride 1% solution
    Lidocaine jelly 2%

Therapy. The variety of therapies that have been recommended for this disease indicates that a highly successful treatment is lacking. If an underlying iron or folate deficiency is detected, it should be corrected. The ulcerations are usually treated topically. Tetracycline suspension (250 mg/5 mL) "swished and swallowed" four times daily helps in some patients. Patients in whom tetracycline therapy fails are treated with topical steroids in a gel (e.g., fluocinonide [Lidex] gel) or a special adherent base (e.g., triamcinolone [Kenalog in Orabase]) applied three times daily or with a spray preparation (e.g., beclomethasone [Vanceril] three to four times daily). Intralesional steroids (triamcinolone [Kenalog-10]) are useful in patients with major aphthous ulcerations. Oral prednisone is effective in aphthous stomatitis but should be used for only a short course in patients with severe, incapacitating disease. Colchicine and pentoxifylline (Trental) have also been reported to be helpful in preventing recurrent disease, but the clinical trials were not controlled.

Pain relief can be obtained with topical anesthetics such as dyclonine hydrochloride (Dyclone liquid) or topical lidocaine (viscous Xylocaine) used 20 minutes before meals. These preparations numb the entire mouth, including the taste buds, for 1 to 2 hours and allow for pain-free, albeit taste-free, dining.

Course and Complications. For minor aphthous stomatitis, spontaneous healing occurs within 4 to 14 days. Major aphthous ulcers take as long as 6 weeks to heal. Individual ulcers lasting much longer than that should be examined by biopsy to rule out malignancy. Recurrences are common and range in frequency from occasional to almost continuous. In most patients, the disease eventually remits, but the time course is highly variable—from 5 to 15 years or longer.

Pathogenesis. Although the cause of aphthous stomatitis is not known, it clearly does *not* represent recurrent herpes infection. Factors implicated in the pathogenesis include emotional and physical stress, hormones, infection, and autoimmunity. Emotional stress is reported by some patients to precipitate attacks, but this has not been well studied or documented. Physical trauma (e.g., from biting or tooth brushing) frequently precipitates a recurrence. Hormonal factors have been suggested because of the association in some women of recurrent outbreaks with the premenstrual phase of their menstrual cycle. A pleomorphic L-form of α-hemolytic *Streptococcus sanguis* has been implicated. Investigators have theorized that recurrent lesions are associated with transformation from a stable form of this organism to a pathogenic form. Definite proof of this theory is still lacking, but the same organism has been suggested to play a role in the immune mechanism. An immune mechanism is the most favored cause. Circulating cytotoxic T-lymphocytes against oral mucosa have been identified and appear to play a role. α-Hemolytic streptococci may play a role in the immune pathogenesis by sharing antigenic determinants with epithelial cells, a feature that results in immunologic cross-reactions.

■ ORAL ULCERS—UNCOMMON CAUSES

Numerous uncommon causes of oral ulcerations exist (Fig. 23–2); several are listed in Table 23–1. Causes include autoimmunity, infection, and malignancy.

Autoimmune Diseases

Pemphigus vulgaris and mucous membrane pemphigoid are autoimmune chronic blistering diseases with prominent or predominant mucosal involvement. Ninety percent of patients with *pemphigus vulgaris* have oral involvement, and in 50% the disease begins in the mouth. Fragile blisters are easily broken, so erosions are the usual finding. The erosions are larger than those in minor aphthous stomatitis and are continuously present. Further details of this disease are discussed in Chapter 11. *Mucous membrane pemphigoid* is a subepidermal blistering process confined to mucous membranes. Mucosae of the mouth, eyes, and conjunctivae are most frequently affected. An example of an oral ulcer in this disease is shown in Figure 23–2. Eye involvement may lead to scarring and blindness.

In both diseases, autoantibodies are directed against mucosal epithelia. In pemphigus vulgaris, the antibodies are deposited between the cells in the epithelium; in mucous membrane pemphigoid, as in bullous pemphigoid, the deposition occurs in the basement membrane zone.

Autoimmune diseases:
1. **Pemphigus vulgaris**
2. **Mucous membrane pemphigoid**

Infections

Infectious diseases causing oral ulcerations, in decreasing order of frequency, include viruses (herpesvirus and coxsackievirus), *Treponema* (syphilis), and systemic

Infectious causes:
1. **Virus: herpesvirus, coxsackievirus**
2. **Syphilis**
3. **Systemic fungi**

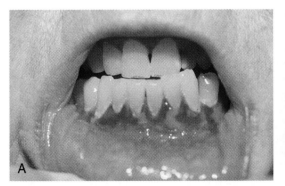
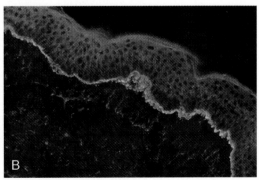

FIGURE 23–2. Oral ulcer. **A,** Mucous membrane pemphigoid. Epithelium—shallow ulcerations. Lamina propria—inflammation. **B,** Immunoglobulin G deposition at the basement membrane zone.

fungi (histoplasmosis). As already mentioned, herpes simplex rarely recurs inside the mouth, but the initial episode often involves the oral mucosa with *herpetic gingivostomatitis.* Erosive gingivitis is characteristic of primary oral herpetic infection and is usually accompanied by lesions on the lips and perioral skin. It is accompanied by fever and regional lymphadenopathy and lasts for 2 to 3 weeks. Infection with coxsackievirus A-4 causes *herpangina,* which appears as a vesicular eruption in the posterior oral cavity lasting 7 to 10 days. Coxsackievirus A-16 causes *hand, foot, and mouth disease,* a distinctive disorder characterized by small vesicles in the posterior portion of the mouth and accompanied by similar lesions on the palms and soles.

The lesion in primary *syphilis* is a *chancre,* which appears as a single, painless, punched-out ulcer and characteristically feels indurated. A dark-field examination of an oral chancre must be interpreted with caution because nontreponemal spirochetes normally colonize the mouth. If doubt exists, a serologic test for syphilis should be performed. If the result is negative, the test should be repeated in 1 month.

Indurated oral ulcerations occur rarely in patients with disseminated systemic fungal infections such as *histoplasmosis.* A biopsy with special stains and cultures confirms the diagnosis.

Cancer

Persistent indurated ulcers must be examined by biopsy.

Malignant tumors inside the mouth can erode and can result in ulcerations. Characteristically, these lesions are indurated. The most common cause is *squamous cell carcinoma,* but lymphomas and leukemias can also cause oral ulcers. A biopsy is diagnostic.

■ THRUSH (Oral Candidiasis)

Thrush is most common in newborns and immunosuppressed patients.

Definition. Thrush is caused by infection of the oral epithelium with *Candida albicans.* The infected epithelium appears white and can be scraped off, leaving an inflamed base (Fig. 23–3).

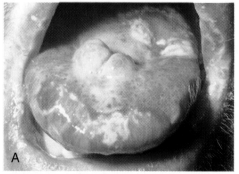 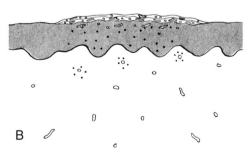

FIGURE 23–3. Thrush. **A,** Epithelium—white, curd-like lesions. Lamina propria—erythema. **B,** Epithelium—hyperkeratoses; hyphae, spores, and inflammatory cells extend into the upper layers of the epithelium. Lamina propria—inflammatory infiltrate.

Incidence. Thrush is most common in newborns, with one third of neonates affected by the first week after birth. In adults, this disorder is uncommon and usually occurs either in denture-wearing patients or in the setting of local or systemic immunosuppression. For example, oral candidiasis is frequent in patients with AIDS, and in these patients it may extend to involve the esophagus. Thrush also occurs in patients with chronic mucocutaneous candidiasis, a rare disorder in which chronic mucous membrane infection is accompanied by skin and nail involvement.

History. Mothers of infected newborns usually have a history of vaginal candidiasis during the latter part of their pregnancy. For older patients acquiring thrush, predisposing factors include the following: dentures; intraoral steroids, such as the aerosolized preparations used in treating asthma; the use of broad-spectrum systemic antibiotics; and systemic immunosuppression from disease or drugs, including systemic corticosteroids.

Predisposing factors:
1. **Dentures**
2. **Steroids**
3. **Antibiotics**
4. **Immunosuppression**

Physical Examination. The lesions appear as white, curd-like papules and patches that sometimes resemble "cottage cheese." Much of this material can be scraped off, leaving an erythematous base. The tongue and buccal mucosa are affected most often. In denture-wearing patients, the mucosal surfaces under the dentures are involved, so the dentures must be removed for the mucosa to be evaluated. The angles of the mouth also may be involved *(angular cheilitis)*, particularly in patients in whom this area remains moist, such as patients with ill-fitting dentures that cause excessive overlap of the upper lip.

The curd-like material can be easily scraped off.

Differential Diagnosis. *Lichen planus* may be confused with thrush. However, thrush is differentiated from this and the other white lesion diseases in that the white material in thrush is easily scraped off.

Laboratory and Biopsy. The diagnostic test is a potassium hydroxide (KOH) examination of material from a scraping. With thrush, one usually has no difficulty in finding hyphae and pseudohyphae. These same elements would be found in the surface epithelium were a biopsy to be done, but because the KOH preparation is diagnostic, biopsy is not required. A culture is not helpful because *C. albicans* may be found in normal flora in the mouth. Candidiasis affecting adults who do not have predisposing factors such as dentures or antibiotics or corticosteroid use should prompt consideration of immunosuppressive conditions such as AIDS.

The KOH examination is diagnostic.

Therapy. Infants are treated with nystatin suspension by applying 1 mL (100,000 units) to each side of the mouth four times daily for 5 to 7 days. Adults can be treated with a "swish and swallow" nystatin suspension in a dose of 5 mL (500,000 units) four times daily. An alternative topical therapy is clotrimazole (Mycelex) troches dissolved in the mouth five times daily for 1 to 2 weeks. Itraconazole (Sporanox) solution can also be used in a "swish and swallow" regimen. Other, systemic therapies include fluconazole (Diflucan) and ketoconazole (Nizoral) taken for 1 to 2 weeks.

In denture-wearing patients, candidal colonization of the dentures also must be treated. Acrylic dentures can be soaked overnight in a dilute (1:10) sodium hypochlorite (Clorox) solution, and a 0.12% chlorhexidine solution (Peridex) can be used for soaking metal plates.

Course and Complications. In newborns, thrush often clears spontaneously, but healing is hastened with therapy. In immunosuppressed patients, the disease can become recurrent and chronic. The most chronic infections are encountered in

```
┌─────────────────────────────────────────────────────────┐
│                                                         │
│                  THERAPY OF THRUSH                      │
│        ─────────────────────────────────────           │
│                                                         │
│   • Infants and children:                               │
│        None                                             │
│        Nystatin suspension: 2 mL (200,000 units) QID    │
│        Fluconazole oral suspension: 2–3 mg/kg/day       │
│   • Adults:                                             │
│        "Swish and swallow"                              │
│            Nystatin suspension: 5 mL (500,000 μL) QID   │
│            Itraconazole solution: 10 mL (100 mg) BID    │
│        Oral                                             │
│            Fluconazole: 100 mg daily                    │
│            Ketoconazole: 200 mg daily                   │
│                                                         │
└─────────────────────────────────────────────────────────┘
```

patients with the syndrome of chronic mucocutaneous candidiasis who are deficient in cellular immunity for *C. albicans*. Even in these patients, however, systemic therapy results in clearing, although recurrences usually follow cessation of therapy.

Complications are uncommon. In severely immunosuppressed patients, esophageal involvement can occur; rarely, the infection spreads systemically, causing disseminated candidiasis, which frequently is a fatal infection.

Pathogenesis. The pathogenesis of candidal infections is discussed in Chapter 13.

■ LICHEN PLANUS

Definition. Oral lesions in lichen planus occur alone or in association with skin lesions. The oral lesions are characterized by inflammation and hyperkeratosis, which clinically appears as white lesions, most commonly in the form of reticulated papules and lines that assume a lace-like pattern (Fig. 23–4). *Erosive lichen planus* is a less common variant. The origin of lichen planus is unknown.

> Lichen planus is the most common cause of white lesions in the mouth.

Incidence. Lichen planus is probably the most common cause of white lesions in the mouth. It has been found in 0.5% to 1% of patients in dental clinics. The highest incidence occurs in adults ages 40 to 60 years.

> Drugs can be causative.

History. Drugs can also cause a lichen planus type of eruption in the mouth. Most often implicated are quinidine, quinacrine, sulfonylureas, and tetracycline.

Usually, no symptoms are associated with the hyperkeratotic type of oral lichen planus. Erosive lichen planus is painful and may make eating difficult. If the patient has accompanying skin lesions, they usually are pruritic.

> The reticulated (lace-like) pattern is characteristic.

Physical Examination. Patches of oral lichen planus usually appear as white lines and puncta in a reticulated (lace-like) pattern. Occasionally, these patches become confluent, producing a solid plaque. Blisters and erosions occur less often and are the result of an intense dermal inflammatory reaction occurring at the dermal-epidermal junction.

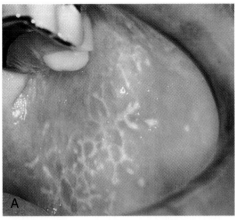

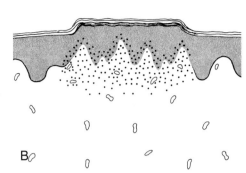

FIGURE 23–4. Lichen planus. **A,** Epithelium—reticulate, lace-like pattern of lines and papules. Lamina propria—erythema. **B,** Epithelium—hyperkeratosis; degeneration of the basal cell layer. Lamina propria—dense, band-like inflammatory infiltrate.

The most common site of involvement is the buccal mucosa, which is bilaterally affected in virtually 100% of patients. The tongue, gingiva, and lips may also be affected. Skin lesions (described in Chapter 12) accompany oral lichen planus in 10% to 40% of cases.

Differential Diagnosis. *Candidiasis* is distinguished from lichen planus by the ease with which white material can be scraped off and by finding hyphae on KOH examination in candidiasis. The two conditions can coexist, so a scraping is often worthwhile because the candidal component is easily treatable. *Leukoplakia* should be considered in patients with the plaque form of lichen planus—a biopsy enables one to distinguish between the two. Mucous patches in *secondary syphilis* are usually accompanied by other manifestations of this disease (e.g., rash, fever, lymphadenopathy), and the disease is diagnosed with a serologic test for syphilis.

Biopsy is diagnostic.

Laboratory and Biopsy. The diagnosis is generally made clinically for lesions in the usual reticulate pattern. If doubt exists or if the patient has plaques, blisters, or erosions, a biopsy is diagnostic. The histologic findings are similar to those in lichen planus in the skin. Even a thin keratinized layer represents *hyper*keratosis in areas that are not normally keratinized, such as the buccal mucosa. In addition, a dense, band-like inflammatory infiltrate in the papillary dermis obscures the basement membrane zone and is accompanied by degenerative changes in the basal cell layer. If the reaction is intense, separation may occur at this area and may result in blisters and erosions.

Therapy. Oral lesions in lichen planus tend to be even more resistant to therapy than skin lesions. Asymptomatic involvement requires no therapy. In patients with symptoms (e.g., those with erosive disease), various agents have been tried with limited success. Some patients benefit from twice-daily applications of a potent (e.g., Lidex) topical steroid gel or ointment. Long-term use, however, predisposes to candidiasis and causes tissue atrophy. Intralesional triamcinolone (Kenalog) in concentrations of 5 mg/mL can be injected into local lesions, sometimes with long-lasting effect. Systemic corticosteroids are effective but should generally be avoided for this chronic disease. Topical tretinoin (Retin-A) gel 0.025% applied twice daily occasionally helps. A higher success rate is achieved with the orally

---

THERAPY OF ORAL LICHEN PLANUS

- Topical therapy
    Steroids (e.g., fluocinonide gel 0.05%)
    Tretinoin gel 0.025%
    Cyclosporine solution
- Intralesional steroids
- Systemic therapy (reserved for extremely severe disease)
    Prednisone
    Acitretin
    Cyclosporine

The course usually is chronic.

administered retinoid, acitretin, in a dose of 25 mg daily. This drug is associated with many side effects, so its use should be reserved for patients with severe, refractory disease. Such patients have also been successfully treated with oral cyclosporine. Improvement has also been reported with the use of a cyclosporine "swish and spit" regimen in a dose of 5 mL (500 mg) three times daily. The extraordinary expense of this therapy can be reduced by applying smaller amounts of the medication directly to the lesions.

Course and Complications. The course is measured in terms of months to decades. In patients with white lesions, approximately 50% experience remittance within 2 years, and of these, approximately 20% experience recurrence. The course is more prolonged in patients with blistering and erosive disease.

Patients with erosive oral lichen planus are at risk for developing squamous cell carcinoma.

Secondary candidal infection occurs in some patients with oral lichen planus. Cases of squamous cell carcinoma have been reported in association with oral lichen planus. Although this complication is uncommon, it appears to be more than coincidental. Therefore, the cases of patients with chronic erosive oral lichen planus should be followed; if an indurated lesion develops, a biopsy should be performed to rule out squamous cell carcinoma.

Pathogenesis. The pathogenesis of lichen planus is discussed in Chapter 12.

■ LEUKOPLAKIA

Definition. *Leukoplakia* literally means "white plaque" (Fig. 23–5). Some clinicians simply use that as the definition of the disease, defining leukoplakia as "a white patch or plaque that cannot be characterized clinically or pathologically as any other disease." Others use the term *leukokeratosis* to describe a white patch that is histologically benign and reserve the term *leukoplakia* for a white patch or plaque in which epithelial dysplasia is present pathologically. We prefer the second definition. Either way, the important point to remember is that for white plaques on mucous membranes, a dysplastic change should be considered a possible cause.

Smoking is a frequent cause.

The white color is due to macerated hyperkeratosis, which in most cases is caused by chronic irritation. Smoking is the most frequent origin, but physical irritation from dentures or ragged teeth may also be causative.

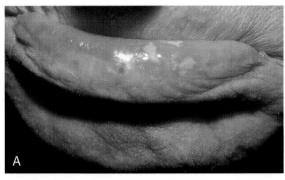
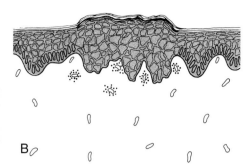

FIGURE 23-5. Leukoplakia. **A,** Epithelium—white patch or plaque. Lamina propria—erythema. **B,** Epithelium—hyperkeratosis; acanthosis with dysplasia. Lamina propria—superficial inflammation with lymphocytes and plasma cells.

Incidence. Leukoplakia is an uncommon disorder primarily affecting middle-aged and elderly adults. The incidence depends, of course, on the definition. The disease is about one tenth as common when dysplastic histologic changes are required criteria.

History. The onset is gradual and usually asymptomatic. Accordingly, leukoplakia is sometimes an incidental finding during a routine physical examination. Some patients seek medical attention because of irritation, which may be the original cause of the problem. Many patients are smokers or have used smokeless tobacco.

Physical Findings. Leukoplakia appears as a white patch or plaque on the mucous membrane. The surface may be flat or verrucous, and the color varies from pure white to gray. It can be located anywhere in the mouth. The tongue is a common location, but leukoplakia can occur on the tonsils, pharynx, or larynx. Leukoplakia may also be found on genital mucosa.

All white lesions should be palpated for induration. Induration and ulceration are important physical findings that strongly suggest carcinoma (Fig. 23–6). Sometimes only part of a white plaque is indurated, and this area should be examined by biopsy to rule out cancer.

Differential Diagnosis. The differential diagnosis of white lesions in the mouth is given in Table 23–1. The reticulated form of oral *lichen planus* is usually clinically distinctive. Mucous patches in *secondary syphilis* are accompanied by other manifestations of that disease, including skin rash and constitutional symptoms. *White sponge nevus* is a hereditary condition that begins in childhood and results in a white lesion that appears "spongy." *Leukokeratosis* is a diagnosis of exclusion that clinically does not fit another known entity and histopathologically shows no dysplastic changes. The diagnosis then often rests with the biopsy.

Oral hairy leukoplakia affects the sides of the tongue with white papules and plaques that sometimes have a filiform ("hairy") surface (Fig. 23–7). This disorder occurs almost exclusively in patients with AIDS and may be the first sign of HIV infection. Ultimately, as many as 30% of patients with AIDS are affected with oral hairy leukoplakia. It is asymptomatic, not premalignant, and is now known to be caused by infection with Epstein-Barr virus. Treatment with acyclovir and other antiviral agents can cause the condition to regress.

Laboratory and Biopsy. The histopathologic findings include hyperkeratosis, acanthosis, and underlying inflammation in the lamina propria composed of lympho-

All white plaques should be palpated; indurated areas must be examined by biopsy to rule out cancer.

Diagnosis depends on the biopsy.

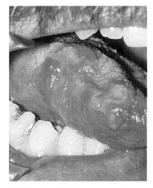

FIGURE 23-6. Squamous cell carcinoma of the tongue. The surface of this large nodule is white (hyperkeratotic) and ulcerated, and the base feels hard and indurated.

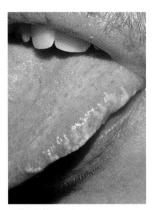

FIGURE 23–7. Oral hairy leukoplakia is associated with AIDS.

Squamous cell carcinoma develops in 30% of patients with "dysplastic leukoplakia."

cytes and plasma cells (plasma cells are common in inflammatory reactions of mucous membranes). In leukoplakia, the epithelial dysplastic changes are similar to those found in actinic keratosis and include cellular pleomorphism, increased numbers of mitotic figures, and derangement of the usual orderly architectural pattern of stratified epithelium. The dysplastic changes may be mild, moderate, or severe. When they are severe (carcinoma in situ), the entire thickness of epithelium is involved with marked dysplastic changes. Invasion of these cells into the underlying lamina propria signifies squamous cell carcinoma.

Therapy. The goals of therapy are to eliminate the cause and surgically remove persistent lesions. Smoking or the use of smokeless tobacco should be eliminated, and sources of physical trauma should be corrected. Lesions may then spontaneously resolve, particularly if they were only mildly dysplastic. For lesions that are persistent or more severely dysplastic, active intervention is recommended. Superficial mucosal lesions can be removed with cryosurgery, carbon dioxide laser ablation, or shave excision. Medical therapies include topical bleomycin and systemic retinoids. Lesions suggestive of squamous cell carcinoma should be excised.

Course and Complications. Spontaneous involution may occur, especially if the aggravating factors are withdrawn. Some lesions may become stationary, whereas others progress to squamous cell carcinoma.

The frequency of development of squamous cell carcinoma in lesions of leukoplakia depends in part on the definition. If dysplasia is among the diagnostic criteria, approximately 30% of leukoplakia lesions will progress to squamous cell carcinoma. If the broader definition (not requiring dysplasia) is used, invasive carcinoma will occur in only 3% to 6%.

Pathogenesis. Usually, leukoplakia appears to be induced by chronic, mild irritation from physical, chemical, or inflammatory processes. Smoking is the most frequent and important cause. Chemical agents in smoking include polycyclic hydrocarbons and phenolic oils. Heat may also contribute. Physical trauma from ill-fitting dentures, long-term use of toothpicks, and irritation from jagged teeth can also cause leukoplakia. Most recently, human papillomavirus infection has been implicated in the pathogenesis of some cases of leukoplakia.

THERAPY OF LEUKOPLAKIA

- Cessation of tobacco use
- Elimination of sources of physical trauma
- Ablation of superficial lesions
        Cryosurgery
        Carbon dioxide laser
        Shave excision
- Topical bleomycin
- Systemic retinoids
- Excision (if cancer is suspected)

■ UNKNOWN (Fig. 23–8)

This 33-year-old man presented with a lesion on the lower lip that started with a "cigarette burn" 1 year earlier. He remained a heavy smoker. On examination, you see an ulcer with a white border.

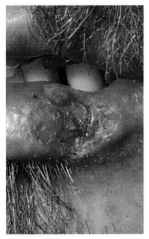

FIGURE 23–8. Unknown.

How would you complete the physical examination?

Palpate the lesion and feel for local lymph nodes. This lesion felt firm and indurated. The patient's head and neck were examined for lymphadenopathy, but none was found.

What is your most likely diagnosis?

For a chronic mucous membrane ulcer, squamous cell carcinoma is the favored diagnosis. The suspicion is heightened by the finding of induration.

How would you confirm it?

A biopsy is required. In this case, it confirmed the diagnosis of squamous cell carcinoma. The lesion was totally excised subsequently.

Important Points

1. Smoking is a risk factor for the development of mucous membrane squamous cell carcinoma.
2. Biopsy is required for all chronic ulcers, especially if these lesions are indurated.

R E F E R E N C E S

General

Conkin RJ, Blasberg B: Common inflammatory diseases of the mouth. Int J Dermatol *30:* 323–335, 1991.

Rogers RS, Randle HW, Powell FC: Oral mucosal diseases. J Am Acad Dermatol *13:*504–506, 1985.

Ulcers

Brice SL, Jester JD, Huff JC: Recurrent aphthous stomatitis. Curr Probl Dermatol *3:*107–127, 1991.

Katz J, Langevitz P, Shemer J, et al.: Prevention of recurrent aphthous stomatitis with colchine: an open trial. J Am Acad Dermatol *31:*459–461, 1994.

Wahba-Yahav AV: Pentoxifylline in intractable aphthous stomatitis: an open trial. J Am Acad Dermatol *33:*680–682, 1995.

Wray D, Ferguson MM, Hutchcon AW, et al.: Nutritional deficiencies in recurrent aphthae. J Oral Pathol *7:*418–423, 1978.

Lichen Planus

Boyd AS, Neldner KH: Lichen planus. J Am Acad Dermatol 25:593–619, 1991.

Eisen D, Ellis CN, Duell EA, Griffiths CEM, Voorhees JJ: Effect of topical cyclosporine rinse on oral lichen planus. N Engl J Med 323:290–294,1990.

Hersle K, Mobacken H, Sloberg K, Thilander H: Severe oral lichen planus: treatment with an aromatic retinoid (etretinate). Br J Dermatol 106:77–80, 1982.

Laurberg G, Geiger J-M, Hjorth N, et al.: Treatment of lichen planus with acetritin: a double-blind, placebo-controlled study in 65 patients. J Am Acad Dermatol 24:434–437, 1991.

Miles DA, Howard MM: Diagnosis and management of oral lichen planus. Dermatol Clin 14:281–290, 1996.

Sigurgeirsson B, Lindelöf B: Lichen planus and malignancy: an epidemiologic study of 2071 patients and review of the literature. Arch Dermatol 127:1684–1688, 1991.

Thrush

Epstein JB, Polsky B: Oropharyngeal candidiasis: a review of its clinical spectrum and current therapies. Clin Ther 20:40–57, 1998.

Kirkpatrick CH, Alling DW: Treatment of chronic oral candidiasis with clotrimazole troches: a controlled clinical trial. N Engl J Med 299:1201–1203, 1978.

Phillips P, De Beule K, Frechette G, et al.: A double-blind comparison of itraconazole oral solution and fluconazole capsules for the treatment of oropharyngeal candidiasis in patients with AIDS. Clin Infect Dis 26:1368–1373, 1998.

Leukoplakia

Epstein JB, Gorsky M, Wong FL, Millner A: Topical bleomycin for the treatment of dysplastic oral leukoplakia. Cancer 83:629–634, 1998.

Kramer IRH, Lucas RB, Pindberg JJ, et al.: Definition of leukoplakia and related lesions: an aid to studies on oral precancer. Oral Surg 46:518–539, 1978.

Resnick L, Herbst JS, Raab-Traub N: Oral hairy leukoplakia. J Am Acad Dermatol 22:1278–1282, 1990.

Silverman S, Gorsky M, Lozada F: Oral leukoplakia and malignant transformation: a follow-up study of 257 patients. Cancer 53:563–568, 1984.

Van der Waal I, Schepman KP, van der Meij EH: Oral leukoplakia: a clinicopathological review. Oral Oncol 33:291–301, 1997.

8

DIAGNOSIS BY

REGION AND

SYMPTOM

■

REGIONAL DIAGNOSIS

■

24

Many skin conditions have a predilection for certain areas of the body. Taking this into account may be helpful diagnostically. Table 24–1 lists the growths and rashes most often encountered in each region. The disorders are listed in estimated decreasing order of frequency. Table 24–1 is not exhaustive, but it can provide another starting point for dermatologic diagnosis. The reader is referred to the earlier chapters for discussion and further differential diagnosis of each of the entities listed.

TABLE 24–1 ■ REGIONAL DIAGNOSES

Growths	Rashes
	Scalp
Nevus	Seborrheic dermatitis (dandruff)
Seborrheic keratosis	Psoriasis
Pilar cyst	Tinea capitis
	Folliculitis
	Face
Nevus	Acne
Lentigo	Acne rosacea
Actinic keratosis	Seborrheic dermatitis
Seborrheic keratosis	Contact dermatitis (cosmetics)
Sebaceous hyperplasia	Herpes simplex
Basal cell carcinoma	Impetigo
Squamous cell carcinoma	Pityriasis alba
Flat wart	Atopic dermatitis
Nevus flammeus	Lupus erythematosus
	Trunk
Nevus	Acne
Skin tag	Tinea versicolor
Cherry angioma	Psoriasis
Seborrheic keratosis	Pityriasis rosea
Epidermal inclusion cyst	Scabies
Lipoma	Drug eruption
Basal cell carcinoma	Varicella
Keloid	Mycosis fungoides
Neurofibroma	Secondary syphilis
	Genitalia
Wart (condyloma acuminatum)	Herpes simplex
Molluscum contagiosum	Scabies
Seborrheic keratosis	Psoriasis
	Lichen planus
	Syphilis (chancre)
	Groin (Inguinal)
Skin tag	Intertrigo
Wart	Tinea cruris
Molluscum contagiosum	Candidiasis
	Pediculosis pubis
	Hidradenitis suppurativa
	Psoriasis
	Seborrheic dermatitis
	Extremities
Nevus	Atopic dermatitis
Dermatofibroma	Contact dermatitis
Wart	Psoriasis
Seborrheic keratosis	Insect bites
Actinic keratosis	Erythema multiforme
Xanthoma	Lichen planus (wrists and ankles)
	Actinic purpura (arms)
	Stasis dermatitis (legs)
	Vasculitis (legs)
	Erythema nodosum (legs)

TABLE 24–1 ■ REGIONAL DIAGNOSES *(Continued)*

Growths	Rashes
	Hands (Dorsa)
Wart	Contact dermatitis
Actinic keratosis	Scabies (interdigital)
Actinic lentigo	
Squamous cell carcinoma	
Keratoacanthoma	
	Hands (Palmar)
Wart	Nonspecific dermatitis
	Atopic dermatitis
	Psoriasis
	Tinea manuum
	Erythema multiforme
	Secondary syphilis
	Feet (Dorsa)
Wart	Contact dermatitis (shoe)
	Feet (Plantar)
Wart (plantar)	Contact dermatitis (shoe)
Corn	Tinea pedis
Nevus	Nonspecific dermatitis
	Psoriasis
	Atopic dermatitis

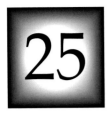

C H A P T E R

25 DIAGNOSIS BY SYMPTOM

FEVER AND RASH
ITCHING PATIENT
SUN SENSITIVITY
SKIN SIGNS OF CANCER
SKIN SIGNS OF AIDS

■ FEVER AND RASH

A wide spectrum of diseases can present with fever and rash, including infections, drug reactions, collagen vascular diseases, and vasculitis. These causes are listed in Table 25–1 according to the primary cutaneous lesions: macules and papules, purpura, nodules and plaques, vesicles and bullae, and pustules. Some of these diseases (e.g., meningococcemia) are life-threatening and require prompt diagnosis and treatment.

The methods used to diagnose the cause of fever and rash are similar to those used for fever of unknown origin. Clues are sought in a complete history and physical examination. The type of eruption is particularly important, as noted in Table 25–1.

Diagnostic laboratory tests are directed by the history and physical examination. Simple procedures such as a potassium hydroxide preparation, a Gram stain, and a Tzanck smear should not be overlooked. These "bedside" tests can quickly establish an infectious cause. A skin biopsy with appropriate stains and cultures may be diagnostic. Further workup is dictated by the clinical setting.

■ ITCHING PATIENT

Because itching is a common symptom, it is often not diagnostically discriminatory. Table 25–2 lists two general categories in which itching is important: skin rashes in which itching is a *prominent* complaint and systemic conditions causing generalized pruritus without primary skin lesions. For the itching patient, therefore, one must first decide whether the itching is caused by a skin disorder or a systemic disorder.

For skin disorders, primary lesions are present, and the type of primary lesion is used to identify the cause. Of the skin disorders listed, scabies is missed most often because of its nonspecific eczematous appearance and the difficulty of find-

TABLE 25–1 ■ FEVER AND RASH

Macules and Papules (Erythematous Rashes)

Infections
  Viral
    Measles (rubella, rubeola)
    Adenovirus
    Echovirus
    Infectious mononucleosis
  Bacterial
    Staphylococcus—toxic shock syndrome
    Streptococcus—erysipelas, rheumatic and scarlet fever
    Typhoid fever
    Typhus—endemic
    Rat-bite fever
  Treponemal
    Erythema migrans (Lyme disease)
    Secondary syphilis
  Fungal
    Cryptococcosis
Drug reaction
Connective tissue disease
  Systemic lupus erythematosus
  Dermatomyositis
  Juvenile rheumatoid arthritis
Erythema multiforme
Kawasaki syndrome

Purpura

Infections
  Viral
    Enterovirus
    Dengue
    Hepatitis
  Bacterial
    Gonococcemia
    Meningococcemia
    Pseudomonas septicemia
    Bacterial endocarditis
  Rickettsial
    Typhus—epidemic
    Rocky Mountain spotted fever
  Erlichiosis
  Fungal
    Candidal septicemia
Drug reaction
Vasculitis

Connective tissue disease
  Systemic lupus erythematosus
  Rheumatoid arthritis
Thrombotic thrombocytopenic purpura

Nodules and Plaques

Infections
  Bacterial
    Tuberculosis
  Fungal
    Histoplasmosis
    Blastomycosis
    Coccidioidomycosis
Lymphoma
Erythema nodosum
Sweet's syndrome

Vesicles and Bullae

Infections
  Viral
    Herpes simplex (primary, disseminated)
    Herpes zoster (disseminated)
    Coxsackie (hand-foot-mouth syndrome)
    Varicella
  Rickettsial
    Rickettsialpox
  Bacterial
    Staphylococcal scalded skin syndrome
Erythema multiforme

Pustules

Infections
  Viral
    Herpes simplex and zoster
    Varicella
  Treponemal
    Congenital syphilis
  Bacterial
    Gonococcemia
  Fungal
    Candidal septicemia
    Blastomycosis
Pustular psoriasis

---

ing a mite. Dermatitis herpetiformis is also overlooked because the intensely pruritic vesicles are excoriated, leaving only nonspecific crusts.

In pruritus resulting from systemic disease, primary skin lesions are absent, although excoriations may be found. Patients with generalized pruritus require a complete medical history and physical examination. Screening tests include a complete blood count with differential count, liver and renal function tests, thyroid profile, and chest radiograph. Frequently, however, a systemic cause is not found.

TABLE 25-2 ■ PRURITUS

Primary Lesions (Skin Disease)	No Primary Lesions (Systemic Disease)
Macules Urticaria pigmentosa (hives when stroked) Erythroderma (Sézary's syndrome) Drug eruptions	*Endocrine* Hyperthyroidism Diabetes mellitus* Hypothyroidism*
Papules and Plaques Scabies Lichen planus Atopic dermatitis Psoriasis Eczematous dermatitis Insect bites Miliaria (heat rash) Drug eruption Dry skin	*Hepatic* Biliary obstruction *Renal* Uremia *Hematologic* Lymphoma (esp. Hodgkin's disease) Polycythemia vera Leukemia* Anemia*
Vesicles Chicken pox Dermatitis herpetiformis	*Carcinomas* Lung Gastrointestinal Breast
Urticaria	*Neuropsychogenic* Delusions of parasitosis Neurodermatitis *Infections* Intestinal parasites

*Not well documented.

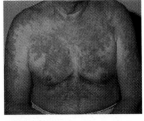

FIGURE 25-1. Photosensitivity in patient with systemic lupus erythematosus. (From Helm KF, Marks JG: Atlas of Differential Diagnosis in Dermatology. New York, Churchill Livingstone, 1998, p 35.)

■ SUN SENSITIVITY

Table 25-3 outlines the small but important differential diagnosis for patients with photosensitivity. The eruption characteristically occurs on sun-exposed skin: the face, the "V" of the neck, and the dorsal aspects of the arms and hands. A clear history of exacerbation by sunlight is present in all these diseases except porphyria cutanea tarda.

Lupus erythematosus (Fig. 25-1), phototoxic drug eruption, and polymor-

TABLE 25-3 ■ SUN SENSITIVITY

Macules, Papules, Plaques

Lupus erythematosus*
Drug eruption*
    Phototoxic—thiazide, quinidine, griseofulvin, tetracycline
    Photoallergic—sunscreens, fragrances
Polymorphous light eruption—idiopathic*

Hives

Solar urticaria

Bullae

Porphyria cutanea tarda

*Most common causes.

TABLE 25-4 ■ SKIN SIGNS OF CANCER

Dermal Nodules

Metastases—carcinoma, lymphoma, leukemia, myeloma

Erythema, Macular and Generalized

Flushing—carcinoid
Exfoliative erythroderma—cutaneous lymphoma

Erythema, Localized Plaques or Nodules

"Cellulitis"—inflammatory breast carcinoma
Subcutaneous fat necrosis—pancreatic carcinoma

Erythema with Scaling Patches

Erythema gyratum repens—carcinoma
Neurolytic migratory erythema—glucagonoma
Dermatomyositis—carcinoma

Pigmentation, Macular and Generalized

Addisonian pigmentation—ACTH/MSH-producing tumor
Slate-gray pigmentation—melanoma

Pigmented Patches and Plaques

Acanthosis nigricans—carcinoma
Eruptive seborrheic keratoses (Leser-Trélat)—carcinoma

Bullae

Sweet's syndrome—leukemia
Paraneoplastic pemphigus—lymphoma, thymoma

Scaling (Acquired Ichthyosis)

Lymphoma (especially Hodgkin's disease)

Excoriations (from Generalized Pruritus)

Lymphoma (especially Hodgkin's disease)

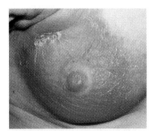

FIGURE 25-2. Inflammatory breast carcinoma.

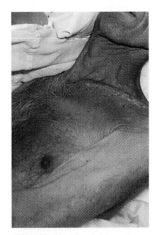

FIGURE 25-3. Addisonian hyperpigmentation in a patient whose lung cancer ectopically produces polypeptides with melanocyte-stimulating activity.

phous light eruption are the most frequent causes of photosensitivity. Lupus erythematosus has a diagnostic biopsy with positive immunofluorescence, and patients with systemic lupus have positive serologic tests. The diagnosis of a phototoxic drug eruption is suggested by history and is confirmed by resolution of the eruption when the offending medication is discontinued. Polymorphous light eruption is a diagnosis of exclusion. It is an idiopathic disorder in which eczematous papules and plaques develop within 24 hours after sun exposure.

■ SKIN SIGNS OF CANCER

Numerous internal cancers have cutaneous manifestations that may be a clue to an underlying malignancy (Table 25–4). These lesions are produced by three mechanisms: infiltration of the skin with the cancer, changes in the skin produced by secretory products from the tumor, and unknown. The two most common infiltrative presentations of metastatic cancer are *hard* dermal nodules and chest "cellulitis" from inflammatory breast carcinoma (Fig. 25–2). Examples of tumors whose secretory products cause skin changes include carcinoid tumors that produce certain vasoactive substances that cause the classic flush and tumors (most commonly small cell carcinomas of the lung) that produce polypeptides with melanocyte-stimulating activity (Fig. 25–3). The necrolytic skin lesions that develop

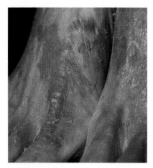

FIGURE 25–4. Necrolytic migratory erythema in a patient with a glucagonoma.

in patients with glucagon-secreting pancreatic tumors (Fig. 25–4) may be due to the accompanying low levels of circulating amino acids that are normally needed for skin maintenance and repair. Acanthosis nigricans (Fig. 25–5) and acquired ichthyosis (Fig. 25–6) are examples of skin signs of cancer in which the pathogenesis is unknown.

■ SKIN SIGNS OF AIDS

Skin disorders are frequent in patients with AIDS. A generalized erythematous exanthem may accompany a febrile illness that occurs 3 to 6 weeks after the primary inoculation with HIV. This symptomatic primary infection occurs in only approximately 10% to 20% of patients and is not diagnostic of early HIV infection. Skin signs are more frequent and more diagnostic later in the course of the disease. Immunosuppression predisposes to the infections and probably also to some of the neoplastic manifestations. For example, infection with type 8 herpes simplex virus is strongly associated with Kaposi's sarcoma, and human papillomavirus 16 has been implicated in oral squamous cell carcinoma. The cause of the miscellaneous disorders in patients with AIDS is unknown.

As noted in Table 25–5, some of the mucocutaneous findings are diagnostic for AIDS, as defined by the Centers for Disease Control and Prevention. HIV-infected individuals are diagnosed as having AIDS if they have any of the following mucocutaneous AIDS-indicator conditions: Kaposi's sarcoma; herpes simplex ulcers lasting more than 1 month; candidiasis of the esophagus or pulmonary tree;

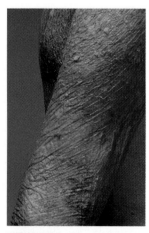

FIGURE 25–5. Acanthosis nigricans of the axilla in a patient with lung cancer.

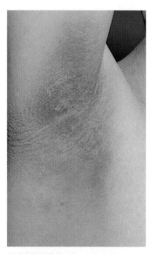

FIGURE 25–6. Acquired ichthyosis is associated with lymphoma and also with AIDS.

TABLE 25–5 ■ SKIN SIGNS OF AIDS

Infection

Viral
Herpes simplex, chronic ulcerative*
Herpes zoster, severe
Oral hairy leukoplakia
Genital warts
Molluscum contagiosum

Fungal
Candidiasis (esophageal, tracheal, pulmonary)*
Papules and nodules from systemic fungal infection*
Seborrheic dermatitis (*Pityrosporum*), severe

Bacterial
Staphylococcal abscesses, recurrent and severe
Papules, nodules, abscesses from mycobacterial infection*
Bacillary angiomatosis

Neoplasms
Kaposi's sarcoma*
Oral and rectal squamous cell carcinoma
Lymphoma

Miscellaneous
Psoriasis, explosive and severe
Acquired ichthyosis
Pruritic papules/folliculitis

*AIDS-indicator conditions (see text).

or extrapulmonary (e.g., skin) coccidioidomycosis, cryptococcosis, histoplasmosis, cytomegalovirus infection, or infection with a mycobacterial organism.

Of the disorders listed in Table 25–5 that are not diagnostic for AIDS, oral hairy leukoplakia is the most suggestive because 83% of these patients develop AIDS within 3 years. For the other nondiagnostic disorders, the possibility of AIDS should be raised, especially if a patient has more than one of them. For confirmation of HIV infection, blood testing is performed with the informed, written consent of the patient.

R E F E R E N C E S

Fever and Rash

Schlossberg D: Fever and rash. Infect Dis Clin North Am 10:101–110, 1996.

Pruritus

Bernhard JD: Mechanisms and Management of Pruritus. New York, McGraw-Hill, 1994.
Kantor GR, Lookingbill DP: Generalized pruritus and systemic disease. J Am Acad Dermatol 9:375–382, 1983.

Photosensitivity

Barber LC, Bickers DR: Photosensitivity Diseases: Principles of Diagnosis and Treatment. 2nd ed. Philadelphia, BC Decker, 1989.

Skin Signs of Cancer

Bergfeld WF: Cutaneous signs of internal malignancy. Postgrad Med 79:75–80, 1986.
Lookingbill DP, Spangler N, Sexton FM: Skin involvement as the presenting sign of internal carcinoma. J Am Acad Dermatol 22:19–26, 1990.
Lookingbill DP, Spangler N, Helm KF: Cutaneous metastases in patients with metastatic carcinoma: a retrospective study of 4020 patients. J Am Acad Dermatol 29:228–236, 1993.

Skin Signs of AIDS

Centers for Disease Control: 1993 revised classification system for HIV infection and expanded surveillance case definition for AIDS among adolescents and adults. MMWR Morb Mortal Wkly Rep 41:1–20, 1992.
Dover JS, Johnson RA: Cutaneous manifestations of human immunodeficiency virus infection: part I and part II. Arch Dermatol 127:1383–1391; 127:1549–1558, 1991.
Spira R, Mignard M, Doutre M-S, et al.: Prevalence of cutaneous disorders in a population of HIV infected patients. Arch Dermatol 134:1208–1212, 1998.
Zalla MJ, Su WPD, Fransway AF: Dermatologic manifestations of human immunodeficiency virus infection. Mayo Clin Proc 67:1089–1108, 1992.

■ INDEX

Note: Page numbers followed by (i) refer to illustrations; those followed by (t) refer to tables. Page numbers in **boldface** refer to main discussions.